**Revision Notes in
Intensive Care Medicine**

Revision Notes in Intensive Care Medicine

Stuart Gillon
Specialty Registrar in Intensive Care Medicine,
Guy's and St Thomas' NHS Foundation Trust,
London, UK

Chris Wright
Consultant in Intensive Care Medicine,
Queen Elizabeth University Hospital,
Glasgow, UK

Cameron Knott
Consultant in Intensive Care Medicine & Medical Donation Specialist,
Austin Hospital & Austin Clinical School,
The University of Melbourne,
Heidelberg, Victoria, Australia

Mark McPhail
Speciality Registrar and Honorary Clinical Lecturer,
Liver Intensive Therapy Unit,
Kings College Hospital NHS Foundation Trust,
London, UK

Luigi Camporota
Consultant in Intensive Care Medicine,
Guy's and St Thomas NHS Foundation Trust,
London, UK

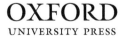

OXFORD
UNIVERSITY PRESS

OXFORD
UNIVERSITY PRESS

Great Clarendon Street, Oxford, OX2 6DP,
United Kingdom

Oxford University Press is a department of the University of Oxford.
It furthers the University's objective of excellence in research, scholarship,
and education by publishing worldwide. Oxford is a registered trade mark of
Oxford University Press in the UK and in certain other countries

Published in the United States of America by Oxford University Press
198 Madison Avenue, New York, NY 10016, United States of America

British Library Cataloguing in Publication Data

Data available

Library of Congress Control Number: 2015960795

ISBN 978–0–19–875461–9

Printed in Great Britain by
Ashford Colour Press Ltd, Gosport, Hampshire

Dedication

The authors would like to thank their families for the support provided and patience shown through the many hours it took to put this book together.

To Chloe, Leena, Claire, Lawrie, Ann, Rachel, Anabel, Hamish, Joshua, and all others. Thank you.

Contents

Abbreviations

2,3-DPG	2,3-diphosphoglyceric acid	**DCD**	donation after circulatory death
AC	activated charcoal	**DIC**	disseminated intravascular coagulation
ACS	abdominal compartment syndrome	**DO$_2$**	oxygen delivery
ACT	activated clotting time	**ECD**	extended criteria donation
AKI	acute kidney injury	**ECMO**	extracorporeal membrane oxygenation
ALF	acute liver failure	**EOLC**	end-of-life care
APACHE	acute physiology and chronic health evaluation	**ERCP**	endoscopic retrograde cholangiopancreatography
APC	activated protein C	**EVAR**	endovascular aneurysm repair
APRV	airway pressure release ventilation	**f**	frequency
APTT	activated partial thromboplastin time	**FFP**	fresh frozen plasma
ARDS	acute respiratory distress syndrome	**F$_i$O$_2$**	fractional inspired O$_2$
ATLS	advanced trauma life support	**FRC**	functional residual capacity
ATN	acute tubular necrosis	**GCS**	Glasgow coma score
AVN	atrio-ventricular node	**GFR**	glomerular filtration rate
BAL	broncho-alveolar lavage	**Hb**	haemoglobin
CABG	coronary artery bypass grafting	**HFNC**	high-flow nasal cannulae
CAM-ICU	confusion assessment method for ICU	**HFOV**	high-frequency oscillatory ventilation
CCOT	critical care outreach team	**HIT**	heparin-induced thrombocytopenia
CPB	cardiopulmonary bypass	**HRS**	hepato-renal syndrome
C$_{dyn}$	dynamic compliance	**HUS**	haemolytic uraemic syndrome
CIT	cold-ischaemia time	**IABP**	intra-aortic balloon pump
CKD	chronic kidney disease	**IAP**	intra-abdominal pressure
CMRO$_2$	cerebral oxygen consumption	**ICM**	intensive care medicine
CO	cardiac output	**ICP**	intracranial pressure
CPAP	continuous positive airway pressure	**ICU**	intensive care unit
CPB	cardiopulmonary bypass	**IMCA**	independent mental capacity advocate
CPET	cardiopulmonary exercise testing	**INR**	international normalized ratio
CPP	cerebral perfusion pressure	**ISS**	injury severity score
CSF	cerebrospinal fluid	**IVD**	intraventricular drain
C$_{static}$	static compliance	**MAP**	mean arterial pressure
CTG	cardiotocography	**MDRO**	multidrug-resistant organisms
CVC	central venous catheter	**MELD**	model for end-stage liver disease (score)
DBD	donation after brain death	**MET**	medical emergency team
DBP	diastolic blood pressure	**MTC**	major trauma centre

MV	minute volume	**RSI**	rapid sequence induction
NAC	n-acetylcysteine	**SAH**	subarachnoid haemorrhage
NAVA	neurally adjusted ventilatory assist	**SAPS**	simplified acute physiology score
NIV	non-invasive ventilation	**SBP**	systolic blood pressure
NMS	neuroleptic malignant syndrome	**SBT**	spontaneous breathing trial
PACU	post-anaesthesia care unit	**SCD**	sickle cell disease
P_aCO_2	arterial partial pressure CO_2	**SD**	standard deviations
P_AO_2	alveolar partial pressure O_2	**SIRS**	systemic inflammatory response syndrome
P_aO_2	arterial partial pressure O_2	**SLE**	systemic lupus erythematosis
PAOP	pulmonary artery occlusion pressure	**SMR**	standardized mortality ratio
P_{ATM}	atmospheric pressure	**SOFA**	sequential organ failure assessment
PCI	percutaneous coronary intervention	**SVR**	systemic vascular resistance
P_iO_2	inspired partial pressure O_2	**TBI**	traumatic brain injury
PEEP	positive end expiratory pressure	**TEG**	thromboelastogram
PEFR	peak expiratory flow rate	**TIPSS**	transjugual intrahepatic porto-systemic shunt
PERT	patient emergency response team	**TISS**	therapeutic intervention scoring system
POD	paracetamol overdose	**TPP**	trans-pulmonary pressure
P_{Peak}	peak pressure	**TTP**	thrombotic thrombocytopenia purpura
P_{Plat}	plateau pressure		
PT	prothrombin time	**TTS**	track and trigger system
PTSD	post-traumatic stress disorder	**UPS**	uninterruptable power supply
RAI	relative adrenal insufficiency	**VH**	variceal haemorrhage
RASS	Richmond agitation and sedation score	**Vd**	dead space
		V/Q	ventilation/perfusion
RER	respiratory exchange ratio	**Vt**	tidal volume
ROC	receiver operator curve	**WCC**	white cell count
ROTEM	rotational thromboelastometry	**WIT**	warm ischaemia time
RRT	renal replacement therapy	**WPW**	Wolf–Parkinson–White syndrome
RRT	rapid response team		

Introduction

Intensive care medicine (ICM) is a specialty on the rise. Borne of the need for respiratory support in the polio epidemics of the mid-twentieth century, ICM has evolved from an ad hoc extension of anaesthetic practice to one of the most rapidly growing and advancing areas of healthcare.

ICM is integral to the care of the seriously ill and injured patient, working in partnership with traditional medical and surgical specialties to deliver increasingly complex and ambitious interventions. The significant decrease in morbidity and mortality associated with, for example, major trauma, severe sepsis, and acute severe asthma, owes much to the evolution of ICM as a specialty.

Additionally, ICM is key to perioperative medicine: complex, invasive surgical procedures that significantly derange physiology are only routinely survivable with high-quality, intensive, post-operative care. Many patients previously deemed too frail to undergo life-prolonging surgery, can now expect a safe and smooth perioperative journey due to the expertise within the intensive care unit (ICU).

The role of ICM extends beyond the walls of the ICU. Mobile intensive care teams identify and support patients deteriorating on general wards. This external role is not limited to the hospital: ICM has made large contributions to pre-hospital and transfer medicine.

Finally, a greater appreciation of the impact of critical illness on patients and their families has led to the development of rehabilitation and follow-up services within intensive care. This necessitates a different range of skills amongst staff.

Not only is ICM increasing in terms of breadth of practice, it is increasing in its depth of understanding and complexity of intervention. Consider respiratory failure as an example. Over a relatively short period of time, simple bag-in-bottle ventilators have evolved into complex, multimodal systems with an array of adjustable parameters. This technological advance has been accompanied by huge strides in the understanding of the pathophysiology of respiratory failure and how this is affected by positive pressure ventilation. Various ventilation 'strategies' have come and gone. Numerous adjunctive pharmacological therapies have been proposed. And other forms of mechanical support, such as oscillation and extracorporeal oxygenation, have joined traditional ventilators.

This expansion in breadth and depth requires delivery by an expert multi-disciplinary team. ICM has always relied upon the input of enthusiastic doctors, nurses, pharmacists, physiotherapists, dieticians, and other professionals. But the explosion in scope of ICM has meant that, in many regions, on-job learning is no longer sufficient and formal training is either highly desirable or mandated. Numerous professional bodies have formed to provide guidance and oversight; curricula have been developed, remarkably similar between regions in their content; and systems of assessment, to judge competency and ensure quality, have been introduced.

It is for professionals working through these programmes of training and undertaking these tests of competency that this book is intended.

The content of *Revision Notes in Intensive Care Medicine* is largely guided by the three major English language medical exams related to ICM: the Fellowship of the College of Intensive Care Medicine (FCICM), set by the college of Australia and New Zealand and undertaken by candidates from that region; the British Fellowship of the Faculty of Intensive Care Medicine (FFICM); and the European Diploma of Intensive Care (EDIC). We have sought to provide a broad overview of the curricula but with particular focus on those areas that appear to be common examination subjects (it should be noted that, at the time of writing, none of the authors have any role in the setting or assessment of these exams; our involvement has been solely as candidates or in supporting colleagues who are candidates).

Despite the medical origins of this publication, we believe it to be highly relevant to the other professions. The National Competency Framework produced by the British Association for Critical Care Nursing has many similarities to the medical curricula mentioned above; comparable critical care frameworks have been proposed for pharmacists. In addition, many universities offer postgraduate ICM qualifications up to Masters level. *Revision Notes in Intensive Care Medicine* would provide a useful companion to these programmes.

We have aimed to incorporate the ever-expanding evidence-base underpinning ICM practice. We have not imposed any in-depth analysis of these papers. Rather we have sought to contextualize what we believe to be the key papers, and would encourage readers to explore the original publications themselves and to draw their own conclusions regarding the quality and validity of the evidence.

Finally, we must acknowledge the changing face of medical education, in particular the rise in prominence of online resources, and consider the role of the book. There are those who would argue that in the Internet age the book, less dynamic and less frequently updated than website resources, is of little or no use. We would, however, (perhaps unsurprisingly) disagree. The book provides a palpable structure to training, and a solid base upon which to build revision. The vast majority of the content will not change: the principles of physics, physiology, and pharmacology are unlikely to be revoked prior to the next edition. And whilst new evidence will emerge, new technologies will evolve, and existing practices will adapt over the lifetime of this book, these developments are best understood in the context of current understanding of the bigger picture. *Revision Notes in Intensive Care Medicine* provides this base and context.

We wish all readers the very best in their training and careers, and welcome all feedback on this inaugural edition.

CHAPTER 1

Respiratory

CONTENTS

1 Respiratory pathophysiology

1.1 Oxygenation, hypoxaemia, and tissue hypoxia

- Hypoxaemia relates to low *arterial* oxygen tension and occurs due to pathology in the transfer of oxygen from the atmosphere to the left side of the heart.
- Hypoxia may relate to any tissue and may be the consequence of either inadequate arterial oxygen tension or inadequate delivery of arterial oxygen to the end organ.
- The causes of hypoxaemia and inadequate oxygen delivery will be described sequentially.

1.1.1 Hypoxaemia and the oxygen cascade

- The sequence of events in the transfer and transport of oxygen from the external environment to arterial blood is illustrated by the oxygen cascade (Fig. 1.1).
- The oxygen cascade demonstrates the sequential reduction in oxygen tension that occurs with each step under normal physiological conditions.
- The oxygen cascade is a useful tool when discussing the processes underlying hypoxaemia, as it provides a systematic means of exploring the many causes of inadequate arterial oxygenation.

1.1.2 Mechanisms of hypoxaemia

- There are several mechanisms of hypoxaemia:
- Low inspired oxygen:
  - Related to atmospheric pressure and F_iO_2 (Table 1.1).
  - Potential clinically relevant causes are:
    - The reduced atmospheric pressure at altitude, relevant in aeromedical work.
    - Hypoxic gas mixtures, which may occur in the event of oxygen supply failure.
- Alveolar hypoventilation:
  - Reduction in global ventilation leads to decrease in ventilation/perfusion (V/Q) and consequential hypoxia.

- ■ Characterized by a normal A–a gradient (Table 1.1) and correction by delivery of high F_iO_2.
- ● Diffusion impairment:
  - ■ Potential causes include:
    - ▪ Increase in the thickness of alveolar membrane (e.g. fibrotic lung disease).
    - ▪ Decrease in capillary transit time and therefore insufficient opportunity for oxygen diffusion and uptake (e.g. hyperdynamic state of severe sepsis).
    - ▪ Reduction in pulmonary capillary blood volume (e.g. hypovolaemia).
- ● Ventilation/perfusion (V/Q) mismatch and shunt:
  - ■ In health, regional V/Q varies from 0.6 (at the bases) to 3 (at the apices); overall V/Q is, however, approximately 1. Almost all blood returning to the left heart is oxygenated.
  - ■ Reduction in ventilation relative to perfusion in a given lung unit results in reduction in V/Q. Physiological *hypoxic pulmonary vasoconstriction* will reduce flow to poorly ventilated units however, some blood flow persists. Blood passing through low V/Q units bypasses (or 'shunts') gas exchange and is returned to the left heart poorly oxygenated.
  - ■ At low shunt fractions, increase in F_iO_2 may compensate for the reduced ventilation and provide adequate arterial oxygenation; at >30% shunt fraction, however, increase in F_iO_2 will not improve arterial oxygenation.
  - ■ A 'true shunt' occurs if blood passes from right to left of the heart via a route with no contact with gas. This may be intra-pulmonary, in lung units with zero ventilation (e.g. dense consolidation) or intra-cardiac (e.g. right to left flow across a septal defect). As there is no opportunity for shunted blood to participate in gas exchange, increase in F_iO_2 will not improve systemic oxygenation.
  - ■ The shunt fraction may be calculated using the equation outlined in Table 1.1.

Table 1.2 outlines factors that allow determination of the underlying mechanism of hypoxaemia.

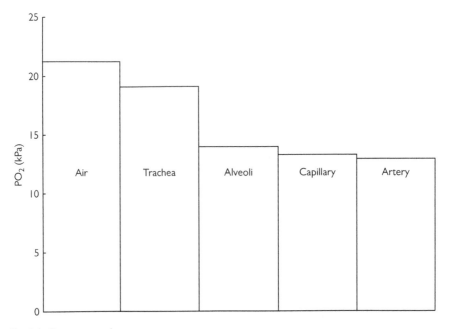

Fig. 1.1 Oxygen cascade

Table 1.1 Oxygen Cascade

Physiological process	Key equations	Normal PO_2 (kPa)	Potential pathological processes
Inspired gas	$PO_2 = FO_2 \times P_{ATM}$ Determined by: fraction of oxygen (F_iO_2) within the gas mix (0.21 in room air) and atmospheric pressure (P_{ATM}) (101.3 kPa at sea level). Rarely a consideration out with high altitude communities and aeromedical work. FiO_2 easily manipulated within the ICU.	21	Altitude, hypoxic gas mixture
Trachea	$PO_2 = F_iO_2\left(P_{ATM} - P_{H2O}\right)$ Gas entering the trachea is humidified. Calculation of the PO_2 must therefore account for the effect of humidity within the gas mix and thus the saturated vapour pressure of water (6.3 kPa at 37°C) is subtracted from P_{ATM}. This results in a small drop in PO_2.	19	Nil
Alveoli	Alveolar Gas Equation $P_AO_2 = \left(FO_2\left(P_{ATM} - P_{H2O}\right)\right) - \dfrac{P_ACO_2}{\text{Respiratory quotient}}$ Within the alveoli, CO_2 makes a far greater contribution to the gas mix (a normal P_ACO_2 being around 5.3 kPa). The effect of CO_2 on P_AO_2 is determined via the Alveolar Gas Equation. There is virtually no gradient between alveolar and arterial CO_2 therefore P_ACO_2 and P_aCO_2 are used interchangeably for the purposes of calculation. The CO_2 production relative to O_2 delivery must be accounted for by addition of the respiratory quotient which is routinely taken to be 0.8.	14	Hypoventilation of any cause (see Section 1.2)

continued

Table 1.1 *continued*

	Physiological process		Key equations	Normal PO_2 (kPa)	Potential pathological processes
Pulmonary capillary	Diffusion	Oxygen diffuses across the alveolar membrane into the pulmonary capillaries. The rate of diffusion (Q) is determined by Fick's law and is dependent upon concentration gradient ($P_1 - P_2$), surface area for diffusion, membrane thickness, and diffusion co-efficient (which is in turn related to solubility and molecular weight of the gas). Any pathology which alters any of these factors (e.g. emphysema – reducing the surface area-; pulmonary oedema, increasing membrane thickness) may impair diffusion and cause hypoxia.	Fick's Law $$Q = \frac{A}{T} \times D(P_1 - P_2)$$ Alveolar–arterial gradient $$A - a\ gradient = P_AO_2 - P_aO_2$$	13	Pulmonary oedema, pulmonary fibrosis
Artery	Admixture/ Shunt	Oxygenated blood from the pulmonary circulation mixes with de-oxygenated blood in the left side of the heart. Normally this 'venous admixture' is small (<3% of total blood flow), arising physiologically from bronchial and the thebesian veins. Pathological increase in the venous admixture may originate within the heart (intra-cardiac) or within the pulmonary vasculature (intra-pulmonary). Intra-cardiac shunt occurs secondary to any right to left flow across the septum (e.g. VSD with elevated right heart pressures). Intra-pulmonary shunt occurs in areas of lung perfused but not ventilated (e.g. consolidation; collapse secondary to endobronchial obstruction; atelectasis secondary to position, effusion, pneumothorax).	Shunt equation $$\frac{Q_S}{Q_T} = \frac{C_CO_2 - C_aO_2}{C_CO_2 - C_vO_2}$$ Oxygen content equation $$C_{O2} = \left(S_pO_2 \times Hb \times 1.34\right) + 0.003 P_aO_2$$		Intra-pulmonary ventilation-perfusion mismatch and shunt: pneumonia, pleural effusion, pneumothorax, ARDS. Intra-cardiac shunt: ASD, VSD

PO_2—partial pressure oxygen; P_aO_2—partial pressure oxygen in alveoli; P_aO_2—partial pressure oxygen in artery; PCO_2—partial pressure carbon dioxide; F_iO_2 – fractional inspired oxygen; P_{ATM}—atmospheric pressure; Q—flow across membrane; A—area of diffusion; D—diffusion coefficient; T—thickness of membrane; D—diffusion coefficient; Q_t—total flow; Q_s—shunt flow; C_cO_2—capillary oxygen content; C_aO_2—arterial oxygen content; C_vO_2—venous oxygen content. ASD—atrial septal defect; VSD—ventricular septal defect; Hb- Haemoglobin.

Table 1.2 Factors differentiating different modes of hypoxaemia

	Corrects with increased F$_I$O2?	Normal A–a gradient?	Normal shunt fraction?
V/Q Mismatch	Yes, if <30%	No	No
True shunt	No	No	No
Diffusion impairment	Yes	No	Yes
Alveolar hypoventilation	Yes	Yes	Yes
Low inspired oxygen	Yes	Yes	Yes

1.1.3 Oxygen carriage

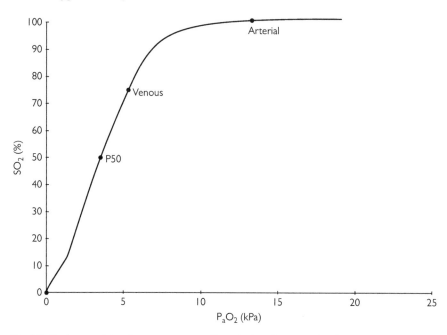

Fig. 1.2 Oxyhaemoglobin dissociation curve. Typical values for arterial and venous blood are indicated; P50 represents the P$_a$O$_2$ at which Hb is 50% saturated, the value of which will alter with right and left 'shifts' of the curve (section 1.1.3).

- Oxygen has low solubility in plasma and therefore relies upon binding to haemoglobin for carriage.
- Every erythrocyte contains 2–3 million haemoglobin molecules (Hb), each capable of binding four oxygen molecules. Hb exhibits allosteric properties, the affinity of Hb increases with every molecule of oxygen it binds. This leads to the classic oxy-haemoglobin dissociation curve (Fig. 1.2).
- Factors that lead to a 'left-shift' of the dissociation curve (and thereby increase the affinity of Hb for O$_2$) include decrease in temperature, P$_a$CO$_2$ or 2,3-diphosphoglyceric acid (DPG), and increase in pH.
- Factors that lead to a 'right-shift' include increase in temperature, P$_a$CO$_2$, DPG, a decrease in pH.

1.1.4 Oxygen delivery

- Oxygen delivery (DO_2) is dependent upon:
    - The transfer of oxygen from atmosphere into blood (as described by the oxygen cascade).
    - The carriage of oxygen in blood, primarily bound to haemoglobin (Hb).
    - Systemic blood flow as determined by cardiac output (CO).
- These factors are illustrated in the oxygen delivery (flux) equation:

$$DO_2 = CO((SaO_2 \times Hb \times 1.34) + 0.003P_aO_2)$$

1.1.5 Hypoxia

- Hypoxia may relate to any tissue. It reflects a failure of oxygen delivery due an abnormality in one of the components of the oxygen delivery equation (section 1.1.4). Mechanisms of hypoxia are classically described as:
    - Hypoxaemic hypoxia—low *arterial oxygen tension* (occurring for any of the reasons described in section 1.1.2).
    - Anaemic hypoxia—low *haemoglobin* (or impaired haemoglobin, e.g. methaemoglobinaemia and carbon monoxide poisoning) and therefore failure of oxygen carriage.
    - Stagnant hypoxia—low *cardiac output*.
    - Cytotoxic hypoxia—abnormal cellular utilization of oxygen leads to failure of aerobic respiration despite adequate oxygen delivery (e.g. cyanide poisoning).

1.2 Physiological ventilation and hypercapnia

Ventilation is the movement of gas in and out of the lungs, allowing clearance of excreted CO_2 and replenishment of O_2 within the alveoli.

CO_2 is around 22 times more soluble than O_2. Consequently, its transfer from plasma to alveoli is not significantly affected by the numerous factors dictating the efficiency of O_2 transfer in the opposite direction. Indeed, at constant metabolic rate, the plasma CO_2 is affected only by ventilatory clearance. Hence, alveolar minute ventilation and P_aCO_2 are directly related.

1.2.1 Ventilation volumes

- Figure 1.3 demonstrates the volumes associate with ventilation. Average values for these volumes are given.
- Minute volume (MV) is the product of Vt and frequency (f).

1.2.2 Alveolar ventilation and dead space

- Not all of the tidal volume (Vt) is involved in gas exchange; dead space contributes a variable proportion of each breath:
    - Anatomical dead space—the conducting airways (e.g. pharynx, trachea, and majority of bronchial tree) do not contribute to gas exchange and therefore constitute dead space. Approximately 2 ml/kg. Reduced by endotracheal intubation as the tube has less volume than the pharynx. Fowler's method is used to measure anatomical dead space in experimental conditions.
    - Alveolar dead space—volume of tidal breath that enters alveoli which are ventilated but not perfused. Negligible in health. Increased in disease (e.g. pulmonary embolism, low cardiac output state).
    - Physiological dead space—the combination of anatomical and alveolar dead space. May be calculated by means of the Bohr equation. A clinically applicable version of the Bohr equation is:

$$\frac{V_D}{V_T} = \frac{P_aCO_2 - P_eCO_2}{P_aCO_2}$$

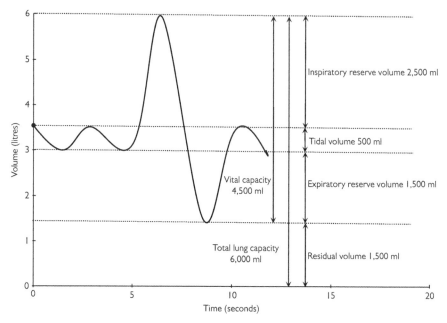

Fig. 1.3 Lung volumes with approximate values for a 70-kg adult.

where V_D = dead space volume; V_T = tidal volume; P_eCO_2 = end tidal partial pressure of CO_2.

- Dead space and mechanical ventilation:
  - The contribution of dead space in the mechanically ventilated patient varies significantly depending upon the relative contribution of frequency and Vt to a given MV.
  - Consider: dead space 150 ml, Vt 600 ml, f 10/min. Total MV: 600 x 10 = 6,000 ml. Alveolar MV: (600 – 150) x 10 = 4,500 ml.
  - Consider now: dead space 150 ml, Vt 200 ml, f 30/min. Total MV: 200 x 30 = 6,000 ml. Alveolar MV: (200 – 150) x 30 = 1,500 ml.
  - Therefore, whilst the total MV is the same in both scenarios, the high f, low Vt configuration leads to a significantly lower alveolar MV with resultant lower CO_2 clearance.

1.2.3 Minute ventilation, carbon dioxide, and oxygen

- The *impact* of alveolar minute ventilation upon arterial gases is illustrated in Figs 1.4 and 1.5.
- In health, the primary determinant of minute volume is P_aCO_2 (Fig. 1.6.). Central chemoreceptors in the medulla detect the change in pH associated with changes in P_aCO_2.
- P_aO_2 only becomes an important determinant of minute ventilation in hypoxia (Fig. 1.7).

1.2.4 'Hypoxic respiratory drive'

The administration of supplemental oxygen may be associated with a rise in P_aCO_2, particularly in the context of chronic lung disease. There is a commonly held belief that this is due

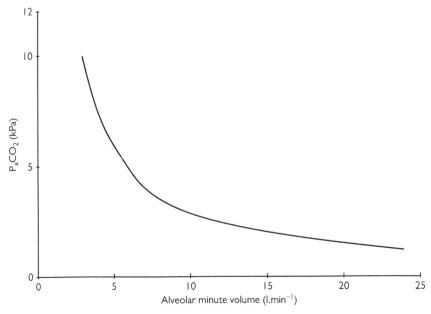

Fig. 1.4 Relationship between alveolar minute ventilation and P_aCO_2. Doubling of alveolar minute volume leads to halving of P_aCO_2.

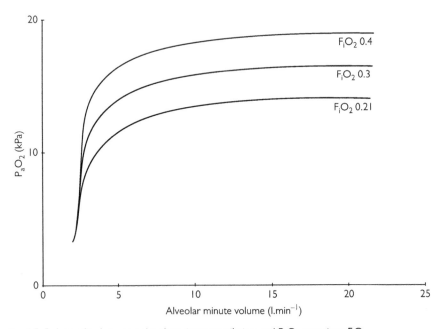

Fig. 1.5 Relationship between alveolar minute ventilation and P_aO_2 at various F_iO_2.

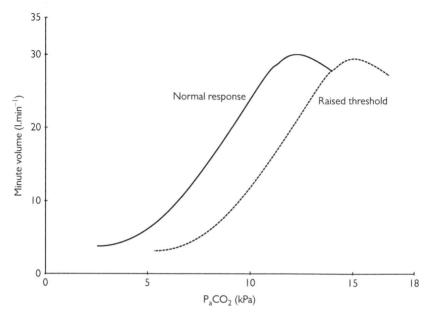

Fig. 1.6 P_aCO_2 as a determinant of minute ventilation. Minute volume rises linearly with rising P_aCO_2 except at extreme hypercapnia where the respiratory drive is blunted. The curve may be shifted, for example, by chronic hypercapnia and administration of opiates.

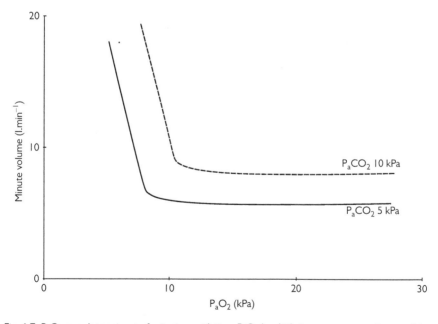

Fig. 1.7 P_aO_2 as a determinant of minute ventilation. P_aO_2 has little impact upon respiratory drive unless hypoxaemic. Hypercapnia shifts the curve leading to initiation of respiratory drive at a higher P_aO_2.

to 'hypoxic respiratory drive': that the chronically hypercapnic patient adapts by converting the primary determinant of minute volume from carbon dioxide to oxygen content. Thus, administration of oxygen leads to a decrease in minute volume and resultant hypercapnia. This is true only in a minority of patients. Oxygen administration associated hypercapnia is more likely to be due to:

- Worsening ventilation–perfusion matching due to supplemental oxygen diffusing to poorly ventilated lung units.
- The Haldane effect: deoxyhaemoglobin is a better buffer of CO_2 than oxyhaemoglobin. Increasing P_aO_2 results in a greater proportion of CO_2 being transported dissolved in plasma.

1.2.5 Mechanics of ventilation

- Compliance:
  - Defined as the change in lung volume per unit change in pressure (usually represented in $ml.cmH_2O^{-1}$).
  - Both the lungs and the chest wall contribute to respiratory compliance. When combined, the reciprocals are added (the reciprocal of compliance is called 'elastance'). Normal values produce:

$$\frac{1}{C_{total}} = \frac{1}{C_{thorax}} + \frac{1}{C_{parenchyma}} = \frac{1}{200} + \frac{1}{200} = \frac{1}{100}$$

$$\therefore C_{total} = 100 \, ml.cmH_2O$$

- Static compliance (C_{static}):
  - Measured when gas flow is absent.
  - It is calculated either by performing an 'end-inspiratory hold manoeuvre' on the ventilator, or adding an inspiratory pause to allow estimation of plateau pressure (P_{Plat}) (inspiratory airway pressure in the absence of gas flow):

$$C_{Static} = \frac{Vt}{P_{Plat} - PEEP}$$

  - Static compliance is typically decreased by lung parenchymal disease (e.g. ARDS, pneumonia, or pulmonary fibrosis), chest wall disease (e.g. kyphoscoliosis, obesity, or circumferential burns), or raised intra-abdominal pressure.
- Dynamic compliance (C_{dyn}):
  - Measured during rhythmic breathing, C_{dyn} is determined by peak pressure (P_{Peak}) rather than plateau pressure.

$$C_{dyn} = \frac{Vt}{P_{Peak} - PEEP}$$

  - P_{Peak} is higher than P_{Plat}. P_{Peak} represents both the compliance of the lung and chest wall, plus the pressure required to overcome airway resistance. As a consequence C_{dyn} is lower than C_{static}.
  - Normally dynamic compliance is only 2–3 $ml.cmH_2O^{-1}$ lower than static compliance. A larger discrepancy arises in the context of obstructive airway disease where higher pressure is required to overcome increased airway resistance.

- Whole lung compliance:

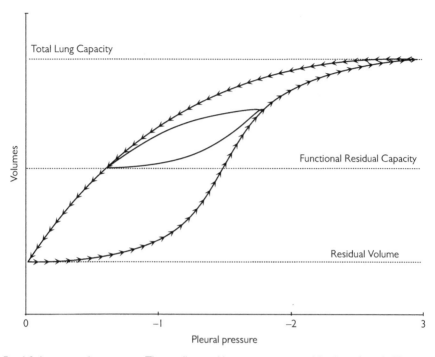

Fig. 1.8 Lung compliance curve. The small central loop represents a tidal volume breath. The larger outer loop represents a vital capacity breath and demonstrates the low compliance encountered at low and high lung volumes.

- If a whole lung compliance curve is created, by charting change in volume against change in pressure, a sigmoid relationship is demonstrated (Fig. 1.8).
- A low compliance region is found at low airway pressures and volumes, where alveoli may be collapsed and require significant force to overcome surface tension. This is followed by a region of maximum compliance; greater volume increase is achieved for a given rise in pressure. Finally, when volume approaches total lung capacity, compliance falls.
- This observation is clinically relevant in setting the optimal level of PEEP.
- Time constants:
  - The rate of inflation of the lung—or units within the lung—depend on the pressure applied, its compliance, and resistance.
  - The time constant of a given unit is defined as the product of compliance and resistance; it reflects how quickly that unit can react to changes in pressure.
  - The lung consists of multiple 'units' of differing compliance and resistance (and therefore different time constants).
  - At end inspiration, pendelluft ventilation occurs and gas moves from units with short time constant (fast units) to units of long time constant (slow units).
  - In health, there is little difference in time constant between units. In disease, particularly inflammatory processes such as ARDS, there may be significant difference.

2 Respiratory monitoring

2.1 Monitoring of oxygen

2.1.1 Pulse oximetry

- A safe, rapid, non-invasive, continuous, and readily available means of determining oxygen saturation (SpO_2).
- Utilizes the Beer–Lambert principle to determine the relative concentrations of oxy- and deoxy-haemoglobin in the arterial blood.
- Two infra-red light emitting diodes (of wavelengths 660 nm and 940 nm) cycle on and off several hundred times per second.
- Light at 940 nm undergoes greater absorption by oxyhaemoglobin than by deoxyhaemoglobin; the opposite is true for light at 660 nm.
- Comparison of the relative absorbance at these two wavelengths allows SpO_2 to be calculated. Accuracy is impaired by movement artefact, nail polish, hypoperfusion, and venous congestion.
- The technology was calibrated on healthy volunteers and is, therefore, less reliable at SpO_2 below 80%.

2.1.2 Oxygenation scores

- P_aO_2:F_iO_2 (P:F) ratio:
  - A simple means of accounting for the impact of F_iO_2 on P_aO_2.
  - Commonly utilized in trials and is a component of the definition of acute respiratory distress syndrome to assess the severity of the syndrome.
  - Normally the P:F ratio exceeds 60 kPa (13.3/0.21 = 63.3 kPa).
  - P:F ratio is, however, affected by many factors, including the F_iO_2 (the relationship between P:F ratio and F_iO_2 is not linear) and airway pressure; and depends on multiple factors, including the cardiac output, the intra-pulmonary shunt fraction, and the arterial-to-venous difference in oxygen content.
- Alveolar–arterial (A–a) gradient:
  - Calculated by subtracting the P_aO_2 from the P_AO_2 (obtained from the alveolar gas equation; Table 1.1)
  - Takes into account both the F_iO_2 and any hypoventilation when describing the degree of hypoxia
- Oxygenation index (OI):
  - Takes into account the mean airway pressure
  - Calculated as:

$$OI = \frac{F_iO_2 \times \text{mean airway pressure}}{P_aO_2} \times 100$$

  - Expresses the pressure required to maintain a given P_aO_2/F_iO_2 ratio and thereby allows comparison of patients with same PaO_2/F_iO_2 ratio but different ventilator pressures
  - The higher the OI, the worse the lung injury
- Lung injury score (Murray score):
  - A means of determining the degree of lung injury in acute respiratory distress syndrome.
  - Primarily used in trials; may be an adjunct to decision-making for extracorporeal support.
  - Calculated from the number of involved quadrants on the chest X-ray, the P:F ratio, the level of PEEP, and the static compliance.

2.2 Monitoring of carbon dioxide

2.2.1 Capnometry and capnography

- The monitoring of end tidal CO_2 ($ETCO_2$) has become a standard of care in the intubated patient.
- Capnometry refers to the monitoring of $ETCO_2$; capnography refers to the graphical display of the waveform of $ETCO_2$ against time.
- Capnometry typically utilizes infrared technology:
  - A detector is placed within the breathing circuit (in-line capnometry).
  - Or a sample of gas is continuously streamed from the circuit for analysis (side-stream capnometry)
  - $ETCO_2$ provides a variety of information, particularly if displayed as capnography, including a value for $ETCO_2$ (P_eCO_2) (Fig. 1.9 and Table 1.3).

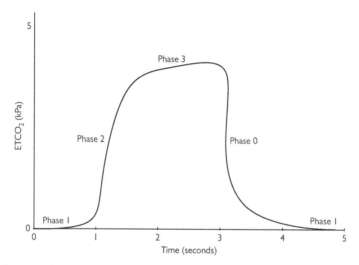

Fig. 1.9 Capnography trace. Phase 0—inspiratory downstroke representing beginning of inspiration. Phase 1—inspiratory baseline representing inspired gas which should be devoid of CO_2. Phase 2—expiratory upstroke, initially representing dead space with no CO_2 then becoming alveolar gas. Phase 3—alveolar plateau.

Table 1.3 Role of capnography

Airway	• Confirmation that the tracheal tube is within the airway at the time of intubation
	• Confirmation that the tracheal tube remains within the airway throughout period of ventilation
	• Confirmation of tube patency and continuity of the ventilator circuit
Breathing	• Provides respiratory rate
	• The graphical display may demonstrate a pattern typical of a particular pathology (e.g. bronchospasm leads to a slow rising stage 2 and 3)
	• Allows determination of dead space: increasing discrepancy between P_eCO_2 and P_aCO_2 (normally <0.7 kPa) suggests increasing dead space (see Section 1.2.2)
Circulation	• Confirms presence of circulation. Particularly useful in the context of cardiac arrest where presence of a capnography trace suggests effective CPR is being performed.
	• Sudden drop in P_eCO_2 suggests fall in cardiac output (e.g. massive pulmonary embolus)

3 Respiratory support

3.1 Oxygen therapy

3.1.1 Hudson mask

- Face mask that delivers *low flow* oxygen (typically between 5 and 8 litres of flow; lower flows may not clear exhaled CO_2 from the mask, leading to CO_2 rebreathing).
- F_iO_2 estimated to lie between 0.4 (at 5–6 litres) and 0.6 (7–8 litres).
- F_iO_2 however varies significantly depending upon patient's minute volume:
  - With normal work of breathing and respiratory rate, the proportion of oxygen flow relative to entrained air will be relatively high and therefore the F_iO_2 will be relatively high.
  - If work of breathing and respiratory rate are increased, the proportion of oxygen flow relative to entrained air will fall and so too will the F_iO_2.
  - There is no means of measuring the F_iO_2.
- Humidified systems are available.

3.1.2 Reservoir bag mask

- This is a *low flow* system in which the addition of a bag to the Hudson mask provides a reservoir of oxygen.
- This overcomes, to some degree, the issue described with standard Hudson masks: even with high work of breathing, oxygen is drawn from the reservoir bag in preference to entrainment of room air; a higher F_iO_2 may be achieved.
- The mask must be well fitted to prevent entrainment of air and benefit from the reservoir.
- At 10 litres flow, an F_iO_2 of around 0.7 can be expected.
- Gas supply cannot be humidified.

3.1.3 Fixed performance mask

- The fixed performance mask utilizes the Venturi effect to create a *high flow* system, which overcomes the issue of variable F_iO_2 affecting the low flow systems.
- The flow of oxygen is forced through a fixed aperture leading to acceleration of flow and entrainment of a fixed proportion of room air; the F_iO_2 is therefore fixed and independent of respiratory effort.
- The F_iO_2 may typically be set at 0.24, 0.28, 0.35, 0.4, or 0.6.
- Humidified circuits utilizing the Venturi effect are available.

3.1.4 Nasal cannulae

- Simple nasal cannulae provide an unobtrusive means of delivering low flow oxygen to the nose.
- Deliver oxygen at 2–4 litres per minute, equating to an F_iO_2 of 0.24–0.35 (although, like the Hudson mask, the F_iO_2 varies with respiratory effort).
- No facility to humidify therefore can lead to drying of mucous membranes.

3.1.5 High flow nasal cannulae

- High flow nasal cannulae (HFNC) utilize the Venturi effect and are capable of delivering up to 60 litres of flow per minute, with an F_iO_2 of between 0.21 and 1.0.
- HFNC systems are capable of humidifying and warming inspired gas.
- Patients may eat, drink, talk cough, and expectorate with the HFNC; compliance is therefore improved in comparison to mask based devices.

- At high flow, HFNC may produce a degree of positive end expiratory pressure, particularly to the soft tissues of the nasopharynx.
- Comparison of HFNC with face mask and non-invasive positive pressure ventilation in a group with hypoxaemic respiratory failure demonstrated no difference in the need for intubation, but an apparent reduction in 90-day mortality for the HFNC group.

FURTHER READING

Frat J-P, Thille AW, Mercat A, et al. High-flow oxygen through nasal cannula in acute hypoxemic respiratory failure. *New England Journal of Medicine* 2015; 372:(23)2185–96.

3.2 Basic principles of mechanical ventilation

Mechanical ventilation is complex with significant variation in nomenclature between different manufacturers. Several fundamental principles however apply universally.

3.2.1 Terms and definitions

For terms and definitions relating to mechanical ventilation see Table 1.4.

Table 1.4 Basic principles of mechanical ventilation

Inspiration	Active ventilator process; positive pressure is applied to the airways. This is the reverse of physiological conditions in which negative pressure causes inspiration.
Expiration	Passive process; elastic recoil of lung, rib, and soft tissue.
Tidal volume (Vt)	Volume of gas inspired/expired every respiratory cycle.
Frequency (f)	Number of respiratory cycles per minute.
I:E ratio	Ratio of inspiration time to expiration time.
Inspiration time (T_{insp})	Time, in seconds spent in inspiration.
Rise time	The proportion of T_{insp} taken to reach target pressure (or volume).
Positive end expiratory pressure (PEEP)	Airway pressure at the end of expiration.
Peak pressure (P_{Peak})	Maximum airway pressure measured in the respiratory cycle. Usually taken to represent pressure applied to the large airways (and is therefore influenced by airway resistance).
Plateau pressure (P_{Plat})	Airway pressure measured during an inspiratory pause. Usually taken to represent the pressure applied to alveoli.

3.2.2 Modes of ventilation

Many modes exist, which are classically described in terms *control, cycle,* and *trigger*.
- Control—determines the 'target' that the ventilator seeks to achieve; may be:
  - *Volume*—the operator determines the volume to be delivered; P_{aw} is determined by resistance and compliance.
  - *Pressure*—operator determines the pressure; resistance, compliance, and T_{insp} determine Vt.

- Cycle—the variable that terminates inspiratory phase and allows expiration:
    - *Time*—cycling occurs after a designated time period (T_{insp}).
    - *Flow*—cycling occurs when the gas flow decreases to a designated proportion of the peak inspiratory flow (usually at 25%).
    - *Volume*—cycling occurs when a designated volume of gas has been delivered.
    - *Limit*—inspiratory phase is terminated if alarm limits (pressure or volume) are reached.
- Trigger—the variable that initiates inspiration:
    - *Time*—inspiration occurs after a designated time period.
    - *Pressure*—fall in pressure within the ventilator circuit triggers inspiration.
    - *Flow*—alteration in the flow through the circuit (modern ICU ventilators employ a circle circuit with continuous flow of gas, respiratory effort causes a decrease in flow, thereby triggering breath).
    - *Diaphragmatic neural activity*—see neurally adjusted ventilatory assist (NAVA) (Section 3.5.3).

Other important variables include:

- Flow pattern—the flow delivered throughout inspiration may follow one of several different patterns:
    - *Constant (or square) flow*—flow rate increases rapidly and remains constant until the target variable has been achieved (typical of some volume controlled modes).
    - *Decelerating flow*—typical of pressure-controlled modes (and more recent volume-controlled modes), flow falls as alveolar pressure increases. May lead to improved distribution of gas throughout alveoli with differing time constants. The degree of deceleration may be altered in in some ventilators by controlling the *ramp*.
    - *Sinusoidal flow*—typical of spontaneous, unassisted breathing.
- Modern ventilators offer a wide array of brand specific modes that are typically hybrids of 'classic' modes:
    - In simplistic terms, ventilator modes may be broadly divided – dependent upon *trigger* – into mandatory (in which there is no patient involvement) or spontaneous (inspiration is triggered by patient and supported by ventilator).
    - Classical mandatory and spontaneous can be further subdivided, dependent upon the *control* utilized (typically volume or pressure).
    - The control, cycle, trigger, and flow pattern of these 'classic' modes are described in Tables 1.5 and 1.6.
- In reality, on the modern intensive care ventilator, mandatory modes almost always have a spontaneous facility to support the patient as they begin to breath, and spontaneous modes have a mandatory backup that will activate in the event of apnoea.
- Ventilatory modes should, therefore, not be considered as binary spontaneous or mandatory modes but rather to lie on a spectrum.

Table 1.5 Mandatory modes of ventilation

Mode	Control	Cycle	Trigger	Flow pattern
Volume controlled ventilation (VCV)	Volume	Volume	Time	Classically constant; typically decelerating on modern ventilators
Pressure controlled ventilation (PCV)	Pressure	Flow	Time	Decelerating
Pressure regulated volume control (PRVC)	Volume	Flow	Time	Decelerating

Table 1.6 Spontaneous modes of ventilation

Mode	Control	Cycle	Trigger	Flow pattern
Volume assist	Volume	Flow	Flow	Constant
Pressure support	Pressure	Flow	Flow	Decelerating
Neurally adjusted ventilatory assist	Pressure	Neural	Neural	N/a

3.2.3 Management of oxygenation and CO₂ clearance on the ventilator

In the mechanically ventilated patient:
- Oxygenation is determined by:
  - F_iO_2—which may be adjusted from 0.21 (21%; room air) to 1.0 (100%).
  - Mean airway pressure—which is determined by the level of PEEP and the I:E ratio (the greater the proportion of the respiratory cycle spent in inspiration, the greater the mean airway pressure).
- CO_2 clearance is determined by *alveolar* minute volume, therefore:
  - Frequency
  - Tidal volume
  - Volume of dead space

3.2.4 Adverse effects of mechanical ventilation

Mechanical ventilation is associated with numerous complications. These include:
- Anaesthetic and sedation related (agent dependent):
  - Dose-dependent effects: hypotension, loss of respiratory drive, bradycardia.
  - Idiosyncratic reactions: anaphylaxis, malignant hyperpyrexia, hyperkalaemia with suxamethonium.
- Airway related: damage to local structures, inadvertent loss of artificial airway.
- Haemodynamic: positive pressure ventilation may induce cardiovascular instability via decreased preload or increase in right ventricular afterload.
- Ventilator induced lung injury (VILI): excess force applied via the ventilator may prove injurious in a number of ways:
  - Volutrauma: over-distension of lung units with excessive Vt in relation to the resting lung volume. Risk believed to be reduced by limiting Vt between 6 and 8 ml/kg.
  - Barotrauma: damage related to the application of excessive pressure to the lung. Risk believed to be reduced by avoiding P_{Plat} >28–30 cmH₂O.
  - Atelectotrauma: damage related to the shear force generated by repeated open and closure of lung units. Theoretically reduced by utilizing a high PEEP, 'open-lung' strategy.
  - Biotrauma: injury to the alveolar membrane triggers up regulation of cytokines resulting in a systemic inflammatory response and multi-organ failure.
  - Oxygen toxicity: excessive partial pressure of oxygen impairs cellular free radical clearance with potential for tissue injury. May also precipitate absorption atelectasis.
- Ventilator associated pneumonia (VAP): see Chapter 6, Section 7.4.

3.3 Non-invasive and invasive ventilation

Ventilation may be classified by the interface between patient and ventilator.

3.3.1 Non-invasive ventilation (NIV)

- A form of mechanical ventilation delivered via the patient's upper airway by means of an external interface:
  - Oro-nasal mask
  - Nasal mask
  - Helmet/hood
  - Mouthpiece
- The principles of mechanical ventilation described in Section 3.1 apply to non-invasive ventilation:
  - Most machines may be triggered by flow or pressure (and therefore inspiration patient initiated) or by time (mandatory inspiration).
  - Pressure is a more common target but volume modes exist.
- Many NIV machines also offer the option of single level continuous positive airway pressure (CPAP); CPAP may also be delivered by a simple circuit with a valve attached to the expiratory limb.
- For the purposes of this chapter, the term NIV will relate to the use of non-invasive ventilatory support with distinct inspiratory and expiratory pressures; CPAP relates to single level positive pressure without inspiratory ventilatory support.
- There has been an increase in both the indications for, and the frequency of, NIV use over recent years.
- NIV avoids many of the complications associated with invasive ventilation, and allows the patient to cough and clear secretions.
- Out with COPD and cardiogenic pulmonary oedema, the evidence-base is limited.
- The potential benefits, contra-indications, and complications of NIV are outlined in Table 1.7; evidence relating to NIV is summarized in Table 1.8.

Table 1.7 Benefits, contra-indications, and complications of non-invasive ventilation

Potential benefits	Safe, avoids the complications of intubation
	Decreases work of breathing
	Increase in mean airway pressure
Contra-indications	Need for immediate intubation
	Facial or upper airway injury or disease process
	Excess secretions
	Multi-organ failure
	Agitation
	Upper gastrointestinal haemorrhage
Complications	Local skin injury
	Gastric distension
	Nosocomial pneumonia[*]
	Barotrauma[*]
	Haemodynamic instability[*]

*But to a lesser extent than invasive ventilation.

Table 1.8 Evidence relating to non-invasive ventilation

Indication for NIV	Guidance and evidence
Exacerbation of COPD	A large body of evidence supports the use of NIV in this patient group. Significant improvement in mortality when compared with standard medical therapy alone. NICE guidelines recommend as first-line management of COPD-induced hypercapnic respiratory failure not responding to medical management. Previous contra-indications to NIV (severe acidosis, hypercapnic coma) have been revised with a trial in an appropriate clinical area (i.e. critical care) now recommended.
Exacerbation of COPD with additional acute pathology	Benefits of NIV less clear-cut in presence of a secondary acute issue (e.g. bronchopneumonia). More likely to fail in the presence of metabolic acidosis. Clear plans should be made in case of failure (e.g. intubation); trials of NIV should be undertaken in an area capable of escalation.
Asthma	Use of NIV in asthma contentious (Section 8).
Neuromuscular disease	Limited role in acute neuromuscular disorders due to frequent coexistence of airway compromise and tendency to requiring prolonged respiratory support. NIV does, however, have a role in chronic neuromuscular disease either as a supportive measure in deterioration associated with acute superimposed illness, or as a form of symptom relief in progressive disease.
Pneumonia	Somewhat controversial area. Trial of NIV has a reported mortality benefit in context of underlying COPD or immune-compromise. The routine use of NIV out with these patient groups is not recommended. If trial of NIV is deemed appropriate it should be undertaken in critical care.
ARDS	The heterogeneous aetiology of ARDS creates difficulty in generating adequate evidence. NIV can be used in 'mild ARDS'; however, its use is not routinely adopted in moderate or severe ARDS.
Cardiogenic pulmonary oedema	Good evidence that the use of NIV improves outcomes, including mortality and rate of endotracheal intubation. Some debate as to whether CPAP or NIV holds greater benefit: more evidence supporting CPAP. The previous suggestion that NIV increases the rate of myocardial infarction has not been borne out in large-scale analysis. Theoretical benefits include decreased work of breathing, decreased preload and decreased afterload.
Obesity	CPAP is commonly used in the chronic management of obstructive sleep apnoea. Additionally, NIV has a demonstrated benefit in treating hypercapnia associated with obesity hyperventilation syndrome.
Trauma	The use of NIV in combination with effective analgesia in patients with blunt chest trauma and pulmonary contusions has been shown to improve outcomes.
Post-extubation	May be used as a prophylactic adjunct to extubation but it is not advised as a rescue tool for those failing post-extubation. Benefits reported by various studies are conflicting. May reduce hospital mortality, need for re-intubation, incidence of pneumonia, and length of stay. If used as a rescue technique, those who subsequently require re-intubation appear to have worse outcomes than if NIV had not been attempted. This may be due to delay of inevitable intubation.

3.3.2 *Invasive mechanical ventilation*

- Invasive ventilation is delivery of mechanical ventilatory support via an artificial airway.
- The artificial airway (endotracheal or tracheostomy tube) sits below the glottis, thereby protecting the lungs from soiling.
- The role of supraglottic airway devices (e.g. laryngeal mask airway) in intensive care is limited to airway emergencies when an endotracheal tube cannot be placed.
- Indications for invasive mechanical ventilation are outlined in Table 1.9.

Table 1.9 Indications for invasive mechanical ventilation

Airway	Airway compromise (e.g. swelling from burns, compression from tumour)
Breathing	Hypoxia (to increase FRC, maximize F_iO_2, reduce O_2 consumption)
	Hypercapnia (to manipulate alveolar minute ventilation, reduce work of breathing)
Circulation	Significant haemodynamic instability (to reduce O_2 consumption, reduce preload, reduce afterload)
Disability	Coma compromising airway protection (GCS of 8 typically used as trigger for intubation)
	Raised intracranial pressure (to maintain optimal P_aCO_2)
	Refractory seizures
Everything else	To facilitate procedures
	To facilitate transfer

FURTHER READING

BTS. *Guidelines for the Management of Community Acquired Pneumonia in Adults*, 2009. http://www.brit-thoracic.org.uk/guidelines/pneumonia-guidelines.aspx.

Glossop AJ, Shepherd N, Bryden DC, Mills GH. Non-invasive ventilation for weaning, avoiding re-intubation after extubation and in the postoperative period: a meta-analysis. *British Journal of Anaesthesia* 2012; 109(3): 305–14.

McNeill G, Glossop A. Clinical applications of non-invasive ventilation in critical care. *Continuing Education in Anaesthesia, Critical Care & Pain* 2012; 12(1): 33–7.

NICE. *Management of Chronic Obstructive Pulmonary Disease in Adults in Primary and Secondary Care*, 2012. http://guidance.nice.org.uk/CG101/Guidance/pdf/English.

Vital FM, Ladeira MT, Atallah AN. Non-invasive positive pressure ventilation (CPAP or bilevel NPPV) for cardiogenic pulmonary oedema. Cochrane Database Syst Rev. 2013;5:Cd005351.

3.4 Adjuncts to ventilatory support

3.4.1 *Recruitment manoeuvres and PEEP titration*

- A recruitment manoeuvre is a deliberate, transient increase in intrathoracic pressure utilized in the management of ARDS with a view to improving oxygenation and/or compliance.
- Recruitment is based upon the principle that:
  - A number of lung units within the ARDS lung are collapsed.
  - That re-opening of these units would improve oxygenation and compliance.
  - That these units have a 'critical opening pressure', which, if exceeded, will result in re-aeration.

- There is no standardized means of performing a recruitment manoeuvre; for the purpose of exams it advisable to have good understanding of one technique and an awareness of others.
- Broadly, techniques may be categorized into:
  - Sigh breath—a large Vt or high P_{insp} are applied for one breath.
  - Sustained inflation—airway pressures are increased to supranormal levels (e.g. 40 cmH$_2$O) for a period of time (e.g. 40 seconds).
  - Extended sigh—increase in PEEP with same driving pressure over a period of time (usually 2 min) with a resultant increase in peak pressure and therefore recruitment.
  - Incremental PEEP—is a stepwise increase in PEEP with same driving pressure up to P_{Peak} of 45 cmH$_2$O (some authors advocate limit of 60 cmH$_2$O for maximal recruitment) then gradually stepped down over time.
- Successful recruitment is often measured by the change in P_aO_2 or compliance; PEEP needs to be adjusted post-recruitment.
- Recruitment may cause barotrauma and may result in worsening haemodynamic instability.
- There is evidence from trials of improved oxygenation and reduced radiological evidence of atelectasis; there is, however, no demonstrable survival benefit, this may reflect the heterogeneous ARDS population included in clinical trials.

3.4.2 Prone position

Prone ventilation in the patient with moderate-severe ARDS has numerous theoretical advantages, but is not without risk (Table 1.10).

Table 1.10 Advantages, risks, and contra-indications of prone ventilation

Advantages	• Ventilation
	▪ More homogeneous distribution of ventilation due to improvement in thoraco-abdominal compliance
	▪ Alveolar pressure more evenly distributed—vulnerable lung unit less likely to collapse on expiration
	▪ The dependant heart does not compress posterior lung units
	▪ Improved alveolar recruitment
	▪ Better drainage of secretions
	• Perfusion
	▪ More homogenous distribution of perfusion
	▪ In semi-recumbent position perfusion and atelectasis are greatest at bases, proning diverts perfusion to better aerated regions
	▪ Possible reduction in extra-vascular lung water
Risks	• With the turn
	▪ Loss of airway or vascular access
	▪ Injury to spine or shoulders
	▪ Increased need for sedation
	▪ Transient hypoxia
	▪ Arrhythmia or haemodynamic instability
	• Whilst prone
	▪ Oedema or pressure sores to face/thorax/iliac crests
	▪ Conjunctival oedema or haemorrhage
	▪ Retinal damage
	▪ Airway obstruction
	▪ Malfunction of lines or tubes
	▪ Nerve compression
	▪ Persistent hypoxia
	▪ Haemodynamic instability

continued

Table **1.10** *continued*

Contra-indications	• Spinal instability
	• Pregnancy
	• Pelvic fracture
	• Severe haemodynamic instability
	• Raised intracranial pressure
	• Raised intra-abdominal pressure

- Most patients (around 80%) will demonstrate improved oxygenation on turning prone; a trial of at least 4 hours is necessary.
- Initial research into prone ventilation suggested improved oxygenation but no difference in mortality; the period of prone ventilation was short (7 hours) and ventilation did not comply with modern, low-tidal-volume strategies.
- Subsequent publications suggested reduced mortality in the most moderate-severe cases of respiratory failure; similar results were reported in a large multi-centre randomized trial, which employed tight exclusion criteria.
- The precise timing and duration of prone ventilation is unclear. There is, however, general consensus that it should be:
  - Utilized for those with moderate-severe respiratory failure (P:F ratio of <20 kPa).
  - Employed early in the illness (<36 hours).
  - Delivered for between 14 and 20 hours per day.
- Turning a critically ill patient into the prone position is inherently risky. Trials report low rates of complications; this may, however, be related to staff familiarity with the proning technique at investigating centre and might not be applicable to general practice.
- Transition to prone requires a co-ordinated team effort with responsibility allocated for leadership, airway, lines, and drains. Following the turn, attention must be paid to the protection of pressure areas, limbs, and eyes. Beds specifically designed for proning are available but uncommon in standard practice.

FURTHER READING

Gattinoni L, Tognoni G, Pesenti A, et al. Effect of prone positioning on the survival of patients with acute respiratory failure. *New England Journal of Medicine* 2001; 345(8): 568–73.

Gattinoni L, Carlesso E, Brazzi L, Caironi P. Positive end-expiratory pressure. *Current Opinion in Critical Care* 2010; 16(1): 39–44.

Guerin C, Debord S, Leray V, et al. Efficacy and safety of recruitment manoeuvres in acute respiratory distress syndrome. *Annals of Intensive Care* 2011; 1(1): 1–6.

Guérin C, Reignier J, Richard J-C, et al. Prone positioning in severe acute respiratory distress syndrome. *New England Journal of Medicine* 2013; 368(23): 2159–68.

3.5 Alternative forms of ventilator support

3.5.1 High-frequency oscillatory ventilation (HFOV)

- HFOV has most commonly been used in patients with ARDS who failed conventional ventilation.
- The benefit of HFOV as a primary mode of ventilation has, however, been called into question by two, simultaneously published, large randomized controlled trials, one of which demonstrated no difference (OSCAR) and the other, worse outcomes with HFOV (OSCILLATE).

- As a consequence, HFOV is far less frequently utilized—although in some centres it is used as a rescue treatment if extracorporeal support is unavailable or contra-indicated.
- In HFOV, a continuous flow of gas circulates through the circuit (bias flow).
- This is maintained at a designated positive pressure (mean airway pressure) by means of an adjustable expiratory valve.
- The mean airway pressure and F_iO_2 are the primary determinants of oxygenation.
- A piston or reciprocating diaphragm oscillates the airway pressure around the mean at very high frequency (4–15 Hz), this leads to very small 'tidal volumes', significantly less than anatomical dead space.
- Such sub-dead-space tidal volumes do not permit adequate CO_2 clearance to occur by standard means; alternative mechanisms of CO_2 clearance are outlined in Table 1.11.
- Potential benefits and disadvantage of HFOV are outlined in Table 1.12; HFOV settings are described in Table 1.13.

Table 1.11 Mechanisms of gas transport in HFOV

Convection	Some degree of bulk flow occurs in the proximal airways.
Molecular diffusion	Movement of gaseous molecules from area of high concentration to low concentration.
Co-axial flow	Bias flow within the ventilator circuit continues into airways with inwards flow occurring in middle and co-axial outwards flow occurring in the periphery.
Taylor dispersion	Interplay between convective forces and molecular diffusion.
Pendelluft ventilation	Exchange between adjacent lung units of differing time constants.
Cardiogenic mixing	Agitation of lung units adjacent to heart and great vessels enhances molecular diffusion.

Table 1.12 Advantages and disadvantages of HFOV

Advantages	Protective strategy: • Lower Vt therefore less risk of volutrauma • Lower peak pressure therefore less risk of barotrauma • 'Open lung' therefore less risk of atelectotrauma Improved oxygenation: • Recruitment of larger number of aerated lung units • Increased functional residual capacity
Disadvantages	Respiratory: • Less effective CO_2 clearance if inappropriate settings • Risk of dynamic hyperinflation • Unable to measure: MV, $ETCO_2$, F_iO_2 effectively • Cooling and drying of inspired gases Cardiovascular: • Increased vagal activity • Decreased venous return and cardiac output (exacerbated by hypovolaemia) Neurological: • Increased sedation requirements • Potential rise in intracranial pressure

Table 1.13 HFOV settings

Mean airway pressure (MAP)	Conventionally set at 2–5 cmH$_2$O above mean pressure measured on the last conventional ventilation mode. Higher MAP improves oxygenation; excessive MAP risks barotrauma.
F$_i$O$_2$	Titrated to desired P$_a$O$_2$ as with conventional ventilation.
Frequency	Ranges from 4 to 15 Hz. Usually started at 5–6Hz. In contrast to conventional ventilation, decreasing frequency increases CO$_2$ clearance. The lower the frequency however, the larger the changes in pressure per cycle and the greater the risk of lung injury. Frequency should therefore be set at highest which achieves adequate CO$_2$ clearance.
Δ pressure	The magnitude of the mechanical diaphragm oscillation. Resistance and compliance within the respiratory circuit determine the effect this has on the pressure oscillation. Typically, this is clinically titrated to the 'wiggle factor', with δ pressure increased until the patient is seen to 'wiggle' down to the level of the knees.

- Additional strategies include permissive hypercapnia and prone ventilation. A deliberate cuff leak may also be employed to enhance CO$_2$ clearance.

3.5.2 Airway pressure release ventilation (APRV)

- APRV applies a continuous airway pressure identical to CPAP (referred to as P$_{high}$ in APRV mode) and adds a time-cycled release phase to a lower set pressure (P$_{low}$).
- With APRV, spontaneous breathing can be integrated and is independent of the ventilator cycle.
- The Vt (or release volume) with each release breath will depend upon the difference between the set high (inspiratory) and low (expiratory) pressures, the T$_{low}$ and the compliance of the respiratory system.
- A rough initial setting would be:
  - P$_{high}$ equivalent to the plateau pressure (if previously in volume control) or to the peak pressure (if previously in pressure control mode).
  - T$_{high}$ of 4–6 seconds.
  - T$_{low}$ of 0.4–0.6 seconds: the expiratory time should be set so that the inspiratory cycle starts when the expiratory flow is 75% the peak expiratory flow—avoiding lung deflation and maintaining end-expiratory lung volume.
  - The P$_{low}$ is set at 0 cmH$_2$O with no additional inspiratory pressure support.
- APRV provides a means of maintaining high mean airway pressure (thereby enhancing oxygenation) whilst minimizing ventilator associated lung injury.

3.5.3 Neurally adjusted ventilatory assist (NAVA)

- NAVA is a novel form of ventilation for the spontaneously breathing patient.
- A specialized nasogastric tube with a set of electrodes detects the patient's neural breathing demand for a breath by monitoring the electrical signal of the diaphragm (Edi). Edi above a designated level (the sensitivity) will trigger the ventilator; the level of support provided is proportional to the magnitude of Edi detected.
- NAVA thus is reported to provide a more reliable trigger and more physiological means of cycling off in accordance with the neural time. It also has the theoretical benefit of tailoring the level of support to patient requirements on a breath-by-breath basis.

- The level of support is designated as 'gain' and is expressed as $cmH_2O.\mu V^{-1}$ of Edi.
- PEEP and F_iO_2 are the same as in standard modes of ventilation.
- Backup modes of flow triggered pressure support and pressure control ventilation provide a safety net should the NAVA signal be lost.
- NAVA is commonly employed as a weaning tool; the optimal means of weaning NAVA support has yet to be determined; clear outcome benefits have yet to be demonstrated.
- NAVA is ineffective in the absence of a central respiratory drive (e.g. brainstem insult, sedative medications) or in the absence of adequate diaphragmatic signal (e.g. phrenic nerve injury, high spinal cord injury, or peripheral neuropathy).

FURTHER READING

Ferguson ND, Cook DJ, Guyatt GH, et al. High-frequency oscillation in early acute respiratory distress syndrome. *New England Journal of Medicine* 2013; 368(9): 795–805.

Terzi N, Piquilloud L, Rozé H, et al. Clinical review: update on neurally adjusted ventilatory assist–report of a round-table conference. *Critical Care* 2012; 16(3): 225.

Young D, Lamb SE, Shah S, et al. High-frequency oscillation for acute respiratory distress syndrome. *New England Journal of Medicine* 2013; 368(9): 806–13.

3.6 Extracorporeal support of the respiratory system

3.6.1 Indications and contra-indications

- Extracorporeal circuits may be utilized to provide CO_2 clearance and/or oxygenation.
- Indications and contra-indications are outlined in Table 1.14.

Table 1.14 Extracorporeal life-support organization: indications and contra-indications for ECMO

Indications	In hypoxic respiratory failure due to any cause ECMO should be considered when the risk of mortality is 50% or greater, and is indicated when the risk of mortality is 80% or greater.
	• 50% mortality risk can be identified by a P_aO_2/F_iO_2 <20 on F_iO_2 >90% and/or Murray score 2–3
	• 80% mortality risk can be identified by a P_aO_2/F_iO_2 <13.3 on F_iO_2 >90% and Murray score 3–4
	• CO_2 retention due to asthma or permissive hypercapnia with a P_aCO_2 >10.6 kPa or inability to achieve safe inflation pressures (Pplat ≤30 cm HO) is an indication for ECMO
	• Severe air leak syndromes
Contra-indications	There are no absolute contra-indications to ECMO, as each patient is considered individually with respect to risks and benefits. There are conditions, however, that are known to be associated with a poor outcome despite ECLS, and can be considered relative contra-indications.
	• Mechanical ventilation at high settings (F_iO_2 >90%, Plateau pressure >30 cmH_2O) for 7 days or more
	• Major pharmacologic immunosuppression (absolute neutrophil count <400/ml³)
	• CNS haemorrhage that is recent or expanding

Reproduced from the *Extracorporeal Life Support Organisation Guidelines for Adult Respiratory Failure* version 1.3. Copyright (2013) Extracorporeal Life Support Organization, http://www.elso.org/resources/Guidelines.aspx (Accessed on 15th September 2015)

3.6.2 Evidence

- The CESAR study investigated the use of ECMO in severe respiratory failure:
  - Patients were randomized to transfer to a specialist respiratory failure centre for ECMO or standard treatment at current hospital.
  - There was a significant decrease in mortality in the intervention group, although not all patients transferred received ECMO.
  - It has been suggested, therefore, that transfer to a specialist respiratory centre may be the key component of the intervention.

3.6.3 The ECMO circuit

- An ECMO circuit consists of:
  - An access cannula within the venous system
    - Typically inserted via the femoral or jugular vein with the tip lying in the IVC
  - A centrifugal pump
  - An oxygenator:
    - A polymethylpentane membrane that allows transfer of gas from a fresh gas flow to blood
    - A fresh gas supply, of up to 11 litres per minute; fractional oxygen content is set at 1.0 in respiratory ECMO and is varied in cardiac ECMO
  - A return cannula
    - For isolated respiratory support the return cannula lies in the venous system with the tip within the RA: veno-venous (VV) ECMO.
    - For cardiac and respiratory support the return cannula is inserted via the femoral artery into the descending aorta: veno-arterial (VA) ECMO.
    - In patients with a combination of cardiac and respiratory failure in whom the heart is expected to recover more quickly than the lungs, both a venous and arterial return cannula may be inserted, thus providing the operator with additional control as the patient recovers: veno-venous-arterial (V-VA) ECMO.
- VV ECMO
  - The primary determinant of systemic oxygenation is ECMO blood flow relative to cardiac output: the closer the ECMO blood flow to cardiac output, the greater the systemic oxygenation; if circuit blood flow is maximized but oxygenation inadequate, measures may be taken to reduce cardiac output, including beta blockade, hypothermia, and sedation.
  - CO_2 clearance is directly related to ECMO sweep gas flow.
- Extracorporeal CO_2 removal (ECCO$_2$ R):
  - Lower blood flow required than ECMO.
  - No meaningful oxygenation of blood.
  - Smaller cannulae may be used.
  - Requires less specialist input than ECMO and therefore feasible in non-specialist centres.
  - Holds promise in patients with hypercapnic respiratory failure.

3.6.4 Risks of extracorporeal support

- Risks associated with ECMO include:
  - Need for transfer to a specialist centre.
  - Cannulation:
    - Haemorrhage
    - Vascular injury

- ▪ Cardiac injury—guidewires or cannulae
- ▪ Hypotension and arrhythmias on initiation of ECMO
- Extracorporeal circuit:
  - ▪ Infection
  - ▪ Entrainment of air
  - ▪ Exsanguination
  - ▪ Activation of clotting cascade
- Coagulation:
  - ▪ Tendency to use unfractionated heparin to prolong circuit life
  - ▪ Thrombocytopaenia, hypofibrinogenaemia, and acquired Von Wilebrand deficiency increase the tendency to bleed
  - ▪ Thrombus formation may occur within the circuit or within cannulated vessels
- Deranged pharmacokinetics due to increased volume of distribution and sequestration of drug onto extracorporeal material:
  - ▪ Risk of under-dosing antibiotics

FURTHER READING

Extracorporeal Life Support Organisation Guidelines for Adult Respiratory Failure, version 1.3, December 2013.http://www.elso.org/resources/Guidelines.aspx

Peek GJ, Mugford M, Tiruvoipati R, et al. Efficacy and economic assessment of conventional ventilatory support versus extracorporeal membrane oxygenation for severe adult respiratory failure (CESAR): a multicentre randomized controlled trial. *Lancet* 2009; 374(9698): 1351–3.

---

4 Airway management

Airway management is a key component of intensive care. It may be described a series of increasingly complex manoeuvres designed to maintain a patent's upper airway and ultimately to protect the lower respiratory system against soiling.

4.1 Basic airway manoeuvres

4.1.1 Techniques

- The head tilt, chin lift, and the jaw thrust represent the most basic means of achieving airway patency in the patient compromised by low conscious state.
- These are commonly employed in conjunction with airway adjuncts, such as the oro-pharyngeal and naso-pharyngeal airways.
- These facilitate spontaneous respiration or assisted ventilation with a bag valve mask or anaesthetic circuit.

4.1.2 Advantages and disadvantages

- They are quick, simple, and often effective.
- They require minimal training and do not subject the patient to increased risk of harm.
- They do not, however, provide protection against soiling of the lower airways, nor do they allow delivery of high levels of positive pressure ventilation.

4.2 Advanced airway manoeuvres

4.2.1 Endotracheal intubation and rapid sequence induction

- The gold standard airway is the endotracheal tube.
- Indications for endotracheal intubation are outlined in Table 1.9.
- This is classically inserted by the rapid sequence induction (RSI) technique.
- The RSI differs from standard induction in that it is designed to secure the airway in the minimum possible time and prevent aspiration of gastric contents.
- There are numerous indications for RSI (Box 1.1); patients undergoing intubation on the intensive care unit almost inevitably fulfil one of these criteria.

Box 1.1 Indications for rapid sequence induction

- Non-fasted state
- Abdominal pathology (particularly ileus and obstruction)
- Incomplete gastric emptying (secondary to pain, trauma, opiates, critical illness)
- Incompetent lower oesophageal sphincter
- Altered consciousness
- Pregnancy
- Metabolic disturbance

4.2.2 'Classic' rapid sequence induction

The classic approach to RSI is outlined in Table 1.15.

Table 1.15 'Classic' rapid sequence induction

Preparation	Equipment and drugs check. Allocation of roles to team members. Clarification of anticipated difficulties and contingency plans (including failed intubation).
Pre-oxygenation	100% oxygen is administered via a closed circuit for 3–5 minutes, or until *expired* O_2 is >85%.
Cricoid pressure	A pressure is applied to the cricoid cartilage by an assistant to compress the upper oesophagus and thereby prevent reflux of gastric contents. Recommended force is 30 Newtons.
Predetermined dose of induction agent	3–7 mg/kg of thiopental (onset of anaesthesia in one 'arm-brain circulation time').
Predetermined dose of muscle relaxant	1.5 mg/kg of suxamethonium (onset of neuromuscular blockade within 60 seconds, heralded by muscle fasciculation).
No positive pressure ventilation prior to intubation	No bag-mask ventilation is undertaken in order to avoid gastric insufflation.
Intubation of trachea	Via direct laryngoscopy.
Confirmation of correct tube placement	By visualization of tube entering glottis; visualisation of chest movement; presence of breath sounds; presence end tidal CO_2 in >5 breaths. Cricoid pressure may then be removed.

4.2.3 Modified rapid sequence induction

- The approach to RSI is frequently modified in intensive care (Table 1.16); this is due to the nature of the patients:
  - A more unstable population than present to the theatre.
  - Greater risk of decompensation on induction of anaesthesia.
  - In whom immediate wake up in the event of complications is not viable.

Table 1.16 'Modified' rapid sequence induction technique

Preparation	Equipment and drugs check. Allocation of roles to team members. Clarification of anticipated difficulties and contingency plans (including failed intubation).
Pre-oxygenation	Sedation may be required to achieve adequate pre-oxygenation in the confused or agitated patient.
	The use of ketamine (1 mg/kg) in combination with NIV as a means of pre-oxygenating the agitated patient has been described as 'Delayed Sequence Induction'. Ketamine has the advantage of preserved respiratory drive and airway reflexes.
Cricoid pressure	May impair laryngoscopy view and there is no clear evidence that it reduces the risk of aspiration; omitted by many operators.
Predetermined dose of induction agent	Thiopental used less commonly in RSI: it is used infrequently in routine anaesthetics and therefore unfamiliar to many practitioners.
	Dose of induction agent frequently titrated: results in slower onset of anaesthesia but reduced risk of hypotension.
	High dose opiates frequently used as a relatively cardio-stable means of inducing anaesthesia and obtunding sympathetic response to laryngoscopy.
	Ketamine occasionally used as a haemodynamically stable induction agent.
Predetermined dose of muscle relaxant	High-dose rocuronium (>1.0 mg/kg) provides intubating conditions comparable to suxamethonium.
	Rocuronium is associated with fewer side-effects.
	In the critically ill population in whom 'wake up' in the event of complications is not viable, the longer action of rocuronium may facilitate emergency intervention (e.g. surgical airway).
	The selective relaxant binding agent sugammadex provides a rapid means of reversing rocuronium if required.
No positive pressure ventilation prior to intubation	Patients with impaired respiratory function may suffer profound desaturation in the period of apnoea between induction of anaesthesia and intubation.
	Constant flow of oxygen throughout the RSI period, by means of nasal cannula, has been demonstrated to better maintain arterial saturation, in a technique termed *apnoeic oxygenation*.
	Gentle manual ventilation is an accepted alternative.

4.2.4 Failed intubation and other airway emergencies in intensive care

- The risk of airway problems, including failed intubation, is significantly higher in the in ICU and emergency department than in the operating theatre.
- This is probably due to the case mix, availability of skilled staff, levels of assistance, and environmental factors.
- Analysis of adverse events reported to the 4th National Audit Project of the Royal College of Anaesthetists led to numerous recommendations to reduce the risk of airway-related problems on the ICU (Box 1.2).

Box 1.2 Recommendations from the 4th National Audit Project relating to ICU airway management

Capnography

- Capnography should be used for the intubation of all critically ill patients regardless of location.
- Continuous capnography should be used in all ICU patients with tracheal tubes who are ventilator-dependent.
- Training of all clinical staff who work on ICU should include interpretation of capnography.

Planning and checklists

- An intubation checklist should be developed and used for all intubations of critically ill patients.
- Every ICU should have algorithms for the management of intubation, extubation, and re-intubation.
- Patients at risk of airway events should be identified and clearly identifiable to those caring for them. A plan for such patients should be made and documented.
- Obese patients on ICU should be recognized as being at increased risk of airway complications and at increased risk of harm from such events.

Equipment

- Every ICU should have immediate access to a difficult airway trolley.
- A fibrescope should be immediately available for use on ICU.

Training and staffing

- Training of staff who might be engaged in advanced airway management of these potentially difficult patients should include regular, manikin-based practice in the performance of cricothyroidotomy.
- Trainee medical staff who are immediately responsible for management of patients on ICU need to be proficient in simple emergency airway management. They need to have access to senior medical staff with advanced airway skills at all hours.
- Regular audit should take place of airway management problems or critical events on the ICU.

- The standard means of managing failed intubation following RSI is outlined in the Difficult Airway Society algorithm (Fig. 1.10).
- This strategy is designed primarily for the theatre patient in whom cessation of anaesthesia is viable.
- For many patients intubated on the ICU, waking up is not a safe option and under these circumstances, the approach to difficult intubation may require modification.

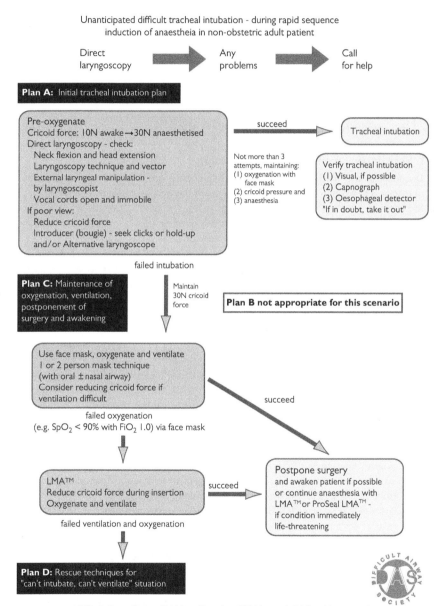

Difficult Airway Society Guidelines Flow-chart 2004 (use with DAS guidelines paper)

Fig. 1.10 Failed intubation algorithm.

Reproduced from *Anaesthesia*, Henderson JJ et al., 'Difficult Airway Society guidelines for management of the unanticipated difficult intubation', 59, pp. 675–94. Copyright (2004) with permission from John Wiley and Sons.

FURTHER READING

Cook T, Woodall M, Harper J. Major complications of airway management in the UK: results of the Fourth National Audit Project of the Royal College of Anaesthetists and the Difficult Airway Society. Part 2: intensive care and emergency departments. *British Journal of Anaesthesia* 2011; 106(5): 632–42.

Henderson JJ, Popat MT, Latto IP, Pearce AC. Difficult Airway Society guidelines for management of the unanticipated difficult intubation. *Anaesthesia* 2004; 59: 675–94.

Sinclair RC, Luxton MC. Rapid sequence induction. *Continuing Education in Anaesthesia, Critical Care & Pain* 2005; 5(2): 45–8.

5 Liberation from the ventilator

5.1 Ventilatory weaning and extubation

- Discontinuation of mechanical ventilation is a two-phase process, consisting of the evaluation of readiness to wean (through readiness testing) and the weaning itself (discontinuation or liberation).
- Readiness testing is the evaluation of objective criteria to determine whether a patient might, successfully and safely, be liberated from the ventilator.
- Weaning may involve either an immediate switch from full ventilator support to breathing without assistance from the ventilator or a gradual reduction in the amount of ventilator support.
- It is useful to distinguish 'weaning'—in which the reduction of assistance given to the patient aims to achieve liberation from the ventilator—from 'titration'—a process aimed at optimizing the level of support in patients not yet deemed suitable for liberation from mechanical ventilation.

5.1.1 Types of weaning

- Patients can be categorized into three groups in relation to the time needed to achieve liberation from ventilator
  - Simple weaning (60% patients): patients who can be extubated after the first weaning test (spontaneous breathing trial or SBT). The main clinical goal is the identification of readiness to wean, through a systematic screening strategy, avoiding delays in extubation.
  - Difficult weaning (30–40% of patients): patients who require up to three SBTs (or as long as 7 days) to be successfully extubated. The reasons for failed weaning have to be explored and corrected. The pathophysiology of weaning failure needs to be understood for the optimal management of the patient.
  - Prolonged weaning (6–15% of patients): this term applies to patients who exceed the limits of difficult weaning.
- In addition, some patients will need mechanical ventilation for more than 21 days and for more than 6 hours per day; these patients are classified as 'long term-weaning'.
- These patients—generally with a tracheostomy –will require an individualized approach to weaning with multi-disciplinary input.
- Regardless of the time required to achieve liberation, the accepted extubation failure rate is 10–20%.
- A re-intubation rate <5–10% may indicate a too conservative approach to extubation, which may lead to delayed liberation in some patients; on the contrary, a re-intubation rate >20–30% may indicate premature extubations.

5.1.2 Stages of weaning

- Stage 1—pre-weaning: main aim is the treatment of the underlying condition and weaning or liberation is not considered or desirable. Titration of ventilation is still possible.
- Stage 2—suspicion: period of diagnostic triggering; physician begins to think that their patient might have a reasonable probability of coming off the ventilator.
- Stage 3: time of measuring and interpreting daily weaning predictors.
- Stage 4: time of decreasing ventilator support (abruptly—through a spontaneous breathing trial or gradually—weaning process).
- Stage 5: extubation (of a weaning-success patient).
- Stage 6: use of non-invasive ventilation (NIV) after extubation.
- Stage 7: re-intubation (if fails).

5.1.3 Criteria for weaning and potential extubation

Weaning criteria are outlined in Box 1.3.

Box 1.3 Criteria for weaning and possible extubation

Airway

- Patent upper airway—if in doubt, this may be confirmed by visualization of airway via laryngoscope or fibrescope and performance of 'leak test'.

Breathing

- Minimal oxygenation support (e.g. F_iO_2 <0.4; PEEP <8 cmH$_2$O)
- Minimal ventilatory support (e.g. pressure support <10 cmH$_2$O)
- Adequate ventilatory drive (on a spontaneous mode of ventilation)
- Ability to clear secretions, and comply with physiotherapy

Circulation

- Haemodynamic stability

Disability

- Sufficient level of consciousness to protect airway

Everything else

- Original pathology prompting intubation resolved
- No procedures requiring sedation or anaesthesia planned in the near future

5.1.4 Weaning predictors

- First, the various indices that predict the likelihood that the patient may be liberated from mechanical support should be assessed (Table 1.17).
- Favourable outcome in this assessment should be followed by a spontaneous breathing trial (SBT).
- The terms applied to the various weaning indices will vary between ventilators.

Table 1.17 Weaning predictors

Indices	Cut-off value
Rapid shallow breathing index (RSBI) = f/Vt	<105 breaths.min^{-1}.l^{-1}
	Only valid if PEEP is = 0 and PS = 0 (flow-by).
P0.1 (airway occlusion pressure)	<(−)5.0 cmH$_2$O
Maximum inspiratory pressure (MIP)	<(-)30 cmH$_2$O (i.e. the more negative the better)
P0.1/MIP	<0.09−0.14 cmH$_2$O
Integrative Weaning Index (IWI)	>25 ml.cmH$_2$O^{-1}.breaths^{-1}.min^{-1}.l^{-1}
(C_{static} × SpO$_2$)/(f/Vt)	

See text in Section 5.1.4 for further explanation. F, frequency; Vt, tidal volume; C_{static}, static compliance.

- Parameters:
  - Rapid shallow breathing index (RSBI)
    - Proposed as a quantitative means of assessing the adequacy of respiratory function to then undertake a spontaneous breathing trial.
    - Measured over 1 minute with ventilator support off:

$$RSBI = \frac{f}{Vt}$$

    where f = frequency (breaths per minute); Vt = tidal volume (litres).
    - P 0.1
      - The negative pressure that occurs 100 ms after a spontaneous inspiratory effort has been detected. Test of respiratory drive, not volitional. Less than −5 (i.e. more negative) indicates increased work of breathing.
    - Maximum inspiratory pressure
      - The negative deflection in the pressure tracing during the patient's active and maximal effort to breathe during an expiratory hold manoeuvre at the end of a relaxed or forced expiration. It is a global assessment of the strength of the inspiratory muscles.
    - P0.1/MIP ratio
      - The relationship between P0.1 and MIP. Relates the work of breathing to the inspiratory muscle power. A higher P0.1 with a lower MIP would imply raised work of breathing with poor inspiratory muscle power and likelihood of pump failure if extubated.
    - Peak cough flow
      - Objectively records cough strength. Can be used serially for neuromuscular weakness or as a predictor for extubation readiness.
  - In patients who perform adequately in weaning prediction tests, a spontaneous breathing trial (SBT) may be undertaken.
  - The patient breathes without pressure support, or PEEP, through their endotracheal tube. The SBT should last *at least 30 minutes*; longer trials should be considered in patients at high risk of extubation failure (Box 1.5).
  - A patient is deemed to have failed the SBT if any of the criteria in Box 1.4 arise.

Box 1.4 Factors suggesting failure of the spontaneous breathing trial

The new onset of any one of the following:
- Physiological assessment:
  - Heart rate >20% of baseline or >140 beats min^{-1}
  - Systolic BP >20% of baseline or >180 mmHg or <90 mmHg
  - Cardiac arrhythmias
  - Respiratory rate >50% of baseline value or >35 min^{-1}
  - Respiratory rate (min)/tidal volume (l) >105 min^{-1} l^{-1}
- Arterial blood gases:
  - P_aO_2< 8 kPa on F_iO_2>0.5 or (SpO_2 <90%)
  - P_aCO_2> 6.5 kPa or increase by > 1 kPa
  - pH <7.32 or fall by >0.07 units
- Clinical assessment:
  - Agitation and anxiety
  - Depressed mental status
  - Sweating/clammy
  - Cyanosis
  - Increased respiratory effort (accessory muscles, facial distress, dyspnoea)

5.1.5 Failure to wean

There are a number of reasons whereby a patient may fail to wean from the ventilator (Table 1.18).

Table 1.18 Failure to wean from ventilator

	Possible causes	Possible approach
Simple weaning	• Delayed awakening due to accumulation of sedative drugs • Excessive level of ventilatory assist • Lack of systematic discussion during rounds • Reduced staffing levels	• Review of sedation • Establish a target sedation score (RASS) • Daily 'sedation holds' (i.e. stop or halve sedatives) if patient over-sedated • Document weaning plan • Standardize and document weaning readiness measurements • Avoid excessive ventilator assistance
Difficult weaning	• Accumulation of sedative drugs • Fluid overload • Left heart failure • Respiratory muscle weakness (myopathy) • Excessive workload due to infection, secretions, unresolved sepsis, etc.	• Review of sedation • Establish a target sedation score (RASS) • Physiotherapy and secretion management • Document weaning plan • Weaning readiness measurements • Echo • Measurement of NT-ProBNP • Optimisation of haemodynamics • Address underlying condition • Review readiness criteria parameters and consider SBT every 24 hours

continued

Table 1.18 *continued*

	Possible causes	Possible approach
Prolonged weaning	• Severe chronic heart failure • Severe chronic respiratory insufficiency • Respiratory muscle weakness • Depression • Poor sleep quality, delirium, • Persistence of underlying condition • Recurring sepsis • Neurological dysfunction	• Consider tracheostomy • Measurement of NT-ProBNP • Optimization of haemodynamics and fluid balance • Optimization of cardiac failure • Address underlying condition • Arrange MDT involvement, including physiotherapy, dieticians, neurology, etc. • Correct metabolic alkalosis • Address sleep, agitation, delirium, and pain

5.1.6 Extubation failure

Extubation failure is pragmatically defined as the need for re-intubation within 48 hours (72 hours if NIV is used).

Box 1.5 Risk factors for extubation failure

- Age >65 years or underlying chronic cardiorespiratory disease
- COPD*
- Heart failure/LV dysfunction*
- OSA/obesity*
- P_aCO_2 >6.5 kPa*
- Neuromuscular disorders*
- Positive fluid balance
- Ventilation >6 days

* These patients may benefit from 'prophylactic' NIV immediately post-extubation if SBT is successful.

5.1.7 Post extubation stridor

Post-extubation stridor occurs in up to 16% of extubations; risk factors are outlined in Table 1.19.

Table 1.19 Risk factors for post extubation stridor

Patient risk factors	Female
	Muscle weakness
	Tracheal infection
	Tracheal stenosis
	Recent airway related surgery
Intensive care related risk factors	Intubation >36 hours
	Excessive cuff pressures
	Large ETT
	Aggressive suctioning
	Nasogastric tube insertion

- Avoidance of risk factors and use of corticosteroids may reduce the incidence of post-extubation stridor.
- In high-risk patients, multiple doses of corticosteroids commenced 12–24 hours prior to extubation are recommended.

5.2 Tracheostomy

5.2.1 Rationale for tracheostomy in intensive care

- There are several indications for performing a tracheostomy on intensive care patients (Box 1.6).
- Tracheostomy confers numerous theoretical advantages over the endotracheal tube (Box 1.7).

Box 1.6 Indications for tracheostomy in the intensive care patient

- Inability to maintain upper airway—either primary airway pathology or neurological impairment
- Prolonged ventilator wean
- Inability to adequately clear respiratory secretions—either excessive secretions or impaired cough mechanism

Box 1.7 Potential advantages of tracheostomy over endotracheal tube

- Shorter tube:
  - Reduced dead space
  - Reduced resistance to gas flow
  - Reduced work of breathing
  - Easier access for suctioning
- Reduced need for sedation:
  - Improved cough and secretion clearance
  - Improved communication
  - Better compliance with physiotherapy
- Avoidance of transglottic tube
  - Improved access for mouth care
  - Potential for speech
  - Potential to eat

Effect of tracheostomy in reducing hospital-acquired pneumonia is unclear as studies are conflicting.

- Whilst there is general consensus on the indications for tracheostomy, the optimal timing of insertion is unclear.
- Studies comparing early (<4 days) versus late (>10 days) tracheostomy insertion in mechanically ventilated critically ill patients have demonstrated no clear difference in outcomes.

5.2.2 Performing the tracheostomy

The contra-indications to, and complications associated with, tracheostomy are outlined in Boxes 1.8 and 1.9.

Box 1.8 Contra-indications to tracheostomy

Local

- Anatomical abnormalities (e.g. tumour, goitre, previous surgery or radiotherapy)*
- Infection over insertion site
- Known or suspected difficult endotracheal intubation*
- Short neck (and difficulty palpating 1st and 2nd tracheal rings)*
- Obesity*
- Unstable spinal injury (preventing hyperextension of neck)*

Systemic

- Coagulopathy
- Significant haemodynamic instability
- Significant respiratory support (e.g. F_iO_2 >0.6; PEEP >10 cmH$_2$O)
- Inability to tolerate changes in P_aCO_2 (e.g. raised intracranial pressure)

* Relative contra-indication: surgical tracheostomy may be more appropriate than percutaneous.

Box 1.9 Complications of tracheostomy

Immediate

- Hypoxia, hypercarbia
- Loss of airway
- Aspiration of gastric contents
- Haemorrhage (ranging from minor oozing to life-threatening arterial haemorrhage)
- Damage to local structures (pneumothorax, surgical emphysema, cricoid cartilage injury, posterior tracheal wall injury, tracheal ring fracture)
- Anaesthesia-related (hypotension, anaphylaxis)

Early

- Infection of stoma
- Displacement of tracheostomy tube with loss of airway
- Occlusion of tracheostomy tube
- Tracheal injury (ulceration, fistula formation)
- Haemorrhage (from mucosal injury or erosion into right brachiocephalic artery)

Late

- Tracheal dilation
- Tracheomalacia
- Tracheal stenosis

- Critical care tracheostomy may be conducted by a percutaneous dilatational technique or by formal surgical means.
- Percutaneous tracheostomies are typically performed by critical care staff on the ICU.
- They are quicker, less expensive, and associated with fewer delays.

- Data regarding outcomes are somewhat conflicting—probably due to variations in surgical technique—but overall percutaneous tracheostomies appear to cause less bleeding and fewer deaths than those inserted surgically.
- The stages of percutaneous tracheostomy are described in Box. 1.10.

Box 1.10 Percutaneous tracheostomy technique

1. Assembly of necessary staff: minimum of one operator, one anaesthetist/airway doctor, and one assistant.
2. Position patient—supine with neck extension.
3. Ultrasound of anterior neck—identification of overlying vascular structures.
4. Anaesthesia/sedation deepened to surgical plane.
5. Identification of 2nd tracheal ring.
6. Infiltration of lignocaine with adrenaline in overlying skin.
7. Airway doctor withdraws ETT until around 2 cm remains below glottis; may be performed under laryngoscopic or bronchoscopic vision. Alternatively the ETT may be replaced by a supraglottic airway device, if risk of aspiration is low.
8. Cannula attached to saline-filled syringe inserted in the midline into the trachea at the level between second and third tracheal rings; aspiration of air suggests entry into trachea.
9. Guidewire passed down cannula.
10. Bronchoscope in the ETT used to confirm presence of guidewire in trachea and midline position.
11. Serial dilators passed over guidewire followed by the tracheostomy.
12. Tracheostomy position confirmed via bronchoscope and return of end tidal CO_2.

5.3 Bronchoscopy

Fibre optic bronchoscopy has a number of roles (Table 1.20).

Table 1.20 Indications for bronchoscopy

Diagnostic	Brocho-alveolar lavage (microbiology, cytology)
	Biopsy (microbiology, cytology)
	Assessment of inhalational injury
	Confirm correct endotracheal tube position
Therapeutic	Removal of bronchial obstruction (sputum, blood, foreign body)
	Placement of bronchial stent
Assist intervention	Fibreoptic tracheal intubation
	Percutaneous tracheostomy
	Positioning of double lumen endotracheal tube
	Positioning of endobronchial blocker

FURTHER READING

Khemani RG, Randolph A, Markovitz B. Corticosteroids for the prevention and treatment of post-extubation stridor in neonates, children and adults. *Cochrane Database of Systematic Reviews* 2009; (3):3.

Epstein SK. Weaning from ventilatory support. *Current Opinion in Critical Care* 2009; 15(1): 36–43.

Young D, Harrison DA, Cuthbertson BH, Rowan K. Effect of early vs late tracheostomy placement on survival in patients receiving mechanical ventilation: the TracMan randomized trial. *JAMA: the Journal of the American Medical Association* 2013; 309(20): 2121–9.

6 Acute respiratory distress syndrome

Acute respiratory distress syndrome (ARDS) is an inflammatory process affecting the lungs. Initial injury precipitates a sequence of events that manifest as impaired oxygenation, impaired compliance, and increased dead space. Histologically, ARDS may be observed as a number of phases: *exudative*, *proliferative*, and *fibrosing*, before final resolution.

6.1 Definition

6.1.1 The Berlin criteria

- The syndrome is defined by the Berlin criteria (Table 1.21).
- In 2012, the Berlin criteria replaced an earlier definition produced by the American-European Consensus Conference on ARDS.
- The new definition clarified the definition of acute, removed the requirement for pulmonary artery catheter measurements, included CT imaging, and integrated ventilator settings.

Table 1.21 Berlin criteria for ARDS

Berlin definition of ARDS	
Timing	Syndrome occurring within 1 week of known clinical insult.
Chest imaging	Bilateral opacities, not explained by effusions or collapse, and in keeping with pulmonary oedema, must be present on the chest X-ray or computed tomography scan.
Origin of oedema	Respiratory failure must not be fully explained by cardiac failure or fluid overload. Objective assessment of cardiac function (i.e. echo) should be conducted if no risk factors for ARDS exist.
Moderate to severe hypoxia	As defined by P_aO_2/F_iO_2 (P:F) ratio, on a ventilator with a PEEP setting of ≥ 5 cmH$_2$O:[*] • P:F <39.9 but >26.6 kPa—mild ARDS • P:F <26.6 but >13.3 kPa—moderate ARDS • P:F <13.3 kP—severe ARDS

[*]Patients may be defined as mild ARDS whilst on CPAP at ≥ 5 cmH$_2$O.

Adapted from *JAMA*, 307, 'The ARDSnet definition taskforce Berlin Definition, 2012. The ARDS Definition Task Force. Acute respiratory distress syndrome: The Berlin Definition', pp. 2526–33. Copyright (2012) with permission from *JAMA*.

6.1.2 Differential diagnosis

The differential diagnosis is outlined in Table 1.22.

Table 1.22 Differential diagnosis of ARDS

Differential diagnosis of ARDS	Discriminating investigation
Cardiogenic pulmonary oedema	Echocardiography; pulmonary artery catheter
Acute eosinophilic pneumonia	Eosinophil count (in blood or BAL)
Cryptogenic organizing pneumonia	BAL with cell count
Diffuse alveolar haemorrhage	Bronchoscopy; BAL

6.2 Aetiology and outcomes

6.2.1 Aetiology

The aetiology of ARDS is broadly divided into *direct* and *indirect* causes (Table 1.23).

Table 1.23 Aetiology of ARDS

Direct	Indirect
Pneumonia	Systemic sepsis
Viral pneumonitis	Major trauma
Chemical (aspiration) pneumonitis	Pancreatitis
Smoke inhalation	Pregnancy-related (eclampsia, amniotic fluid emboli)
Near drowning	Transfusion-related lung injury
Pulmonary contusions	Tumour lysis syndrome
Reperfusion injury	
Thoracic irradiation	

6.2.2 Mortality

- Mortality for mild, moderate, and severe ARDS is quoted as 27, 32, and 47%, respectively.
- Increasing age is associated with greater mortality, as is alcohol abuse.
- ARDS associated with trauma carries a lower mortality than other causes; ARDS associated with sepsis has a higher risk of death.
- ARDS non-survivors typically die *with* respiratory failure rather than *of* respiratory failure: hypoxia tends not to be the mode of death.

6.3 Management of ARDS

ARDS has been the focus of much critical care research. A number of landmark trials have been published and are outlined in Tables 1.24, 1.25, and 1.26. An awareness and understanding of these studies is important.

6.3.1 General management of ARDS

Table 1.24 describes the general strategies for management of ARDS.

Table 1.24 General management of ARDS

Sedation	Improves compliance with mechanical ventilation and reduces oxygen consumption. Must be balanced against the risks of excessive or prolonged sedation.
Neuromuscular blockade	Improves compliance and decreases oxygen consumption. Neuromuscular blockade is, however, associated with complications. There is evidence to suggest that their use in the early stages of severe ARDS (P:F <20 kPa) decreases mortality.
Cardiovascular monitoring	There appear to be no outcome benefits in routine insertion of a pulmonary artery catheter to guide the management of ARDS.
Fluid balance	The use of a 'conservative' fluid strategy—as dictated by a strict fluid management protocol—leads to improved lung function and reduced number of ventilator days but no reduction in mortality, when compared to a 'liberal' fluid strategy.
'House-keeping'	Strict attention should be paid to: • Infection control • DVT prophylaxis • Ulcer prophylaxis • Nutrition

FURTHER READING

ARDSnet. Pulmonary-artery versus central venous catheter to guide treatment of acute lung injury. *New England Journal of Medicine* 2006; 354(21): 2213–24.

ARDSnet. Comparison of two fluid-management strategies in acute lung injury. *New England Journal of Medicine* 2006; 354(24): 2564–75.

The ARDS Definition Task Force. Acute respiratory distress syndrome: the Berlin definition. *JAMA: the journal of the American Medical Association* 2012; 307(23): 2526–33.

Papazian L, Forel J-M, Gacouin A, et al. Neuromuscular blockers in early acute respiratory distress syndrome. *New England Journal of Medicine* 2010; 363(12): 1107–16.

6.3.2 Ventilator strategies in ARDS

Careful attention should be paid to ventilation of the ARDS patient (Table 1.25).

Table 1.25 Ventilator strategies proposed in ARDS

Low tidal volume ventilation	The use of low tidal volumes (6 ml/kg ideal body weight) leads to a significantly lower mortality than high tidal volumes (12 ml/kg). The optimal tidal volume is unknown; 6–8 ml/kg is a common target.
Maintenance of plateau pressure <30 cmH$_2$O	The avoidance of excessive pressure and the target of 30 cmH$_2$O are derived from the same study as tidal volumes. The optimal and safe maximum pressures are unknown.
PEEP	The use of high PEEP is suggested as a means of maintaining open alveoli, and of reducing atelectrauma. Investigations of outcome benefit have produced conflicting results: probably due to the heterogeneity of the ARDS population. Meta-analysis suggests possible improvement in ICU mortality with high PEEP in the severe ARDS subgroup.
Recruitment manoeuvres	The use of recruitment manoeuvres in an attempt to open collapsed alveoli has been shown to improve oxygenation. There is, however, no evidence to demonstrate improved outcomes.
Permissive hypercapnia	Acceptance of hypercapnea and respiratory acidosis as a means of reducing ventilator associated lung injury is common practice. Respiratory acidosis is well tolerated by most patients; at extreme levels it may precipitate sufficient pulmonary vasoconstriction to cause right ventricular dysfunction.
Prone ventilation	See Section 3.4.2.
HFOV	See Section 3.5.1.
ECMO	See Section 3.6.

FURTHER READING

ARDSnet group Ventilation with lower tidal volumes as compared with traditional tidal volumes for acute lung injury and the acute respiratory distress syndrome. The Acute Respiratory Distress Syndrome Network. *New England Journal of Medicine* 2000; 342(18): 1302–30.

Hodgson C, Keating JL, Holland AE, et al. Recruitment manoeuvres for adults with acute lung injury receiving mechanical ventilation. *Cochrane Database of Systematic Reviews* 2009; (2): Cd006667.

Santa Cruz R, Rojas JI, Nervi R, Heredia R, Ciapponi A. High versus low positive end-expiratory pressure (PEEP) levels for mechanically ventilated adult patients with acute lung injury and acute respiratory distress syndrome. *Cochrane Database Systematic Reviews* 2013; 6: Cd009098.

6.3.3 Specific therapies for ARDS

A number of specific therapies, aimed at modifying the disease process, have been proposed for the treatment of ARDS; clinical trials have produced almost universally disappointing results (Table 1.26).

Table 1.26 Specific therapies proposed for ARDS

Steroids	Theoretically beneficial given the inflammatory nature of ARDS. Steroids appear to improve oxygenation and to increase the number of ventilator-free days. Evidence regarding mortality benefit is conflicting and appears to be related to the timing of steroids. Late steroids may improve mortality if given between 7 and 13 days, but appear to increase mortality beyond 14 days. Early steroids (<72 hours) may improve mortality but remain under-investigated.
B$_2$ agonists	B$_2$ agonists have been shown to reduce extravascular lung water and airway pressure; there is, however, no evidence that this results in improved outcome. They may worsen outcomes.
Surfactant	Inhaled exogenous surfactant has the theoretical benefit of replacing the dysfunctional endogenous surfactant produced by the ARDS lung and thus reducing the force required to recruit ateletatic alveoli. No clinical benefit has been demonstrated.
Statins	The anti-inflammatory property of statins has been postulated as potentially beneficial in ARDS. A small trial of statins in ARDS demonstrated improvement in non-pulmonary organ dysfunction. Larger study has shown no benefit.
Inhaled pulmonary vasodilators (e.g. nitric oxide)	Inhaled nitric oxide selectively vasodilates those pulmonary vessels serving the ventilated lung. It has negligible systemic effects. In theory it should improve ventilation-perfusion matching and reduce right ventricular afterload. Whilst the use of nitric oxide consistently improved oxygenation it has not been shown to improve outcomes.

- Other agents proposed in the treatment of ARDS in whom theoretical benefits have not been borne out in clinical trials include: n-acetylcysteine, intravenous prostacycline, macrolide antibiotics and ketoconazole.

FURTHER READING

Afshari A, Brok J, Moller AM, Wetterslev J. Inhaled nitric oxide for acute respiratory distress syndrome and acute lung injury in adults and children: a systematic review with meta-analysis and trial sequential analysis. *Anesthesia and Analgesia* 2011; 112(6): 1411–21.

Craig TR, Duffy MJ, Shyamsundar M, et al. A randomized clinical trial of hydroxymethylglutaryl-coenzyme a reductase inhibition for acute lung injury (The HARP Study). *American Journal of Respiratory and Critical Care Medicine* 2011; 183(5): 620–6.

Davidson WJ, Dorscheid D, Spragg R, Schulzer M, Mak E, Ayas NT. Exogenous pulmonary surfactant for the treatment of adult patients with acute respiratory distress syndrome: results of a meta-analysis. *Critical Care* 2006; 10(2): R41.

Meduri GU, Marik PE, Chrousos GP, et al. Steroid treatment in ARDS: a critical appraisal of the ARDS network trial and the recent literature. *Intensive Care Medicine* 2008; 34(1): 61–9.

Smith FG, Perkins GD, Gates S, et al. Effect of intravenous β-2 agonist treatment on clinical outcomes in acute respiratory distress syndrome (BALTI-2): a multicentre, randomized controlled trial. *Lancet* 2012; 379(9812): 229–35.

7 Inhalational injury

7.1 Mechanisms of injury

7.1.1 Mechanism

Multiple mechanisms of injury coexist:

- Heat (causes oedema, erythema, and ulceration of the mucosa).
- Toxins (e.g. sulphur dioxide, chlorine, ammonia) cause damage by pH or free-radical damage.
- Environmental hypoxia due to oxygen consumption.

7.1.2 Pathophysiology

The pathological process follows a similar pattern to other forms of lung injury:

- Exudative phase (characterized by neutrophil influx, macrophage activation, increased permeability, type 2 pneumocyte dysfunction with resultant decrease in surfactant production).
- Fibrotic phase (fibrosing alveolitis, neoangiogenesis collagen deposition).

7.2 Assessment and management

Initial assessment and management should follow a systematic, advanced trauma life support based approach:

7.2.1 Airway

- Seek evidence of airway involvement (facial or mucosal burns, singeing of nasal hair, hoarse voice, carbonaceous sputum).
- Low threshold for early intubation as airway burns may result in rapidly progressive oedema, which makes later airway intervention impossible.
- Endotracheal tubes should be uncut and secured in such a way that progressive swelling will not cause migration of the tube (wiring to gum or teeth is an option).

7.2.2 Breathing

- Respiratory distress may take time to evolve.
- ABG provides a baseline and allows measurement of carboxyhaemoglobin levels.
- In the ventilated patient, lung protective strategy should be employed.
- Bronchoscopy allows documentation of the injury and evacuation of sputum plugs.
- Consider nebulized salbutamol, heparin, and N-acetyl cysteine.

7.2.3 Circulation

For further information see burns in Chapter 8, Section 3.2.3.

7.3 Specific toxins

7.3.1 Carbon monoxide

- Binds to haemoglobin with 250 times the affinity of oxygen and thus impacts upon oxygen carriage; the oxy-haemoglobin curve is shifted to the left.
- Cellular cytochrome oxidase system is inhibited.
- Combined, tissue hypoxia ensues.
- Pulse oximeters cannot differentiate between oxyhaemoglobin and carboxyhaemoglobin: a blood gas is therefore required.
- Plasma carboxyhaemoglobin (COHb) level >10% potentially problematic.
- Management is with oxygen therapy: 100% oxygen reduces the half-life of COHb from 4 hours to 1 hour.
- As a general rule:
  - COHb >10%: oxygen therapy with high concentration face mask
  - COHb >25%: oxygen therapy and ventilation
  - COHb >40%: comatose, pregnant or failing to respond to conventional therapy—consider hyperbaric oxygen (3 atmospheres pressure reduces half-life to 30 minutes—impractical in most centres and infrequently used)

7.3.2 Cyanide

- Combustion of household materials may liberate cyanide gas.
- Cyanide binds to the ferric ion on cytochrome oxidase, blocking aerobic cellular metabolism.
- Clinical features relate to generalized cytotoxic hypoxia; cyanide poisoning should be considered in any patient with a history of smoke inhalation and unexplained lactic acidosis.
- Treatment includes:
  - Supportive measures
  - Direct binding of cyanide:
    - Intravenous *hydroxycobalamin* or dicobalt edetate
  - Induction of methaemoglobinaemia:
    - The resultant ferric ion provides an alternative binding site for cyanide
    - *Amyl nitrate or sodium nitrite*
  - Sulphur donation
    - Sulphur donors convert cyanide to the inert and renally excreted thiocyanate
    - *Sodium thiosulphate*

8 Acute severe asthma

- Asthma is a chronic disease of the airways associated with airway hyper-reactivity and inflammation.
- Exacerbation of asthma is characterized by mucosal oedema, increase in sputum production, and bronchospasm, the combination of which leads to widespread airflow obstruction.

8.1 Risk factors and severity

8.1.1 Risk factors for fatal asthma

Risk factors for fatal asthma are outlined in Box 1.11.

Box 1.11 Risk factor for fatal asthma

- Previous life-threatening asthma with acidosis or need for ventilation
- Hospital admission for asthma within the last year
- Three or more asthma medications for chronic control
- Heavy beta agonist use
- 'Brittle' asthma
    - Type 1—wide PEFR variability
    - Type 2—sudden severe attacks despite appearing well controlled
- Evidence of adverse psycho-social circumstances (alcohol abuse, non-compliance with treatment, social isolation)

8.1.2 Severity of asthma

Markers of severity are described in Table 1.27.

Table 1.27 Markers of severity in asthma

Degree of severity	Features
Moderate	PEFR 50–75% predicted
Severe	PEFR 33–55% predicted
	Respiratory rate >25
	Heart rate >110
	Low or normal P_aCO_2
	Unable to complete a sentence
Life-threatening	PEFR <33% predicted
	Feeble respiratory effort; silent chest
	Arrhythmias
	Hypotension
	Bradycardia
	Hypoxia (SpO2 <92%; P_aO_2 <8 kPa)
	Hypercapnia
	Altered neurological state

- An arterial blood gas and chest X-ray are indicated in the presence of any feature of life-threatening asthma.

8.2 Management

8.2.1 Medical management of asthma

The medical options in the management of asthma are described in Table 1.28.

Table 1.28 Medical management of asthma

Beta 2 agonists	• Inhaled beta 2 agonists are first-line treatment for acute severe asthma. Salbutamol and terbutaline are equally effective; both are equivalent to inhaled adrenaline and have fewer side-effects. • Inhaled therapy may be delivered by repeated metered dose inhaler or nebulizer. The particle size generated by the former facilitates more favourable distribution within the smaller airways. • Intravenous therapy has no added benefit and should be reserved for those in whom inhaled therapy cannot be effectively delivered.
Anti-cholinergic agents	• Inhaled ipratropium bromide has a synergetic effect with beta agonists and is recommended in acute severe asthma. • Ipratropium may dry secretions increasing tenacity and increasing difficulty in expectoration.
Steroids	• Steroids reduce mortality, early use is recommended. • In the absence of vomiting or gut failure, oral prednisolone (40 mg od) and intravenous hydrocortisone (100 mg qid) are equally efficacious.
Magnesium sulphate	• A single intravenous dose of magnesium sulphate (1.2–2 g) is recommended in severe or life-threatening asthma. • Bronchodilation is believed to be due to inhibition of calcium influx into smooth muscle. • The benefits of repeated dosing are unclear and may precipitate hypermagnesaemia with associated muscle weakness.
Theophylline	• The addition of intravenous aminophylline does not appear to confer any additional benefit to standard therapy. It is associated with increased incidence of side-effects, in particular arrhythmia and vomiting.
Antibiotics	• Routine use of antibiotics in acute severe asthma is not recommended. These should be reserved for cases in whom bacterial infection is suspected.
Helium–oxygen mix	• Heliox is of lower density than air or oxygen. In theory this makes flow within the narrowed airways more likely to be laminar than turbulent (as described by Reynold's number) and thus reduces the resistance to flow. • There is no evidence, however, that heliox improves respiratory function or outcomes.

Adapted, with permission, from British Guideline for the Management of Asthma, *SIGN* 2014.

8.3 Respiratory mechanics in asthma

8.3.1 Airflow limitation

- The respiratory failure associated with asthma is mechanical in nature:
  - Airflow limitation occurs primarily in the small airways.
  - During spontaneous inspiration, negative pressure generated by the diaphragm and thoracic muscles expands these small airways, assisting flow.
  - Return of intrathoracic pressure to neutral during normal, passive expiration causes the small airways to reduce in size.

- Flow limitation therefore occurs primarily in expiration.
- Attempts by the patient to increase expiratory flow by active exhalation increases intrathoracic pressure, potentially exacerbating the small airway obstruction.

8.3.2 Dynamic hyperinflation

- In severe airflow limitation, the expiratory time may be insufficient to allow complete expiration:
  - The residual volume may increase with each breath in a process known as *dynamic hyperinflation* or *gas-trapping*.
  - Hyperinflation shifts the lungs up the compliance curve (Fig. 1.8), decreases compliance, and thereby places the respiratory system at further mechanical disadvantage.
  - Compensatory tachypnoea increases the work of breathing and decreases the time available for expiration.
  - And so ensues a vicious cycle of deteriorating respiratory function.

8.3.3 Dynamic hyperventilation in mechanical ventilation

- Dynamic hyperinflation can be identified in the mechanically ventilated patient by observation of the gas flow against time waveform:
  - Failure of expiratory flow to return to baseline before the ventilator triggers, suggests incomplete expiration and hence dynamic hyperinflation.
  - The degree of hyperinflation may be quantified by measuring *intrinsic PEEP* (or auto PEEP).
  - In the absence of any spontaneous respiratory effort, an *expiratory hold* is performed on the ventilator and end expiratory alveolar pressure allowed to equilibrate with upper airway pressure.
  - The measured pressure minus the PEEP delivered by the ventilator equals the intrinsic PEEP.
  - In the presence of patient respiratory effort, an expiratory hold is not feasible. Under these circumstances, intrinsic PEEP can only be measured by an oesophageal balloon.

8.3.4 Practicalities of mechanical ventilation in asthma

Ventilation in asthma can be difficult; it requires careful monitoring and management (Table 1.29).

Table 1.29 Ventilation and asthma

Non-invasive ventilation	• Traditionally has a limited role in asthma.
	• In theory, IPAP will reduce the work of breathing, whilst EPAP splints open small airways assisting expiration.
	• Should only be undertaken in a critical care area capable of escalation to invasive ventilation if required.
Induction of anaesthesia	• The bronchodilatory effects of ketamine provide potential benefits as an induction agent.
	• Hypotension on induction may be significant as high intrathoracic pressures impede preload.
Maintenance of sedation	• Ketamine may provide sedation and bronchodilation.
	• The inhalational anaesthetic agents halothane, sevoflurane, and isoflurane have bronchodilatory properties. Delivery of anaesthetic agents via intensive care ventilators may be problematic, as is scavenging of waste gases and monitoring of end tidal anaesthetic concentrations.

Table 1.29 *continued*

Dynamic hyperinflation	• Risk reduced by increasing the period of time in expiration:
	  ▪ Prolonged I:E ratio (short inspiratory time, high inspiratory flow rate)
	  ▪ Slow respiratory rate

The role of PEEP	• Intrinsic peep generated by dynamic hyperinflation creates problems with ventilation:
	  ▪ The lungs are shifted up the compliance curve, potentially leading to decreased compliance
	  ▪ The patient will need to generate greater changes in flow or pressure to trigger the ventilator: dysynchrony is more likely
	• Extrinsic, ventilator delivered, PEEP may aid to splint open small airways and promote alveolar emptying.
	• In spontaneous ventilatory modes, extrinsic PEEP may reduce the effort required to trigger ventilation by reducing the negative pressure deflection required by the patient to initiate inspiration.

Airway pressures	• Volume-controlled ventilation in severe asthma typically produces high-peak airway pressures (reflecting resistance to flow within the airways) but normal plateau pressures. The reduction in the difference between peak and plateau pressures (and therefore tidal volumes) may be used as an indication of improving bronchial airway calibre.

FURTHER READING

Scottish Intercollegiate Guidelines Network (SIGN). *British Guideline on the Management of Asthma.* Edinburgh: SIGN; 2014. (SIGN publication no. 141). [cited 05 Sep 2015]. Available from URL: http://www.sign.ac.uk

---

9 Exacerbation of COPD

9.1 General

- Exacerbation of COPD is characterized by increased dyspnoea, sputum production, or cough.
- Up to 80% of exacerbations are precipitated by viral (e.g. rhinovirus, influenza, parainfluenza) or bacterial infection (*Haemophilus influenzae, Moraxella catarrhalis*, and *Streptococcus pneumonia* being most common).
- Differential diagnosis includes pneumonia, pneumothorax, pulmonary oedema, or pulmonary embolus.
- Whilst the mechanisms underlying asthma and COPD differ, the mechanisms of respiratory failure are similar. Many of the principles of management apply to exacerbations of both conditions.

9.2 Management of COPD

9.2.1 Medical management

Medical management is described in Table 1.30.

Table 1.30 Management of acute exacerbation of COPD

Bronchodilators	• Salbutamol and ipratropium improve airflow limitation. • Multi-dose inhaler and nebulizer delivery appear equally efficacious. • There is no clear guidance regarding the use of intravenous bronchodilators in COPD.
Steroids	• Systemic steroids result in more rapid resolution of symptoms and reduction in length of hospital stay but no demonstrable improvement in mortality. • Oral and intravenous routes appear equally efficacious, assuming the oral route is available.
Antibiotics	• Recommended in the presence of increased purulence of sputum or focal chest X-ray change. • Amoxicillin, macrolides, and tetracyclines are acceptable first-line therapy. Local sensitivities and guidance should, however, be followed.
Aminophylline	• A methylated xanthine derivative, aminophylline bronchodilates, increases diaphragmatic activity and acts as a diuretic. • There is no evidence that intravenous aminophylline improves outcome in exacerbations of COPD. • Its use is, however, recommended in cases of bronchospasm refractory to inhaled salbutamol.
Respiratory stimulants	• The use of doxapram as a respiratory stimulant to manage hypercapnic respiratory failure is recommended only if non-invasive ventilation is unavailable.

9.2.2 Non-invasive ventilation

• Non-invasive ventilation (NIV) is the treatment of choice for hypercapnic respiratory failure, which persists despite optimal medical management.
• NIV is discussed in greater detail in Section 3.3.

9.3 Invasive ventilation and COPD

9.3.1 The controversy of mechanical ventilation

• Intubation and invasive ventilation are contentious issues in the context of exacerbations of COPD with an oft cited belief that outcomes are generally poor.
• When compared to other groups with severe respiratory failure, however, COPD patients have a lower mortality and shorter duration of ICU stay.
• Furthermore, long-term follow-up of those requiring invasive ventilation found post-discharge quality of life to be largely maintained and that the vast majority of patients would choose to undergo ventilation again, if required.

9.3.2 Predictors of survival and futility

• Predictors of increased mortality include the need for ventilation for greater than 72 hours and failed extubation attempt.
• A previous need for mechanical ventilation, not related to surgery, appears to be a predictor of survival.

FURTHER READING

Esteban A, Anzueto A, Frutos F, et al. Characteristics and outcomes in adult patients receiving mechanical ventilation: a 28-day international study. *JAMA: the journal of the American Medical Association* 2002; 287(3): 345–55.

Nevins ML, Epstein SK. Predictors of outcome for patients with COPD requiring invasive mechanical ventilation. *CHEST Journal* 2001; 119(6): 1840–9.

NICE. *Management of Chronic Obstructive Pulmonary Disease in Adults in Primary and Secondary Care*, 2012. http://guidance.nice.org.uk/CG101/Guidance/pdf/English.

Wildman MJ, Sanderson CF, Groves J, et al. Survival and quality of life for patients with COPD or asthma admitted to intensive care in a UK multicentre cohort: the COPD and Asthma Outcome Study (CAOS). *Thorax* 2009; 64(2): 128–32.

10 Pneumonia

10.1 Categorization of pneumonia

10.1.1 Community acquired pneumonia

- Community acquired pneumonia (CAP) is an acute infection of the lung parenchyma, evolving in the community or within 48 hours of hospital admission.
- Common organisms are outlined in Table 1.31.

10.1.2 Hospital acquired pneumonia

- Hospital acquired pneumonia (HAP) is defined as pneumonia acquired more than 48 hours following admission.
- Incidence of HAP is increased by chronic lung disease and immunocompromised.
- Causative organisms in HAP differ from CAP, with Gram-negative bacterial most commonly implicated (Table 1.31) in hospital.
- Antibiotic resistance is more common in HAP, particularly in the immunocompromised, those receiving antibiotics within the last 90 day, in hospital for greater than 5 days, and originating from a long-term care facility.
- Local resistance patterns should guide antibiotic choice; however, anti-pseudomonal beta lactams (e.g. pipericillin with tazobactam) or a quinolone (e.g. ciprofloxacin) are commonly used in the treatment of HAP.

Table 1.31 Common causative organisms in CAP and HAP

Community acquired pneumonia	Hospital acquired pneumonia
Streptococcus pneumonia	*Pseudomonas aeruginosa*
Haemophillus influenzae	*Escherichia coli*
Mycoplasma pneumoniae	*Klebsiella pneumoniae*
Legionella	*Acinetobacter spp.*
Chlamydia pneumoniae	

10.1.3 Ventilator-associated pneumonia

- Ventilator-associated pneumonia (VAP) is defined as nosocomial pneumonia occurring in a patient ventilated for greater than 48 hours.
- Intubation is associated with a 21-fold increase risk of pneumonia.

- Proposed mechanisms behind this higher incidence include:
  - Aspiration of oropharyngeal contents around the cuff
  - Colonization of the tracheal tube (biofilm)
  - Haematological spread
- Diagnosis requires the development of new respiratory symptoms associated with new chest X-ray infiltrates.
- Confirmation of VAP requires isolation and quantification of bacteria from the respiratory tract (Table 1.32).
- Numerous means of reducing the incidence of VAP have been suggested (Box 1.12), many of which are routinely combined as bundles of care. The introduction of care bundles in themselves has been suggested to decrease the rate of VAP.

Table 1.32 Respiratory tract sampling in the intubated patient and thresholds for diagnosis of VAP

Sampling technique	Method	Quantitative diagnostic threshold for VAP (colony forming units(CFU)/ml)
Tracheobronchial aspiration	Suction catheter advanced until resistance met; suction applied.	1,000,000 CFU/ml
Non-directed bronchoalveolar lavage	Catheter advanced until resistance met, sterile saline injected and then aspirated.	10,000 CFU/ml
Bronchoalveolar lavage	Fibreoptic bronchoscope wedged into segment, sterile saline injected and aspirated	10,000 CFU/ml
Protected Brush Specimen	Bronchoscope wedged in to segment, sterile brush extended from scope to sample airway.	1,000 CFU/ml

Box 1.12 Strategies for reducing the incidence of VAP

- Reduce the risk of micro aspiration of bacteria:
  - Semi-recumbent position (>30-degree head up)
  - Prone ventilation
  - Monitor cuff pressures (avoid cuff deflation to <30 cmH$_2$0)
  - Supraglottic suction devices
  - Feeding:
    - Entreral feeding increases the risk of VAP
    - The use of post-pyloric feeding tubes does not reduce VAP incidence
    - There is no convincing evidence that pro-kinetics reduce VAP incidence
- Gastric acid:
  - The use of proton pump inhibitors has been demonstrated to increase risk of VAP
- Reduce bacterial colonization:
  - Chlorhexidine mouthwash
  - Selective oral and digestive decontamination (Chapter 6, Section 7.4.5)
  - Use of sterile respiratory equipment
- Minimize duration of ventilation:
  - Aim to extubate as early as possible, daily assessment
  - Daily sedation holds

10.1.4 Healthcare associated pneumonia

- Healthcare associated pneumonia (HCAP) is defined as a pneumonia developing in a non-hospitalized patient who has extensive exposure to healthcare environments (e.g. dialysis or nursing home resident); this has implications for multi-drug resistance.

10.1.5 Immunocompromise

- Pneumonia in the immunocompromised poses an additional challenge.
- The chest X-ray appearance is useful in directing diagnosis (Table 1.33); however, bronchoscopy directed alveolar lavage is the gold standard and often necessary to obtain positive microbiology.

Table 1.33 Differential diagnosis of pneumonia in the immunocompromised patient based on chest X-ray findings

Diffuse infiltrate on the CXR	Focal infiltrate on CXR
Cytomegalovirus	Gram-negative rods
Pneumocystic jiroveci (PCP)	Staphylococcus aureus
Aspergillus	Aspergillus
Cryptococcus	Norcardia
Non-infective cause (drugs, radiation, graft versus host disease)	Cryptococcus
	Non-infective causes

- Invasive ventilation in neutropaenic pneumonia is associated with a particularly high mortality, and a there is typically a higher threshold for intubation (see Section 3.3).

10.2 Assessment and severity scores

- All patients admitted to hospital with CAP should have CXR and routine bloods.
- Microbiological investigation of severe CAP should include blood culture, sputum for Gram stain and culture, urine pneumococcal antigen, urine legionella antigen, and PCR for mycoplasma, where available.
- All patients admitted with CAP should have the severity of illness assessed. The British Thoracic Society recommend the CURB 65 system (Table 1.34); patients with a score of $>/= 3$ should be considered for transfer to a critical care bed.
- The SMARTCOP system (Fig 1.11) is an alternative means of predicting the need for respiratory or haemodynamic support.

Table 1.34 CURB 65 score

Scoring (1 point for each)	30-Day mortality as predicted by CURB 65
Confusion	0–0.7%
Urea >7 mmol/l	1–3.2%
Respiratory Rate >30 per minute	2–13%
Blood Pressure (Systolic) <90 mmHg	3–17%
Age >65 years	4–41.5%
	5–57%

SMART-COP

A tool for predicting which patients with community-acquired pneumonia (CAP) are likely to require intensive respiratory or vasopressor support (IRVS).

CAP confirmed on CXR

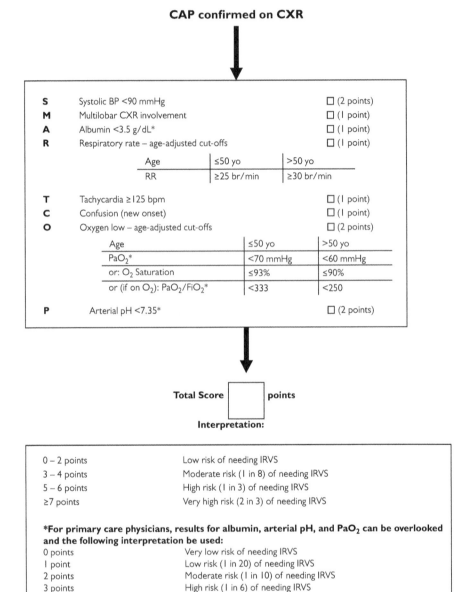

S	Systolic BP <90 mmHg	☐ (2 points)
M	Multilobar CXR involvement	☐ (1 point)
A	Albumin <3.5 g/dL*	☐ (1 point)
R	Respiratory rate – age-adjusted cut-offs	☐ (1 point)

Age	≤50 yo	>50 yo
RR	≥25 br/min	≥30 br/min

T	Tachycardia ≥125 bpm	☐ (1 point)
C	Confusion (new onset)	☐ (1 point)
O	Oxygen low – age-adjusted cut-offs	☐ (2 points)

Age	≤50 yo	>50 yo
PaO_2*	<70 mmHg	<60 mmHg
or: O_2 Saturation	≤93%	≤90%
or (if on O_2): PaO_2/FiO_2*	<333	<250

P	Arterial pH <7.35*	☐ (2 points)

Total Score [ ] points

Interpretation:

0 – 2 points	Low risk of needing IRVS
3 – 4 points	Moderate risk (1 in 8) of needing IRVS
5 – 6 points	High risk (1 in 3) of needing IRVS
≥7 points	Very high risk (2 in 3) of needing IRVS

*For primary care physicians, results for albumin, arterial pH, and PaO_2 can be overlooked and the following interpretation be used:

0 points	Very low risk of needing IRVS
1 point	Low risk (1 in 20) of needing IRVS
2 points	Moderate risk (1 in 10) of needing IRVS
3 points	High risk (1 in 6) of needing IRVS
≥4 points	High risk (1 in 3) of needing IRVS

Fig. 1.11 SMARTCOP score (to convert mmHg to kPa divide by 7.5).

Reproduced from *Clinical Infectious Diseases*, 47, Charles PG et al., 'SMART-COP: a tool for predicting the need for intensive respiratory or vasopressor support in community-acquired pneumonia', pp. 375–84. Copyright (2008) with permission from Oxford University Press

10.3 Management

10.3.1 Antibiotics

- Patients with severe CAP should immediately receive parenteral antibiotics:
  - A beta lactamase-resistant penicillin (e.g. co-amoxiclav) combined with a macrolide (e.g. clarithromycin) is recommended as first line.
  - Second- and third-generation cephalosporins may be a suitable alternative in penicillin allergy (although a small proportion of patients will demonstrate cross reactivity).
  - Duration of treatment should be guided by microbiological results and opinion; at least 7 days is recommended in severe CAP.

10.3.2 Steroids

- In a multi-centre randomized control trial, the use of methylprednisolone was shown to re-duce 'treatment failure' in a group of patients with CAP and high inflammatory markers.
- Treatment failure was defined as:
  - Development of shock
  - Subsequent need for ventilator support
  - Radiographic progression
  - Death

10.3.3 Non-invasive ventilation

- Non-invasive ventilation has a limited role in respiratory failure secondary to CAP.
  - Whilst many exhibit improvement in oxygenation, greater than 50% are likely to fail (particularly if RR >30 or age >40).
  - Trials of NIV should therefore be undertaken in a critical care area.

10.3.4 Invasive ventilation

- Invasive ventilation should employ standard lung protective strategies.
- It should be noted that consolidated lung may not be amenable to ventilation. Accordingly, volume and pressure applied may only impact upon healthy lung, risking iatrogenic injury.

10.4 Complications of pneumonia

10.4.1 Parapneumonic effusion

- Common (up to 50%).
- British Thoracic Society recommend diagnostic tap and if empyema drainage.

10.4.2 Abscess formation

- More common in debilitated patients, those with history of alcohol abuse, and following aspiration.
- Require prolonged antibiotic therapy.

10.4.3 Metastatic infection

- Particularly common with *Staphylococcus aureus* and *Streptococcus pneumoniae*.
- May affect joints, meninges and endocardium.

10.4.4 Legionella-specific complications

- Encephalitis
- Pericarditis

- Pancreatitis
- Hyponatraemia
- Deranged liver function
- Thrombocytopaenia

FURTHER READING

Bouadma L, Deslandes E, Lolom I, et al. Long-term impact of a multifaceted prevention program on ventilator-associated pneumonia in a medical intensive care unit. *Clinical Infectious Diseases: an official publication of the Infectious Diseases Society of America* 2010; 51(10): 1115–22.

British Thoracic Society. *Guidelines for the Management of Community Acquired Pneumonia in Adults*, 2009. http://www.brit-thoracic.org.uk/guidelines/pneumonia-guidelines.aspx

Charles PG, Wolfe R, Whitby M, et al. SMART-COP: a tool for predicting the need for intensive respiratory or vasopressor support in community-acquired pneumonia. *Clinical Infectious Diseases: an official publication of the Infectious Diseases Society of America* 2008; 47(3): 375–84.

Lim WS, van der Eerden MM, Laing R, et al. Defining community acquired pneumonia severity on presentation to hospital: an international derivation and validation study. *Thorax* 2003; 58(5): 377–82.

Torres A, Sibila O, Ferrer M, et al. Effect of corticosteroids on treatment failure among hospitalized patients with severe community-acquired pneumonia and high inflammatory response: a randomized clinical trial. *JAMA: the journal of the American Medical Association* 2015; 313(7): 677–86.

---

11 Pulmonary embolus

11.1 Risk factors and presentation

- Pulmonary embolus (PE) describes the obstruction of the pulmonary arterial system by thrombus, fat, air, or tumour.

11.1.1 Risk factors

- Risk factors for thrombus related disease are described by Virchow's triad:
  - Venous stasis
  - Hypercoagulability
  - Endothelial injury
- All critically ill patients are at risk and should receive mechanical and pharmacological prophylaxis unless contra-indicated.

11.1.2 Presentation

- The clinical manifestations of pulmonary embolus (PE) are vague:
  - Tachycardia
  - Hypotension
  - Tachypnoea
  - Hypoxia
  - All are common in critical care; high index of suspicion is required
- Approximately 10% of patients with acute pulmonary embolus will die within 3 months of diagnosis.

11.1.3 Risk stratification

- Pulmonary emboli which cause the systolic blood pressure to drop below 90 mmHg or 40 mmHg below baseline for 15 minutes or more, are defined as 'massive'.
- All other PTE are categorized as 'sub-massive'.
- A number of factors are associated with an increased risk of death:
  - RV dysfunction, identified either by echocardiogram or CT scan (2–3-fold increase in mortality)
  - The presence of thrombus in the RV
  - Co-existing deep vein thrombosis
  - Elevated troponin
  - Elevated brain naturetic peptide
  - Elevated lactate
  - Hyponatraemia
- The mortality of untreated PTE is estimated at between 20 and 30%; death is usually the result of a second embolic event.

11.2 Pathophysiology

11.2.1 Hypoxaemia

- The degree of hypoxia is variable; mechanisms are described in Box 1.13.
- Obstruction of the pulmonary arterial tree and low cardiac output state creates an acute ventilation–perfusion mismatch with significant rise in alveolar dead space; a rise in minute volume is therefore required to achieve adequate CO_2 clearance.

Box 1.13 Mechanisms of hypoxaemia in pulmonary embolus

- V/Q mismatch:
  - Obstruction to flow leads primarily to an increased V/Q with rise in deadspace.
  - If a large vessel is obstructed, blood will be diverted through other, patent pulmonary vessels, flow will therefore exceed ventilation in these lung units, and a degree of shunt will occur.
- Depletion of surfactant leads to atelectasis.
- Reperfusion injury to the endothelium.
- Acute rise in right heart pressure may result in right to left flow of blood through existing atrial or ventricular septal defect creating an intra-cardiac shunt.
- Reduction in cardiac output causes reduction in venous oxygen saturation (due to increased systemic oxygen extraction, this therefore increases the impact of venous admixture).

11.2.2 Acute cor pulmonale

- Mechanical obstruction and reactive pulmonary vasoconstriction leads to a sudden increase in right ventricular (RV) afterload.
- The RV copes poorly with sudden increase in afterload: the consequence is dilation and impaired systolic function.
- The left and right ventricles exhibit 'interdependence' owing to the fixed volume of the pericardial sack: RV dilation impinges on the LV leading to impaired LV filling and potentially low cardiac output.
- RV coronary perfusion is determined by the mean arterial pressure—RV pressures (this differs from coronary perfusion in the higher pressure LV which cannot occur during systole and

is therefore dependent upon diastolic blood pressure); PTE causes elevation of RV pressures, hence elevated mean arterial pressure is required to maintain coronary perfusion.

- If mechanical ventilation is required to support respiratory function, this too will increase RV afterload, further impeding RV function.

11.3 Supportive management

11.3.1 Hypoxaemia

- Hypoxia is treated in the first instance with supplemental oxygen.
- Mechanical ventilation may be required for refractory hypoxia or unsustainable work of breathing.

11.3.2 Cor pulmonale and shock

- Management of shock depends upon optimization of RV loading and coronary perfusion.
- Volume resuscitation may provide some improvement in cardiac output; excess fluid administration will, however, further distend the RV with a detrimental effect on systolic function and coronary perfusion.
- Noradrenaline may be required to maintain MAP and coronary perfusion.
- Pulmonary vasodilators have an uncertain role; options include:
  - Intravenous (e.g. milrinone, prostacyclin)
  - Enteral (sildenafil)
  - Inhaled (nitric oxide, prostacyclin)

11.4 Specific management

11.4.1 Anticoagulation

- First-line therapy is therapeutic anticoagulation.
- Low molecular weight heparin (LMWH) and fondiparinux are at least as effective as unfractionated heparin (UH) in reducing recurrence of thrombus or death.
- The convenience of the LMWH and fondaparinux make these the treatment of choice in most patients; the exceptions to this rule are:
  - Massive PTE—in which there is little experience with any anticoagulant other than UH
  - If thrombolysis is being considered—in which the risk of bleeding is less with UH
  - If there is risk of significant bleeding—the shorter half-life and reversibility of UH makes it preferable
  - If absorption of subcutaneous drugs is believed to be impaired—IV UH is preferable

11.4.2 Thrombolysis

- In PTE with hypotension, systemic thrombolysis has been demonstrated to reduce mortality.
- The use of thrombolysis for 'moderate' pulmonary emboli, in the absence of hypotension, has been shown to reduce the incidence of pulmonary hypertension and length of hospital stay but has not been demonstrated to reduce mortality.

11.4.3 Caval filter

- Caval filters provide mechanical protection from recurrent PTE.
- They are typically placed in the inferior vena cava under radiological guidance.
- Filters have a role when anti-coagulation is contra-indicated, if PTE has recurred despite therapeutic anti-coagulation, and in those in whom cardiorespiratory function has been so impaired by the initial PTE that a further embolic event is likely to prove fatal.

11.4.4 Embolectomy

- Embolectomy may be considered for massive PTE, where thrombolytic therapy is contra-indicated.
- Embolectomy may be performed by catheter or surgical technique.
- Catheter options include: rheolytic, in which pressurized saline is used to disrupt the thrombus; rotational, in which a rotating device is used to disperse clot; suction; or ultrasound.
- Surgical embolectomy requires a hospital with cardiothoracic facilities.
- Outcomes following catheter and surgical embolectomy have not been compared.

FURTHER READING

Meyer G, Vicaut E, Danays T, et al. Fibrinolysis for patients with intermediate-risk pulmonary embolism. *New England Journal of Medicine* 2014; 370(15): 1402–11.

NICE. *Venous Thromboembolism—Reducing the Risk*, 2010. http://guidance.nice.org.uk/CG92

Sharifi M, Bay C, Skrocki L, Rahimi F, Mehdipour M. Moderate pulmonary embolism treated with thrombolysis (from the 'MOPETT' Trial). *The American Journal of Cardiology* 2013; 111(2): 273–7.

---

12 Pleural disease

12.1 Pleural effusions

Pleural effusion describes the presence of fluid between the parietal and visceral pleura.

12.1.1 Analysis of pleural fluid

- Protein level
    - >30 g.l^{-1} = exudate
    - <30 g.l^{-1} = transudate
    - If plasma protein normal
- Light's criteria
    - More sensitive and particularly useful if plasma protein low (as is often the case in the ICU)
    - Suggestive of exudate, if any of the following criteria fulfilled:
        - Pleural to serum protein level >0.5
        - Pleural to serum LDH level >0.6
        - Pleural LDH level >2/3 upper limit of normal serum LDH level
- Findings suggestive of an empyema
    - pH <7.2
    - Glucose <3.3
    - Bacteria on microscopy
    - Fluid LDH >1,000

12.1.2 Aetiology

- Transudates:
    - Consequence of increased capillary hydrostatic pressure, or decreased plasma oncotic pressure:
        - Failure of heart, liver, kidneys

- Hypothyroidism
- Meig's syndrome (the right-sided effusions associated with ovarian tumours)
- A small proportion (<5%) of pulmonary tumours

- Exudates:
  - Consequence of increased capillary permeability or decreased lymphatic absorption from the pleural space:
    - Pulmonary infections: pneumonia, tuberculosis, empyema
    - Pulmonary malignancy: bronchial carcinoma, mesothelioma
    - Connective tissue disease: rheumatoid arthritis, systemic lupus erythematous
    - Systemic inflammation: pancreatitis

12.1.3 Management

- Drainage is indicated if:
  - Contributing to respiratory failure
  - Infected (i.e. empyema)
- Complex, organized effusions may be managed by:
  - Radiologically guided drainage to optimize drain position (ultrasound or CT)
  - Instillation of tissue plasminogen activator +/− DNAase may be used to break down complex effusions
  - Video-assisted thoracoscopic surgery (VATS) may be required for formal surgical decortication

12.2 Pneumothorax

12.2.1 Aetiology

- Spontaneous (primary)
- Secondary
  - Emphysema
  - Cancer
  - Tuberculosis
  - ARDS
- Iatrogenic
  - Bronchial or pleural biopsy
  - Central line or pacemaker insertion
- Traumatic
- Ventilator associated lung injury

12.2.2 Management

- Small pneumothoracies (<2 cm on X-ray) with no associated respiratory difficulty may be managed conservatively, with observation; administration of a high F_iO_2 may speed absorption of air from the pleural space.
- Larger pneumothoracies, and those associated with respiratory difficulty, should be drained by intercostal drain +/− suction (high-volume, low-pressure system).

12.2.3 Refractory pneumothoracies

- Refractory or recurrent pneumothoracies may benefit from:
  - Medical pleurdesis
  - VATS pleurectomy
  - Open thoracotomy with pleurectomy

12.3 Bronchopleural fistula

12.3.1 Aetiology

- Post-pulmonary surgery
- Post-pneumonia
- Cancer (particularly bronchial, also thyroid and oesophageal)
- Penetrating trauma
- ARDS

12.3.2 Management options

- Chest drain insertion; avoidance of suction.
- Minimization of airway pressure:
  - Avoidance of positive pressure ventilation, where possible
  - Lowest pressures required, if mechanical support required
  - High frequency oscillatory ventilation
  - Extracorporeal membrane oxygenation
  - Double lumen tubes and selective lung ventilation
- Definitive closure:
  - Bronchoscopy:
    - Stents
    - Glue
    - Bronchial blocker
  - Segmentectomy/lobectomy

FURTHER READING

Hooper C, Lee YG, Maskell N. Investigation of a unilateral pleural effusion in adults: British Thoracic Society pleural disease guideline 2010. *Thorax* 2010; 65(Suppl 2): ii4–17.

Lois M, Noppen M. Bronchopleural fistulas: an overview of the problem with special focus on endoscopic management. *CHEST Journal* 2005; 128(6): 3955–65.

MacDuff A, Arnold A, Harvey J. Management of spontaneous pneumothorax: British Thoracic Society pleural disease guideline 2010. *Thorax* 2010; 65(Suppl 2): ii18–31.

Oxford Medical Education '*Pleural Effusion*' and '*Pneumothorax*', http://www.oxfordmedicaleducation.com/respiratory/

---

13 Massive haemoptysis

13.1 General

13.1.1 Definition

- Massive haemoptysis is defined as blood loss within the airways at a rate that poses an immediate threat to life.
- This may be as little as 200 ml/24 hours.

13.1.2 Source

- The majority of cases from bronchial vessels (90%), although pulmonary (5%) and non-pulmonary systemic (5%), are alternative sources.
- The likely cause is dependent upon geographical location (Table 1.35).

Table 1.35 Causes of haemoptysis in developed and developing regions

Developed regions	Developing regions
<ul><li>Neoplasm</li><li>Inflammation<ul><li>Chronic bronchitis</li><li>Fungal lung disease</li><li>Vasculitis</li><li>Cystic fibrosis</li><li>Other bronchiectasis</li></ul></li><li>Coagulopathy</li><li>Iatrogenic</li></ul>	<ul><li>Tuberculosis</li><li>Lung abscess</li><li>Neoplasm</li></ul>

13.2 Management

13.2.1 Priorities

- Death from massive haemoptysis is by asphyxiation rather than exsanguination.
- The priorities are, therefore, to secure the airway, preserve gas exchange, then volume resuscitation.

13.2.2 Intervention

- Large-bore endotracheal tube to facilitate bronchoscopy.
- Preserve gas exchange:
  - Placing the bleeding side down
  - Isolating the lungs with bronchial blockers or a double lumen tube
- Volume resuscitation.
- Correction of coagulopathy.
- Tranexamic acid.
- Consideration of anti-tussives.

13.2.3 Definitive management

- Bronchoscopy potentially allows identification of the bleeding point and definitive intervention.
- Bronchoscopic options include:
  - Balloon tamponade
  - Direct injection of haemostatic drugs
  - Isolation of bleeding lobe with a bronchial blocker
- CT angiogram with subsequent radiological embolization provides a possible alternative definitive management.

CHAPTER 2

Cardiovascular

CONTENTS

1 Shock

1.1 Background

1.1.1 Definition

- Shock is a multifactorial syndrome in which cardiovascular dysfunction results in a reduction in tissue oxygen delivery to a level below that required to meet metabolic demands.
- This imbalance between oxygen delivery and demand results in tissue hypoxia and lactic acidosis, which, if not promptly reversed, leads to progressive cellular injury, multiple organ failure, and death.
- Tissue oxygen delivery is dependent upon the complex balance between blood flow and perfusion pressure, at both global and local levels.
- This complex balance of perfusion and blood flow is represented in a clinical context by two end parameters, the manipulation of which forms the basis of cardiovascular management in the intensive care:
  - Blood pressure
  - Oxygen carriage
- *Blood pressure* is the end product of a number of independent cardiovascular factors (Fig. 2.1) and is the most frequently used parameter to define shock.
  - A systolic blood pressure (SBP) below 90 mmHg is commonly considered to represent shock.
  - Mean arterial pressure (MAP) is, however, a better indicator of vital organ perfusion; the exception is the left ventricular myocardium which is only perfused in diastole and therefore relies upon adequate diastolic blood pressure (DBP).
- Shock may however occur in the presence of a normal blood pressure: tissue perfusion is dependent not only upon adequate blood pressure, but also adequate flow and *oxygen carriage*.

- Oxygen carriage is represented by the oxygen flux equation in which cardiac output (CO) is a key factor:

$$DO_2 = CO(SpO_2 \times Hb \times 1.34) + (0.003\ P_aO_2)$$

- Examination of the determinants of blood pressure and oxygen carriage reveals four primary cardiovascular parameters (preload, myocardial contractility, heart rate, and systemic vascular resistance) which may contribute to a state of shock; this forms the basis of the categorization of shock (section 1.2).

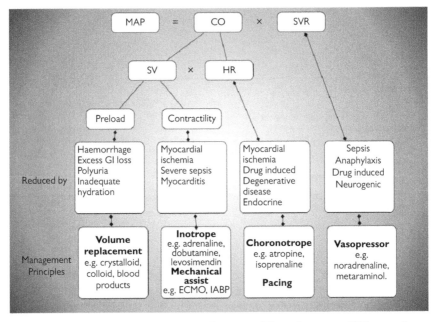

Fig. 2.1 Aetiology of shock. MAP, mean arterial pressure; CO, cardiac output; SVR, systemic vascular resistance; SV, stroke volume; HR-heart rate.

1.2 Classification of shock

- The development of shock is related to the alteration of one or more of the four main components that regulate cardiovascular performance:
  - Preload (dependent upon the circulating blood volume and tone of the venous capacitance system, which regulate the venous return to the heart)
  - Heart rate
  - Myocardial contractility
  - Systemic vascular resistance (as determined by arteriolar tone)
- Shock can be classified into three categories based on aetiology.

1.2.1 Hypovolaemic shock

- Hypovolaemia is the most common cause of shock. Inadequate circulating volume results from:
  - Blood loss (trauma, gastrointestinal bleeding, ruptured aortic aneurysm, etc.)
  - Fluid loss (diarrhoea, vomiting, burns)
  - Third space fluid sequestration (bowel obstruction, pancreatitis, and cirrhosis)

1.2.2 Cardiogenic shock

- Cardiogenic shock is a state of inadequate tissue perfusion due to myocardial pump dysfunction. It is often diagnosed by the presence of:
  - A systolic blood pressure of <90 mmHg or a mean arterial pressure (MAP) <65 mmHg for ≥1 hour that is not responsive to fluid administration.
  - A cardiac index <2.2 l/min/m².
  - Elevated end-diastolic filling pressure (pulmonary-artery occlusion pressure, PAOP >18 mmHg), and pulmonary oedema.
  - However, the absence of pulmonary congestion and hypotension at initial clinical evaluation does not exclude a diagnosis of cardiogenic shock.

1.2.3 Distributive (vasodilatory) shock

- In distributive shock, contrary to the other types of shock, the tissue hypoxia is contributed to by an ineffective tissue oxygen extraction and the loss of vasoregulatory control leading to inappropriate vasodilatation and maldistribution of blood flow within the micro-circulation.
- Cardiac output is typically preserved or increased.
- Causes of distributive shock include:
  - Severe sepsis
  - Neurogenic shock after cerebral or spinal cord injury, leading to loss of vasomotor tone and bradycardia
  - Anaphylaxis
  - Drug reactions
  - Adrenal failure
  - Conditions associated with the formation of peripheral shunts, such as chronic liver failure and Paget's disease

1.2.4 Further classification: hyperdynamic and hypodynamic

- The three categories of shock can be grouped, according to their haemodynamic profiles, into two types, depending on whether the cardiac output is decreased (hypodynamic) or increased (hyperdynamic):
  - Hypodynamic shock (hypovolaemic and cardiogenic) is characterized by:
    - Low cardiac output
    - Inadequate blood flow or volume
    - High-resistance vasoconstricted state, with cool, clammy peripheries, weak/ thready pulse with prolonged capillary refill time
  - Hyperdynamic shock is characterized by:
    - High cardiac output
    - Inability of the cells to extract and utilize oxygen
    - Low-resistance vasodilated state, with warm, dilated peripheries, bounding pulses, and tachycardia

2 Cardiovascular assessment and monitoring

2.1 Clinical parameters

2.1.1 Clinical

Assessment should begin with clinical parameters, as outlined in Table 2.1.

Table 2.1 Clinical manifestations of shock

System	Clinical	Investigations
Neurological	Confusion, agitation, decreased conscious state	
Cardiovascular	Ischaemic chest pain, tachycardia, hypotension.	ST changes on ECG
Renal	Low urine output	Elevation in plasma creatinine
Respiratory	Low SpO$_2$, increased RR	Increase in dead space
Other	Cool peripheries, prolonged capillary refill time	Elevation in plasma lactate, fall in SvO$_2$

2.2 Biochemical parameters

- The measurement of three easily obtainable biochemical parameters can indirectly assess global tissue oxygenation and perfusion in patients with shock:
  - Mixed and central venous oxygenation
  - Arterial blood lactate
  - Difference between arterial and mixed venous partial pressure of CO_2 ($\Delta_{a-v}pCO_2$).

2.2.1 Venous oxygen saturation

- Central venous oxygen saturation (ScvO$_2$) is measured in blood drawn from a central venous catheter in the superior vena cava; mixed venous oxygen saturation (SvO$_2$) is measured in blood from a pulmonary artery catheter port in either the right ventricle or pulmonary artery.
- Reduction in venous oxygen saturation suggests an increase in oxygen extraction in the peripheral tissues, due to decreased oxygen delivery.
- In the context of steady oxygen demand, *decreased* venous oxygen saturation occurs secondary to a fall in one of the components of the oxygen flux equation (Section 1.1.1).
- *Increase* in venous saturation suggests impaired oxygen extraction; this may occur with the mitochondrial dysfunction of severe sepsis and in the uncoupling of the cellular respiration associated with particular toxins (cyanide and salicylates).
- Normal value for ScvO$_2$ (65%) is typically lower than that of the SvO$_2$ (70%):
  - Due to relatively higher oxygen extraction by organs draining into the superior vena cava in comparison to those draining into the inferior vena cava.
  - This relationship may reverse in the context of shock, during which oxygen extraction from the viscera increases disproportionately to oxygen extraction from the brain.

2.2.2 Lactate

- Inadequate tissue oxygen delivery leads to anaerobic metabolism and a subsequent lactic acidosis.
- Elevated lactate is a non-specific finding and may be secondary to a number of other mechanisms (Table 2.2).
- Tracking of plasma lactate provides information regarding severity of illness and adequacy of resuscitation.
- The measurement of lactate is a key component of the Surviving Sepsis Guidelines.

Table 2.2 Classification of lactic acidosis (as described by Cohen and Woods 1976)

	Mechanisms	Associated disease process
Type A Lactic Acidosis	Clinical evidence of inadequate tissue oxygen delivery	Low cardiac output; low oxygen content; severe anaemia; extreme muscular activity (sprinting, seizures); regional hypoperfusion (ischaemic gut or limb).
Type B Lactic Acidosis	B1 Underlying disease	Acute hepatic failure; ketoacidosis; leukaemia; lymphoma; AIDS.
	B2 Drugs and toxins	Metformin; methanol; adrenaline; salbutamol; antiretroviral drugs.
	B3 Inborn errors of metabolism	Pyruvate dehydrogenase deficiency

Data from Cohen RD and Woods HF, *Clinical and Biochemical Aspects of Lactic Acidosis*, 1976.

2.2.3 Difference between the venous and arterial and pCO₂ ($\Delta_{v\text{-}a}pCO_2$)

- $\Delta_{v\text{-}a}pCO_2$ is measured as the difference between contemporaneous measurements of central venous or mixed pCO_2 and the arterial pCO_2.
- $\Delta_{a\text{-}v}pCO_2$ reflects the adequacy of blood flow to remove the tissue CO_2, and therefore is an expression of cardiac output.

2.3 The arterial waveform

2.3.1 General

- Placement of the arterial catheter is one of the most common interventions in the intensive care unit; the waveform assists in interpretation of the shock state (Table 2.3).
- A catheter is inserted into a peripheral or central artery; this allows arterial blood to be in contact with a column of fluid in a monitoring line, which is in turn in contact with a pressure transducer (which converts mechanical energy into an electrical signal).
- The column of fluid is connected to a pressurized bag of normal saline; a valve allows an infusion of 3–4 ml per hour of fluid down the line to maintain catheter patency.
- The transducer kits are specifically designed (in terms of length, diameter, and material) to provide optimal *damping* of the pressure waveform:
    - An 'underdamped' trace will display an inaccurately high systolic blood pressure and an inaccurately low diastolic blood pressure (but mean arterial pressure should be accurate).
    - an 'overdamped' trace will delay an inaccurately low systolic blood pressure and an inaccurately low diastolic blood pressure (but mean arterial pressure should be accurate).
- Typically, the facility exists to draw samples from the arterial catheter for frequent arterial blood analysis.
- Basic information provided by the arterial waveform includes:
    - Pulse rate
    - Beat to beat measurement of:
        - Systolic blood pressure
        - Diastolic blood pressure
        - Mean arterial pressure

2.3.2 Morphology of the arterial waveform

- The shape of the arterial waveform is determined by numerous factors:
    - The stroke volume.
    - The force of ejection from the left ventricle (contractility).

- The ability of the central arterial tree to distend and accommodate ejected blood (capacitance).
- The rate of dissipation of blood from the central arteries into peripheral circulation (peripheral resistance).
- Systolic blood pressure is influenced by stroke volume and level of capacitance:
    - In the context of stable capacitance, increase in stroke volume will lead to increase in systolic blood pressure.
    - As capacitance decreases (e.g. as arteries develop arteriosclerosis with increasing age), systolic blood pressure will rise.
- Diastolic blood pressure is determined by the ability of proximal vessels to recoil and maintain pressure within the system in the absence of left ventricular output and the resistance to this blood flow by peripheral arteries:
    - The reduced capacitance of arteriosclerosis is also associated with decreased elastic recoil, and therefore a reduction in diastolic blood pressure.
    - Reduction in peripheral vascular resistance (e.g. with sepsis) allows a pressure drop from the central compartment to a lower final level (which manifests as a lower diastolic blood pressure).

2.3.3 The dicrotic notch

- Represents closure of the aortic valve (and hence end of systole).
- Typically occurs at one-third into the pressure wave descent when aortic pressure (AoP) exceeds left ventricular pressure (LVP); if peripheral resistance is reduced (e.g. sepsis), AoP>LVP later in the cycle and the dicrotic notch shifts down the curve.

2.3.4 Cardio-respiratory interactions

- Discussed under 'fluid responsiveness', Section 2.5.

2.3.5 Pulse contour analysis

- Discussed under 'cardiac output monitoring', Section 2.4

Table 2.3 Changes in the arterial waveform in response to shock states

	Mean arterial pressure	Diastolic blood pressure	Pulse pressure	Pulse pressure variation	Dicrotic notch
Hypovolaemia	↓	↑	↓	↑	–
Impaired ventricular function	↓	↑	↓	–	–
Vasodilation	↓	↓	↑	–	Downwards shift

FURTHER READING

Nirmalan M, Dark PM. Broader applications of arterial pressure wave form analysis. *Continuing Education in Anaesthesia, Critical Care & Pain* 2014; **14**(6): 285–90.

2.4 Cardiac output monitoring

In the search for the aetiology of a shock state, or in the ongoing monitoring and circulatory optimization of the critically ill patient, it may be desirable to measure (and monitor the changes of) cardiac output. Numerical values for cardiac output may be obtained by minimally invasive or invasive means.

2.4.1 Pulmonary artery catheter

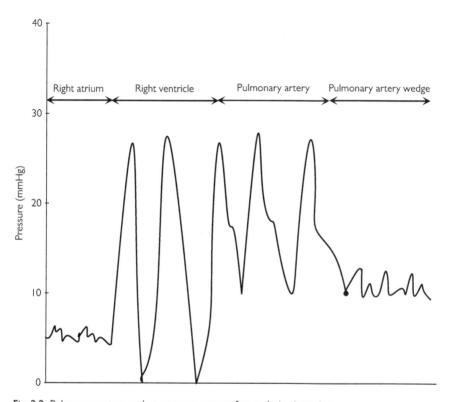

Fig. 2.2 Pulmonary artery catheter: pressure waveforms during insertion.

- A venous catheter is inserted by means of a sheath into a central vein and 'floated' via a balloon at the tip through the right heart chamber into the pulmonary arterial circulation.
- Insertion may be assisted by fluoroscopy or, more commonly, by monitoring the pressure changes as it moves through the various chambers (Fig. 2.2).
- Generally considered the 'gold standard' of cardiovascular monitoring, indications are outlined in Table 2.4.
- Measured and derived parameters are outlined in Table 2.5.
- Recently fallen out of favour, as a number of large, prospective trials have shown no outcome benefit with PAC use, and an increase in adverse events and resource consumption in the PAC group. Recognized complications are listed in Table 2.6.
- The validity of assessing a monitoring device by means of a randomized controlled trial is, however, questioned. Many clinicians still consider it superior to other forms of cardiovascular monitoring and it remains a standard of care in many centres, particularly for cardiac patients.

Table 2.4 Indications for pulmonary artery catheter insertion

Determination of:	Aetiology of the shock state
	Cardiogenic vs. non-cardiogenic pulmonary oedema
Diagnosis of:	Pulmonary hypertension
	Intra-cardiac shunt
Monitoring of:	Oxygen delivery
	Fluid balance
	Response to vasoactive drugs
	Central temperature

Table 2.5 Pulmonary artery catheter parameters. Calculation of CaO_2 is described in Chapter 1, Table 1.1.

	Variable		Normal values
Direct measurements	Right atrial pressure (RAP)		2–6 mmHg
	Right ventricular pressures (RVP)		sys 20–30 mmHg dia 0–5 mmHg
	Pulmonary artery pressures (PAP)		sys 20–30 mmHg dia 8–12 mmHg mean 10–20 mmHg
	Pulmonary artery wedge pressure (PAWP)		4–12 mmHg
	Cardiac output (CO)		4–8 litres.min^{-1}
Derived variables	Cardiac index (CI)	$\dfrac{CO}{BSA}$	2.5–4 litres.min^{-1}
	Systemic vascular resistance (SVR)	$\dfrac{MAP - RAP}{CO}$	800–1,200 dynes.s.cm^{-5}
	Pulmonary vascular resistance (PVR)	$\dfrac{mPAP - LAP}{CO}$	37–250 dynes.s.cm^{-5}
	Oxygen delivery (DO$_2$)	$CO\left(SpO_2 \times Hb \times 1.34\right) + \left(0.003\, P_aO_2\right)$	
	Oxygen consumption (VO$_2$)	$10\left(CaO_2 - CVO_2\right) \times CO$	

Table 2.6 Complications associated with the pulmonary artery catheter

Complications associated with insertion	Arterial puncture
	Pneumothorax/haemothorax
	Arrhythmias
	Air embolus
	Valvular damage
Complications associated with catheter in situ	Misinterpretation of information
	Catheter knotting within right ventricle
	Pulmonary artery rupture
	Infection
	Thrombus

- Cardiac output is measured by means of thermodilution:
  - A saline bolus, of known volume and temperature, is injected through a port 10 cm proximal to the tip.
  - A thermistor at the tip monitors the resultant change in blood temperature; cardiac output is derived by means of the Stewart–Hamilton equation:

$$CO = \frac{k\left(\text{core temperature} - \text{indicator temperature}\right) \times \text{volume of indicator}}{\text{Change in blood temperature}}$$

  - Cardiac output measurement is traditionally conducted intermittently by manual boluses of saline.
  - Alternatively, continuous monitoring systems are available in which a heating element is integrated into the proximal portion of the catheter, intermittently heating passing blood and thereby generating frequent, automatic temperature washout curves from which cardiac output may be monitored.
- Measurement may be rendered inaccurate by:
  - Tricuspid regurgitation
  - Intra-cardiac shunt
  - Slow injection of fluid
  - Impairment of thermistor function due to proximity to vascular wall

2.4.2 Trans-pulmonary dilution and pulse contour analysis techniques

- The PiCCO and LiDCO systems are both examples of trans-pulmonary dilution monitors; PiCCO utilizes cold saline as the dilutional marker, whilst LiDCO uses lithium.
- Trans-pulmonary dilution:
  - A tracer (either cold saline or lithium) is injected into the venous system.
  - A sensor is integrated into the arterial line (or external to the arterial line) and measures blood temperature or lithium concentration over a period of time, generating a washout curve that reflects cardiac output.
  - If cold saline is used (PiCCO), cardiac output may then be derived from the Stewart–Hamilton equation (Section 2.4.1).
  - If lithium is used as a marker (LiDCO), a slightly different method, based upon the principle of the *conservation of mass*, is utilized to calculate cardiac output.
  - Measurement of cardiac output combined with heart rate, blood pressure, and body surface area allow derivation of:
    - Cardiac index
    - Stroke volume/stroke volume index
    - Systemic vascular resistance/systemic vascular resistance index
  - Rendered inaccurate by:
    - Severe aortic regurgitation
    - Intra-aortic balloon pump
    - ECMO (both veno-venous and veno-arterial)
- Pulse contour analysis:
  - Following 'calibration' (to determine a conversion factor that equates changes in stroke volume with changes in pulse pressure), analysis of the arterial pressure waveform against an algorithm allows continuous cardiac output monitoring.
  - Additional parameters include:
    - Stroke volume
    - Stroke volume variation (see Section 2.5)
    - dPmax—gradient of the upstroke on the pulse wave, reflective of ventricular contractility

- Rendered inaccurate by:
  - Cardiac arrhythmia
  - 'Damped' arterial line
  - Pacing
  - Intra-aortic balloon pump (IABP)
- PiCCO
  - Requires a central venous catheter and a specialized, thermistor-tipped arterial line inserted into a large artery (usually femoral; axillary an alternative).
  - A volume of cold saline is injected into a CVC port via a temperature sensor; change in blood temperature is measured by a dedicated femoral or axillary arterial line.
  - In addition to cardiac output, this PiCCO thermodilution technique offers a number of additional markers of preload and cardiac performance (Table 2.7).
  - Following initial calibration by thermodilution, analysis of the arterial pressure waveform against an algorithm allows continuous cardiac output monitoring.

Table 2.7 PiCCO parameters

Stroke volume/ cardiac output	Initial calibration via thermodilution, continuous measurement via analysis of the arterial pressure wave form.
Stroke volume variation (SVV) (<12%)	Measurement of the change in stroke volume throughout the respiratory cycle (see assessing volume responsiveness, Section 2.5).
Intrathoracic blood volume index (ITBVI) (800–1000 ml/m²)	Volume of blood within the chest, derived from thermodilution technique; an indicator of preload.
Global end diastolic volume index (GEDI) (650–1000 ml/m²)	Volume of blood within all four cardiac chambers at the end of diastole; an indicator of preload.

- LiDCO
  - Utilizes lithium rather than cold saline as the measured indicator.
  - Uses a standard arterial line—at any site—and does not require a central venous catheter; the lithium may be injected via a peripheral line.
  - Lithium measurement is inaccurate in patients on lithium for therapeutic reasons and in the presence of non-depolarizing neuromuscular blocking agents.
  - Does not provide ITBVI or GEDVI.
- Vigileo/flotrac
  - Attached to a standard arterial line at any site.
  - Requires no calibration and derives the cardiac output from a nomogram based upon age, sex, and weight.
  - Absence of calibration increases ease of use but is likely to render the system less accurate than calibrated pulse contour analysis systems.
  - The vigileo/flotrac allows measurement of PPV and SVV.

2.4.3 Oesophageal Doppler

- The oesophageal Doppler obtains a Doppler ultrasound signal from the descending aorta by means of a probe inserted into the oesophagus. The integral of the resultant velocity–time trace (essentially the area under the curve) indicates the distance travelled by blood each cardiac cycle (the *stroke distance*). This, multiplied by the cross-sectional area of the aorta,

provides a value for stroke volume. The cross-sectional area is estimated from a nomogram based upon age, height, and gender.
- Measured and derived values are described in Table 2.8.
- Numerous assumptions are made:
  - Descending aorta carries 70% of cardiac output (the remaining 30% supplying the vessels of the head, neck, and upper limbs)
  - Cross-sectional area estimate reflects mean systolic diameter
  - Negligible diastolic flow
  - Blood velocity is measured accurately
- Insertion of oesophageal Doppler:
  - Via the nose or mouth, with the tip advanced to between 35 and 40 cm from the teeth
  - The probe is rotated to obtain the optimal waveform: that is the clearest trace, with the highest peak
  - Competence in insertion is reportedly achievable in as few as 12 training sessions
  - The device may remain *in situ* for up to 14 days
- Contra-indications: oesophageal varices or surgery.
- Rendered inaccurate by: aortic regurgitation, coarctation, or aneurysm.
- In the majority of patients, however, measurements of cardiac output have been shown to be accurate.
- Its use in the perioperative setting has been demonstrated to reduce complications and length of stay.

Table 2.8 Parameters derived from the oesophageal Doppler

Parameter	Definition	Comments
Stroke volume (SV)/ cardiac output 4–7 litres/minute	The product of stroke distance (derived from the area under the velocity–time trace) and cross-sectional area of aorta (estimated from nomogram). Assumption that 70% of total stroke volume is carried in descending aorta.	May be used as a value in its own right, to identify stroke volume variation (Section 2.5), or to assess response to fluid challenge.
Flow time corrected (FTc) 330–360 ms	The duration of forward flow in the aorta. Dependent upon heart rate therefore corrected to 60 beats per minute by dividing flow time by square root of cardiac cycle time.	Measure of vasomotor tone. Low FTc suggests vasoconstriction and usually low preload. High FTc suggests a vasodilated state.
Peak velocity (PV) Age 20: 90–120 cm.s^{-1} Age 70: 50–80 cm.s^{-1}	The maximal velocity of blood in the descending aorta. A marker of myocardial contractility. Decreases with age.	Low PV reflects poor myocardial contractility.

2.5 Assessment of preload responsiveness

2.5.1 General

- Preload responsiveness is defined as the ability of the heart to significantly increase stroke volume in response to volume expansion.
- Measurement of preload responsiveness is not appropriate in the resuscitation of massive fluid loss, where volume replacement is clearly required.

- Rather, it is in the resuscitated patient, in whom preload status is unclear, where an assessment of preload responsiveness may be beneficial in the optimization of haemodynamics.
- Assessment of preload responsiveness may be broadly divided into static and dynamic parameters.
- An algorithm for the assessment of fluid responsiveness is outlined in Fig. 2.4.

2.5.2 Static parameters

- Left ventricular end diastolic volume (LVEDV)—as a marker of cardiac myocyte stretch —determines stroke volume (Frank-Starling curve—Fig. 2.3).
- The use of cardiac filling pressures (CVP; RAP) as a determinant of preload status is based upon the assumption that myocardial stretch is proportional to filling pressure.
- This disregards numerous factors that may influence the relationship between venous pressure and left ventricular myocyte stretch, including:
  - Diastolic function of the left ventricle
  - Integrity and function of cardiac valves
  - Pulmonary vascular resistance
  - Intrathoracic pressures
- There is little evidence that any cardiac filling pressure is a reliable predictor of preload responsiveness. There is an argument that extreme values of filling pressures, e.g. PAWP <8 mmHg or >18 mmHg, could reasonably be assumed to represent hypo- and hyper-volaemia.
- Static parameters, such as CVP, may however have a role as:
  - Mean circulatory filling pressure
  - Mean systemic filling pressure
- These are complex concepts; for further explanation, the reader is directed to the relevant review articles listed in further reading (Magder 2006; Henderson 2010).

2.5.3 Dynamic parameters

- Dynamic parameters may be broadly divided into those dependent upon cardio-respiratory interactions and those based upon response to 'fluid challenge'.

2.5.4 Cardio-respiratory interactions

- Intrathoracic pressure varies throughout the respiratory cycle, decreasing during inspiration in normal negative pressure ventilation and increasing during inspiration in the context of artificial positive pressure ventilation.
- A relative decrease in intrathoracic pressure (during inspiration in the spontaneously breathing patient or expiration in the ventilated patient) facilitates the return of blood to the right atrium; it also increases the volume of the pulmonary vasculature, sequestering blood, and reducing return to the left heart.
- Conversely, a relative increase in intrathoracic pressure impedes venous return.
- This respiratory variation may observed as:
  - A 'swing' on the arterial line trace
  - Variation in the stoke volume (SVV)
  - Variation in pulse pressure (PPV)
- The magnitude of respiratory variation is increased in hypovolaemia:
  - PPV or SVV greater than 10–13% predicts preload responsiveness.
  - This only holds true in mechanically ventilated patients, with no spontaneous respiratory effort, receiving tidal volumes of 8–10 ml/kg.
  - PPV and SVV are invalidated by cardiac arrhythmia.

- An alternative cardio-respiratory relationship that predicts volume responsiveness, but remains valid in the presence of arrhythmia, and which may be utilized in a spontaneously breathing patient, is variation in inferior vena cava (IVC) diameter:
  - Hypovolaemia leads to a reduction in the diameter of the IVC at all points in the respiratory cycle and a more marked reduction in IVC diameter when the intrathoracic pressure drops.
  - IVC variation is assessed using an ultrasound probe in the subcostal position.
  - The diameter is measured in expiration and then during rapid nasal inspiration (the 'sniff test').
  - A reduction in diameter of >50% is associated with volume responsiveness.

2.5.5 'Fluid challenge'

- Assesses volume status against the Frank-Starling curve (Fig. 2.3):
  - Optimal filling is regarded as the LVEDV (x axis) at which SV (y axis) is at its maximum.
  - A fluid challenge is administered with a view to increasing LVEDV.
  - The SV (or a surrogate for SV such as MAP) is monitored and an increase designates the patient as being on the upwards slope of the curve (and therefore preload responsive); failure to increase stroke volume in response to fluid suggests the patient is on the plateau or downwards portion of the curve (and therefore fluid non-responsive).
  - A fluid challenge may be administered by means of a *straight leg raise*:
    - Results in transfer of blood from the lower limbs to the thorax and a transient increase in LVEDV (analogous to a 300–500-ml fluid bolus).
    - Advantageous, as those deemed to be fluid non-responders do not receive a futile and potentially harmful increase in LVEDV: returning the legs to the normal position, decreases intrathoracic volume to the pre-challenge state.
    - Those with a positive response to the straight leg raise can subsequently receive fluids.

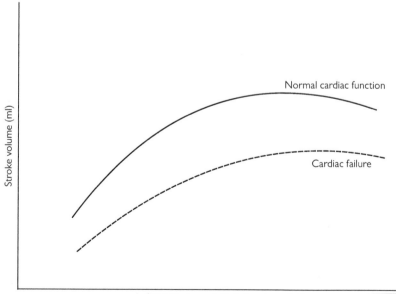

Fig. 2.3 Frank-Starling curve.

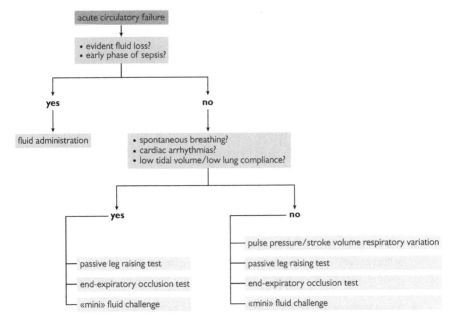

Fig. 2.4 Decision-making relating fluid administration.

Reproduced from *Critical Care*, 17, Monnet and Teboul, 'Assessment of volume responsiveness during mechanical ventilation: recent advances', © 2013 Springer-Verlag Berlin Heidelberg and BioMed Central. (http://ccforum.com/content/17/2/217).

FURTHER READING

Cohen RD, Woods HF. Clinical and Biochemical Aspects of Lactic Acidosis. Oxford: Blackwell Scientific Publications, 1976

The National Heart, Lung, and Blood Institute Acute Respiratory Distress Syndrome (ARDS) Clinical Trials Network. Comparison of two fluid-management strategies in acute lung injury. *New England Journal of Medicine* 2006; 354(24): 2564–75.

Harvey S, Harrison DA, Singer M, et al. Assessment of the clinical effectiveness of pulmonary artery catheters in management of patients in intensive care (PAC-Man): a randomized controlled trial. *Lancet* 2005; 366(9484): 472–7.

Henderson WR, Griesdale DE, Walley KR, Sheel AW. Clinical review: Guyton-the role of mean circulatory filling pressure and right atrial pressure in controlling cardiac output. *Critical Care* 2010; 14(6): 243.

Magder S. Point: the classical Guyton view that mean systemic pressure, right atrial pressure, and venous resistance govern venous return is/is not correct. *Journal of Applied Physiology* 2006; 101(5): 1523–5.

Marik PE, Baram M, Vahid B. Does central venous pressure predict fluid responsiveness?: a systematic review of the literature and the tale of seven mares. *CHEST Journal* 2008; 134(1): 172–8.

Marik PE, Cavallazzi R, Vasu T, Hirani A. Dynamic changes in arterial waveform derived variables and fluid responsiveness in mechanically ventilated patients: a systematic review of the literature. *Critical Care Medicine* 2009; 37(9): 2642–7.

Monnet X, Rienzo M, Osman D, et al. Passive leg raising predicts fluid responsiveness in the critically ill. *Critical Care Medicine* 2006; 34(5): 1402–7.

Monnet X, Teboul J-L. Assessment of volume responsiveness during mechanical ventilation: recent advances. *Critical Care* 2013; 17(2): 217.

Wakeling H, McFall M, Jenkins C, et al. Intraoperative oesophageal Doppler guided fluid management shortens postoperative hospital stay after major bowel surgery. *British Journal of Anaesthesia* 2005; 95(5): 634–42.

2.6 Echocardiography in the intensive care unit

2.6.1 Role of echocardiography

- Echocardiography is an increasingly utilized tool in the management of critical illness (Table 2.9).
- It provides more information regarding the cardio-respiratory system than any other single investigation, although there are barriers to its use (Table 2.10).

2.6.2 Training

A growing belief that basic echocardiography is a key skill for intensive care doctors has led to the introduction of a number of critical care specific echocardiography courses and accreditation pathways. In the UK, accreditation in critical care echocardiography is a joint venture between the Intensive Care Society and the British Society of Echocardiography. It takes the form of a two-stage pathway—Focused Intensive Care Echocardiography (FICE) and advanced accreditation—with an emphasis on approved training course, supervised practice, quality control by means of review of saved images, and assessment.

2.6.3 Windows, modes, and variables

- In transthoracic echocardiography, four basic 'views' are obtained from three different windows:
  - Parasternal long axis
  - Parasternal short axis
  - Apical four chamber
  - Subcostal
- Echocardiography modes include 2-dimensional, m-mode, colour Doppler, and spectral Doppler.
- Commonly assessed variables are described in Table 2.11.

Table 2.9 Role of echocardiography in intensive care

Diagnosis of specific pathologies	Myocardial ischaemia
	Valvular pathologies (stenosis, regurgitation, infective endocarditis)
	Cardiomyopathy
	Pericardial effusion
	Pulmonary pathologies (pulmonary embolus; pleural effusion)
	Aortic pathologies (dissection, co-arctation, aneurysm)
	Differentiation of cardiogenic and non-cardiogenic pulmonary oedema (i.e. ARDS)
Monitoring of haemodynamic management	Determination of shock state (cardiogenic, vasodilatory, hypovolaemic, obstructive)
	Assessment of response to therapy (inotropes, vasodilators, vasopressors)
Procedural	Pericardiocentesis
	Placement of ECMO cannulae
	Placement of intra-aortic balloon pump
	Placement of pulmonary artery catheters

Table 2.10 Advantages and disadvantages to intensive care echocardiography

Advantages	Disadvantages
• Bedside test, avoids need for transfer • Rapid • Low risk • Non-invasive (transthoracic)/minimally invasive (transoesophageal) • Provides unparalleled breadth of cardio-respiratory information	• Requires significant training, limits availability • Risk of misinterpretation of images • Adequate images often difficult to achieve in the critically ill • Not entirely risk-free: transoesophageal echo may lead to dental, airway or oesophageal trauma

Table 2.11 Echocardiography parameters of relevance to intensive care

Variable	Implication
Left ventricular end diastolic volume/diameter	An increase in end diastolic volume or diameter usually represents left ventricular dilatation. Decrease in end diastolic volume suggests impaired ventricular filling (e.g. diastolic dysfunction, pericardial tamponade) or hypovolaemia.
Ejection fraction/ fractional area change/fractional shortening	Markers of left ventricular contractility represented in 3-, 2-, and 1-dimensional measurements, respectively. A decrease suggests global reduction in contractility; an increase is in keeping with a hyperdynamic left ventricle.
Peak velocity/ peak gradient/ mean gradient	Representation of blood flow whilst passing through a valve. Increase in these variables beyond reference range suggests stenosis.
Estimated pulmonary artery systolic pressure	The presence of tricuspid regurgitation allows estimation of pulmonary artery systolic pressure. Modification and simplification of Bernoulli's law states that: $$RVSP = 4\ TRVmax^2$$ where RVSP = right ventricular systolic pressure; TRVmax = maximum velocity of tricuspid regurgitant jet. Assuming no pulmonary valve stenosis, the pulmonary artery systolic pressure is taken to equal RVSP + right atrial pressure (or CVP)
Inferior vena cava diameter/ variability	Measurement of IVC diameter and the reduction with sniff allows estimation of right atrial pressure:

IVC Diameter	Collapse with Sniff	RA Pressure (mmHg)
≤21 mm	>50 %	Normal 3 (0–5)
Intermediate	Intermediate	Intermediate 8 (5–10)
>21 mm	<50 %	High 15 (10–20)

3 Cardiovascular support

3.1 Vasopressors and inotropes

3.1.1 General

- Whilst frequently used interchangeably, the term inotrope and vasopressor are distinct: a positive inotrope being an agent that increases myocardial contractility and vasopressor an agent that increases vascular tone. A positive chronotrope increases heart rate.
- A variety of drugs are available, many with activity affecting both myocardium and vascular tone.
- The choice of agent is dependent upon underlying pathophysiological process and local familiarity.
- Attempts to demonstrate the superiority of one haemodynamic agent over another in terms of outcome have generally been unsuccessful.
- The exception may be the novel inotropic agent *levosimendan*, which has, in a handful of small trials, demonstrated a trend to improved survival in the context of cardiogenic shock.

3.1.2 Commonly used agents

- Commonly used vasopressors and inotropes are described in Table 2.12.

3.1.3 Key studies

- Key studies relating to inotropes and vasopressors, and their use, include:
  - The comparison of noradrenaline and dobutamine with adrenaline alone in patients with septic shock: no difference in efficacy or safety between the groups.
  - The comparison of high versus low blood pressure (65–70 mmHg vs 80–85 mmHg) targets in patients with septic shock: no difference in either 28- or 90-day mortality between groups. However, those with chronic hypertension were less likely to require renal replacement therapy when treated to a higher target MAP.
  - Vasopressin versus norepinephrine infusion in patients with septic shock (VASST): no mortality benefit from the addition of vasopressin.
  - Comparison of dopamine and norepinephrine in the treatment of shock: no mortality difference but higher rate of adverse events (primarily arrhythmia) in the dopamine group.
  - Comparison of beta blocker (esmolol) versus placebo in patients with vasopressor-dependent septic shock (small, single centre trial): apparent decrease in mortality in the beta blocker group, warranting further investigation.
  - In the LIDO study, comparison of levosimendan with dobutamine in patients with low output cardiac failure demonstrated greater improvement in cardiac performance and reduced mortality in the levosimendan group. This mortality benefit was not, however, supported by the larger SURVIVE study.

Table 2.12 Vasopressors and inotropes

Drug	Classification	Mode of action	Preparation and dose range	Pharmacokinetics	Effect upon myocardium	Effect upon vasculature	Comments
Adrenaline	Endogenous catecholamine	Primarily via β receptors at low doses; α receptor activity predominates at high dose.	May be administered as a 1-mg bolus in the cardiac arrest setting. Infusion of adrenaline is used for management of the shock state.	Metabolized by mitochondrial MAO and COMT within the liver, kidneys and blood.	Increased cardiac output, increased heart rate, increased myocardial oxygen consumption.	At low doses, where β effects predominate, peripheral vasculature may dilate. At high dose, vasoconstriction occurs.	A potent inotrope and vasoconstrictor, adrenaline use may be limited by arrhythmia, increase in myocardial oxygen consumption, hyperglycaemia, and increased lactate production.
Noradrenaline	Endogenous catecholamine	Primarily α1 agonist; minimal β activity	Clear solution; 2 mg/ml. Diluted in dextrose.	Metabolism via MAO in nerve endings and COMT in plasma.	Limited inotropic effect. Potential decrease in cardiac output secondary to increased afterload. Increased oxygen consumption.	Peripheral vasoconstriction. Increased systolic and diastolic pressures.	Naturally occurring noradrenaline released from post-ganglionic sympathetic neurones increases myocardial contractility.

Dopamine	Endogenous catecholamine	200 or 800 mg in 5ml.	Effect within 5 min. T ½ (half life) 3 min. Metabolized by MAO and COMT.	At intermediate dose (2.5–10 µg.kg.min⁻¹) β effects predominate leading to increased contractility, HR and CO.	At high doses (>10 µg.kg. min⁻¹), α effects predominate leading to increased vascular resistance.	Low dose (<2.5 µg.kg.min⁻¹) dopamine exerts its effects via dopaminergic receptors leading to dilation of splanchnic circulation. It inhibits Na⁺ resorption in the proximal tubule, causing diuresis. It does *not* prevent renal failure. It cannot cross the blood–brain barrier but may stimulate the chemoreceptor trigger zone which lies outwith.
	Dose dependent: Low dose via dopaminergic receptors; intermediate dose via β receptors; high dose via α receptors.					
Dobutamine	Synthetic catecholamine.	250 mg in 20 ml	T ½ 2 min. Metabolized in plasma by COMT.	β1 effects increase cardiac output by means of increased contractility and heart rate. Increase in myocardial oxygen demand.	β2 effects cause decreased systemic vascular resistance and potentially hypotension.	
	Mixed β1 and β2 activity					

continued

Table 2.12 *continued*

Drug	Classification	Mode of action	Preparation and dose range	Pharmacokinetics	Effect upon myocardium	Effect upon vasculature	Comments
Milrinone	Phosphodiesterase inhibitor (PDE 3)	Inhibition of phosphodiesterase in cardiac and vascular smooth muscle. Resultant increase in intracellular cAMP		Long T ½ exacerbated in renal failure.	Increased contractility. Improved relaxation (lusitropy).	Vasodilation of systemic and pulmonary circulations (inodilator), leading to reduction in afterload; noradrenaline frequently added.	Used primarily in cardiac surgery to facilitate wean from bypass. Marked vasodilation limits role in sepsis. Effective for pulmonary hypertension.
Levosimendan	Calcium sensitizer	Binds to troponin C, blocking interaction with inhibitory troponin I. Prolongs actin–myosin cross-bridge formation. Some PDE 3 inhibition. Promotes K+-ATP channel opening.		T ½ 1.3 hours. Metabolized in liver to two active metabolites (OR 1855, OR 1896) with T ½ of 75–78 hours. Effect further prolonged by renal failure.	Increased cardiac output without increase in myocardial oxygen demand. Improved coronary blood flow. Improved relaxation (lucitropy).	Vasodilation of systemic and pulmonary circulations (inodilator), leading to reduction in afterload; noradrenaline frequently added.	LIDO (double blinded RCT vs dobutamine) demonstrated greater improvement in cardiac output and reduction in PCWP in levosimendin group. Reduced mortality in levosimendin group (RR 0.57 0.34–0.95; p 0.028). Subgroup analysis suggests the benefit may be even greater in those on beta blockers.

Metaraminol	Synthetic catecholamine	Acts primarily via α1 agonism but has some β effect.	Presented as a clear solution of 10 mg in 1 ml. Usually diluted to a concentration of 500 µg per ml and administered in 1ml boluses.	Despite β agonism, cardiac output typically drops on administration due to an increase in afterload.	Increases systemic vascular and pulmonary vascular resistance.	May be administered via a peripheral line. Predictable effect. Popular for peri-procedural use.
Ephedrine	Synthetic catecholamine	Direct and indirect sympathomimetic actions. Action on both β and α receptors. Also inhibits the effect of MAO on noradrenaline.	Clear solution, 30 mg/ml.	Increase in heart rate and myocardial contractility, leading to an increase in cardiac output.	Increases systemic vascular resistance but to a lesser extent than other peripheral vasoactive drugs.	May be administered peripherally. Commonly used in peri-procedural setting. Also acts as a weak respiratory stimulant.
Glucagon/insulin	Endogenous hormone	Glucagon stimulates the production of cAMP via non catecholamine receptors. Insulin improves carbohydrate utilization within myocardial cells, thereby enhancing myocardial energy transfer	Very high doses of insulin must be administered intravenously to achieve the inotropic effect (0.25–0.5 units/kg/hour). This must be accompanied by sufficient glucose and potassium to prevent the associated hypoglycaemia and hypokalaemia.	Increase in myocardial contractility without increase in oxygen demand.	Minimal effect.	Traditionally used in the treatment of beta blocker and calcium channel antagonist overdose, the role of insulin and glucagon is now being extended to other shock states, in particular sepsis.

continued

Table 2.12 *continued*

Drug	Classification	Mode of action	Preparation and dose range	Pharmacokinetics	Effect upon myocardium	Effect upon vasculature	Comments
Vasopressin	Endogenous hormone	Vasopressin acts to vasoconstrict (V1 receptors) and increase water retention (V2 receptors).	Administered as an infusion. Rate between 0.01 and 0.04 units/hour.		Minimal effect	Systemic vasoconstriction.	The effect of vasopressin on the healthy circulation is minimal. The blood pressure raising effect seen in the shock state may be in part due to a relative insufficiency of vasopressin in critical illness.

FURTHER READING

Annane D, Vignon P, Renault A, et al. Norepinephrine plus dobutamine versus epinephrine alone for management of septic shock: a randomized trial. *Lancet* 2007; 370: 676–84.

Asfar P, Meziani F, Hamel J-F, et al. High versus low blood-pressure target in patients with septic shock. *New England Journal of Medicine* 2014; 370(17): 1583–93.

De Backer D, Biston P, Devriendt J, et al. Comparison of dopamine and norepinephrine in the treatment of shock. *New England Journal of Medicine* 2010; 362(9): 779–89.

Follath F, Cleland J.G, Just H, et al. Efficacy and safety of intravenous levosimendan compared with dobutamine in severe low-output heart failure (the LIDO study): a randomized double-blind trial. *Lancet* 2002; 360(9328): 196–202.

Mebazaa A, Nieminen M.S, Packer M, et al. Levosimendan vs dobutamine for patients with acute decompensated heart failure: the SURVIVE Randomized Trial. *JAMA* 2007; 297(17): 1883–91.

Morelli A, Ertmer C, Westphal M, et al. Effect of heart rate control with esmolol on hemodynamic and clinical outcomes in patients with septic shock: a randomized clinical trial. *JAMA* 2013; 310(16): 1683–91.

Russell J.A, Walley K.R, Singer J, et al. Vasopressin versus norepinephrine infusion in patients with septic shock. *New England Journal of Medicine* 2008; 358(9): 877–87.

3.2 Mechanical cardiovascular support

3.2.1 Mechanical ventilation

- The application of positive pressure ventilation (via either mask or tracheal tube) provides a degree of mechanical support to the left heart.
- The mechanisms underpinning this mechanical benefit are poorly understood, and subject to debate; a comprehensive review on the subject is included in Further reading.
- In contrast, increase in intrathoracic pressure will increase the right ventricular afterload, with potentially detrimental impact on RV function.

3.2.2 Intra-aortic balloon pump

- Developed in the 1960s, the intra-aortic balloon pump (IABP) is the most commonly used mechanical specific means of cardiovascular support.
- The physiological benefits of the IABP are outlined in Table 2.13; indications are listed in Table 2.14; complications are described in Table 2.15.
- Despite widespread use, particularly in the management of cardiogenic shock associated with myocardial infarction, there is no evidence of improved outcomes when early revascularization is utilized.

Table 2.13 Physiological benefits of the intra-aortic balloon pump

	Benefit
Primary	Increase myocardial oxygen supply
	Decrease myocardial oxygen demand
Secondary	Increase cardiac output
	Increase coronary perfusion pressure
	Decrease heart rate
	Decrease systemic vascular resistance

- The IABP consists of a catheter-mounted balloon placed in the aorta.
- Inserted via the femoral artery and the tip advanced to a point distal to the left subclavian artery but proximal to the renal arteries.
- Correct position may be confirmed by TOE or on chest X-ray (the radio-lucent tip should sit level with the carina). Malposition may lead to occlusion of aortic branches.
- The catheter is connected to a supply of helium and a pressure transducer. Helium is chosen as the driving gas as its low density permits the rapid flow of gas required for the frequent balloon inflation–deflation required for IABP operation.
- Inflation–deflation is co-ordinated with the cardiac cycle. Either the ECG or the aortic pressure waveform may be used for timing; modern devices will automatically select the clearer of the two signals. The balloon should inflate at the beginning of diastole. This is identified by the mid-point of the t wave on the ECG or the dichroitic notch on the pressure waveform.
- Balloon inflation increases (or augments) aortic root diastolic pressure: this facilitates coronary blood flow during this period of myocardial relaxation. The balloon should deflate immediately before the onset of systole. The upstroke of the pressure waveform, or the beginning of the QRS complex on ECG, are used to identify this event. Rapid deflation creates a vacuum within the aorta, 'sucking' blood down the aorta and reducing afterload.
- In the correctly functioning balloon (see Fig 2.5):
  - Augmented systolic pressure (measured at the aortic root) should be greater than the non-augmented systolic pressure.
  - Augmented diastolic pressure should be less than non-augmented diastolic pressure.
  - Mis-timing of balloon inflation or deflation results in suboptimal augmentation and, if sufficiently out of synch with the cardiac cycle, may worsen cardiac function.

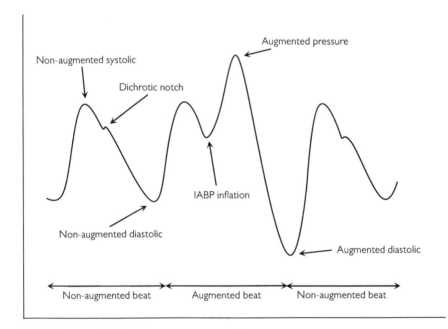

Fig. 2.5 Intra-aortic balloon pump pressure waveform.

- In addition to the timing of inflation–deflation, a ratio of augmented to non-augmented beats should be set.
  - Maximal support is achieved with 1:1 ratio (all beats augmented).
  - Support is weaned by reducing the ratio prior to removal.
  - Systemic heparinization is usually instituted at ratios below 1:1, as the risk of thrombus formation increases at this point.

Table 2.14 Indications and contra-indications for the intra-aortic balloon pump

Indications	Cardiogenic shock
	Unstable, refractory angina
	Support of high-risk general surgical patients
	Wean from cardiopulmonary bypass
	Septic cardiomyopathy
Contra-indications	Aortic regurgitation (any greater than trivial)
	Abdominal aortic aneurysm
	Thoracic aortic aneurysm
	Aortic dissection
	Peripheral vascular disease

Table 2.15 Complications relating to the intra-aortic balloon pump

Related to insertion	Damage to related structures
	Aortic injury
	Arterial haemorrhage
Occurring whilst *in situ*	Thrombosis (heparin should be used if ratio <1:1)
	Lower limb ischaemia
	Gas embolus
	Infection
	Renal failure
	Thrombocytopaenia
	Haemolysis

3.2.3 Extracorporeal membrane oxygenation and cardiac assist devices

- The term cardiac assist device incorporates a range of devices capable of partial or complete replacement of RV, LV, or biventricular function.
- These devices may be extracorporeal or intracorporeal; insertion may be surgical or percutaneous; and the duration of use ranges from days to months.
- In general, these devices are used for cardiogenic shock, refractory to maximal medical management.
- They are currently a bridge to either recovery or definitive treatment (e.g. heart transplant); in the future some devices may become a destination therapy.
- The pumps may be pulsatile—involving pneumatically or electrically driven compression of a blood reservoir—or non-pulsatile—utilizing centrifugal or axial pumps to drive blood flow.
- Complications are listed in Table 2.16; examples in Table 2.17.

Table 2.16 Complications of cardiac assist devices

Short-term	Haemorrhage
	Air embolus
	RV failure (may require biventricular support)
	Cannula obstruction
	Haemolysis
	Arrhythmia
Long-term	Thrombus
	Stroke
	Infection
	Valve failure
	Device failure

Table 2.17 Examples of short term cardiac assist devices

Impella	A catheter-mounted axial flow pump inserted via the femoral artery and passed in a retrograde fashion through aortic valve into left ventricle. Available in a 2,500 ml/min format which may be inserted percutaneously or 5,000 ml/min format, which requires cut-down or surgical placement. Lifespan of 10 days.
Tandem heart	An extracorporeal centrifugal pump inflow catheter inserted via femoral vein, septal puncture performed and catheter passed into left atrium. Outflow catheter inserted into femoral artery, sits in iliac artery. Flow of 5,000 ml/min. Lifespan of 14 days.
Venous-arterial extracorporeal membranous oxygenation (VA-ECMO)	An extracorporeal centrifugal pump has major advantage of also being able to oxygenate blood, thereby supporting cardiovascular and respiratory systems. Venous blood drawn from cannula in vena cava. Arterial blood returned to cannula in aorta. Flows of up to 5,000 ml/min.

FURTHER READING

Luecke T, Pelosi P. Clinical review: positive end-expiratory pressure and cardiac output. *Critical Care* 2005; 9(6): 607.

Thiele H, Zeymer U, Neumann F.-J, et al. Intraaortic balloon support for myocardial infarction with cardiogenic shock. *New England Journal of Medicine* 2012; 367(14): 1287–96.

4 Arrhythmias

4.1 Electrophysiology

4.1.1 Membrane potential

- The electrical potential of any physiological membrane is governed by the relative concentration of charged ions inside and outside the cell, the permeability of the membrane to these ions, and the presence of ionic pumps.
- In cardiac cells, in the resting state, the relative distribution of cations (primarily Na^+, Ca^{2+}, and K^+) and anions (primarily Cl^-) causes the inside of the cell to be negatively charged in respect to the outside.

- Change in the permeability of the membrane to ions (due to the opening of ion channels) leads to a rapid shift in ions down the electro-chemical gradient, depolarization of the membrane, and generation of an action potential.
- Two types of cardiac action potential are described: those of pacemaker cells and those of the general cardiac conduction system.

4.1.2 Pacemaker action potential

The pacemaker action potential is described and illustrated in Table 2.18 and Fig. 2.6.

Table 2.18 Pacemaker action potential

Phase 0	The membrane potential gradually and spontaneously increases (baseline drift) until a threshold potential is reached at which point 'slow L-type Ca^{2+} channels' open, the resultant influx of Ca^{2+} causing depolarization.
Phase 3*	Ca^{2+} channels close; K^+ channels open. K^+ exits the cell down the electro-chemical gradient (K^+ is a predominantly intra-cellular ion) and the cell rapidly repolarizes.
Phase 4	Slow leak of cations into the cell via Na^+ leak, T-type Ca^{2+} channels, and Na^+/Ca^{2+} pump leads to gradual drift of the baseline potential until threshold potential is again reached. The gradient of this drift (and hence the frequency of depolarization) is increased by sympathetic stimulation (which opens Ca^{2+} channels) and decreased by parasympathetic stimulation (which opens K^+ channels).

*There is no Phase 1 or 2 in the pacemaker action potential.

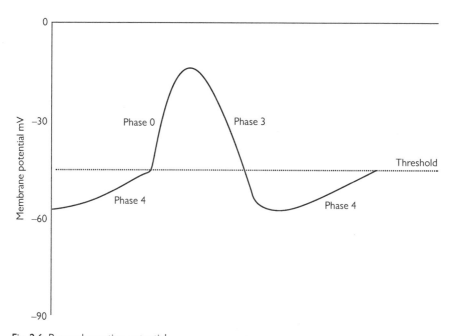

Fig. 2.6 Pacemaker action potential.

4.1.3 Conduction action potential

The conduction action potential is described and illustrated in Table 2.19 and Fig. 2.7.

Table 2.19 Conduction action potential

Phase 0	Threshold potential is reached, 'fast Na⁺ channels open', and the membrane rapidly depolarizes.
Phase 1	Na⁺ channels close, K⁺ channels open; membrane repolarization begins.
Phase 2	L-type Ca^{2+} channels open: influx of Ca^{2+} maintains depolarization by offsetting the repolarizing effects of K⁺ efflux. The influx of Ca^{2+} contributes to activation of the myocardial contractile proteins. It also prevents any further depolarization, creating an absolute refractory period, and therefore protecting cardiac muscle from continuous stimulation and tetany.
Phase 3	Ca^{2+} channels close. K⁺ efflux is unopposed and the membrane repolarizes. This phase represents the relative refractory period during which depolarization may occur but requires a supranormal stimulus.
Phase 4	Ionic gradients are returned to normal by the $3Na^+/2 K^+$ exchange pump

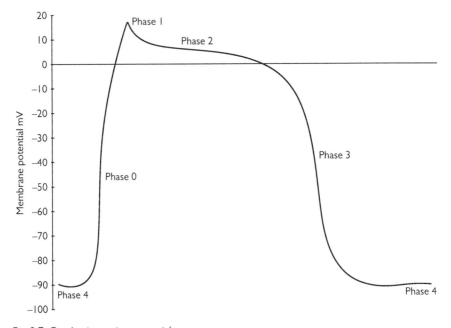

Fig. 2.7 Conduction action potential.

4.1.4 Electrical conduction and arrhythmias

Arrhythmias are common on the intensive care unit, both as the primary reason for referral and as a complication of other critical illnesses. Knowledge of the more common arrhythmias is, therefore, important, as is an understanding of the initial management and stabilization of such conditions.

- Electrical activity normally originates in the sino-atrial node, located at the junction of the superior vena cava and right atrium. The impulse is conducted by the Bachmann Bundle across the atria, the resultant myocardial depolarization represented by the p wave on the ECG. Loss of organized atrial electrical activity leads to atrial fibrillation. Presence of an abnormal re-entrant loop within the atria leads to atrial flutter.

- From the atria, the electrical impulse normally enters the atrio-ventricular node (AVN) where conduction slows momentarily. The resultant delay, represented by the PR interval (120–200 ms) on ECG, is a protective feature that prevents atrial fibrillation being conducted directly to the ventricles. Numerous conduction abnormalities may occur in the AVN. Impaired AVN conduction is most commonly due to ischaemia (particularly right coronary artery) but may also be secondary to infection (localized, e.g. infective endocarditis; systemic, e.g. Lyme disease, syphilis), infiltration (e.g. amyloidosis), or from systemic insults (e.g. drugs, endocrine disorders, raised intracranial pressure, electrolyte disturbance, or hypothermia). It may present in the young due to congenital abnormality, or in the elderly due to age-related degeneration of the conducting system. Impaired AVN conduction may appear on the ECG as prolongation of the PR interval (first-degree heart block), as the intermittent failure of the p wave to conduct to the ventricles (second-degree heart block), or complete failure of p waves to conduct to the ventricles (third-degree heart block).
- Further AVN-related arrhythmia include the atrio-ventricular node re-entrant tachycardia (AVNRT), in which an aberrant conduction loop develops in the AVN leading to a regular, narrow complex tachycardia without p-waves preceding the QRS complexes. Alternatively, aberrant conduction loops may occur secondary to an accessory between the atria and ventricles. The most common syndrome involving an accessory pathway is the Wolf–Parkinson–White syndrome (WPW). For the majority of the time in the WPW heart, the cardiac impulse passes from atria to ventricles via both the AVN and the accessory pathway simultaneously. This is represented by a slurring of the upstroke of the R wave on the ECG (delta wave). Occasionally, the electrical impulse will travel from atria to ventricle via *either* the AVN or the accessory pathway and then travel in a retrograde fashion back into the atria via the other pathway. As a result, a re-entrant loop is established via the accessory pathway and a regular, narrow complex tachycardia ensues.
- On entering the ventricles, the cardiac impulse travels rapidly down the Bundle of His (which divides into the right bundle, left anterior fascicle, and left posterior fascicle), through the Purkinje Fibres and throughout the ventricle. This rapid conduction system allows rapid depolarization of the ventricle and is represented by the relatively narrow QRS complex on the ECG (80–120 ms). Increase in QRS duration suggests that the impulse is not travelling down the rapid conduction system but rather is being transmitted through the far more slowly conducting myocardium. This occurs when there is damage to one component of the ventricular conduction system (bundle branch block) or if the cardiac impulse originates outwith the normal conducting system (e.g. ventricular pacing wire; ventricular 'escape' rhythm due to third-degree heart block). The morphology of the broadened QRS complex allows determination of the location of ventricular conduction abnormality with left and right bundle branch block resulting in characteristic ECG changes.
- Repolarization of ventricular myocardium is represented by the T wave on ECG. Time taken for repolarization may be determined by measuring time from Q wave to T wave (QT interval) (<450 ms when corrected for heart rate). A prolonged QT interval increases the risk that the myocardium may depolarize whilst still in the relative refractory period. This so-called R on T phenomenon can precipitate life-threatening ventricular arrhythmia (classically torsades-de-pointes). Prolongation of the QT interval may be due to genetic abnormalities, secondary to a number of drugs (e.g. macrolide antibiotics, amiodarone, methadone, haloperidol), or endocrine disturbance.

4.2 Bradyarrhythmia

4.2.1 Definition and aetiology

- Bradycardia is defined as a heart rate less than 60 beats per minute (it may be a physiological or a pathological process).
- Causes are outlined in Table 2.20.

Table 2.20 Causes of bradycardia

Intrinsic cardiac	• Ischaemia (particularly right coronary artery distribution) • Age-related degeneration of the conduction system • Infiltrative disease (amyloid, haemochromatosis) • Congenital • Cardiac infection (particularly aortic and mitral valve endocarditis and aortic root abscess)
Systemic	• Pharmacological • Neurological (raised ICP and Cushing's response) • Endocrine (hypothyroidism) • Electrolyte disturbance (hyperkalaemia, hypermagnaesaemia) • Hypothermia

4.2.2 Adverse signs

- The need to intervene is dependent upon:
    - Absolute rate (extreme bradycardia is at risk of evolving into asystole or ventricular fibrillation)
    - Haemodynamic consequences of the bradycardia
- Resuscitation guidelines (Fig. 2.8) describe adverse signs (chest pain, syncope, pulmonary oedema, and hypotension), which represent failure in oxygen delivery to key organs, presumed secondary to the bradycardia-induced low cardiac output state.
- These adverse signs are, therefore, commonly used as a trigger for urgent intervention.

4.2.3 Management

- Bradycardia should be managed as per ALS guidelines (Fig. 2.8).

4.3 Tachyarrhythmia

4.3.1 Significance

- Tachyarrhythmias are tolerated well for short periods of time in the healthy heart.
- In the context of heart disease or critical illness, however, a rapid heart rate can lead to significant decompensation due to:
    - An increase in myocardial oxygen demand.
    - Reduction of relative time in diastole and, therefore, reduces time for both ventricular filling (causing diastolic dysfunction) and left ventricular myocardial perfusion (causing systolic dysfunction).
    - Ventricular filling is further impaired by those tachyarrhythmia in which atrial function is lost or impaired (in particular atrial fibrillation).
    - The combination of the above factors may lead to a low cardiac output state and precipitate myocardial injury or infarction.

4.3.2 Atrial fibrillation

- Common in the intensive care unit and is associated with increased mortality, particularly in sepsis and respiratory failure.
- More common in the elderly (present in 9% of patients >80 years old), and in those with ischaemic heart disease.

Adult bradycardia algorithm

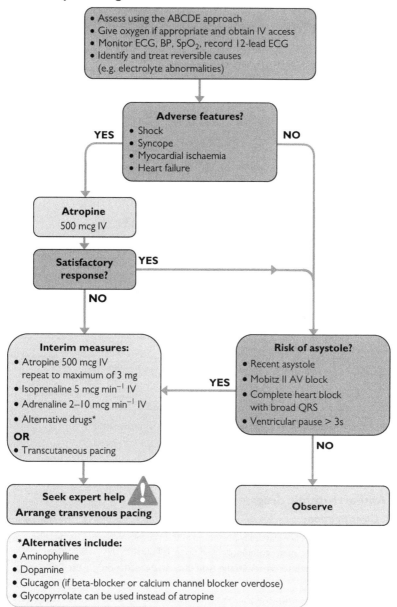

Fig. 2.8 Advanced life-support algorithm for management of bradycardia.

Reproduced with the kind permission of the Resuscitation Council (UK).

4.3.3 Adverse signs

- As with bradyarrhythmia, whilst the absolute rate becomes important at extreme heart rates, it is evidence of other organ compromise, which guides urgency of intervention.

4.3.4 Management

- Management of unstable tachyarrhythmia should follow the ALS protocol (Fig. 2.9).

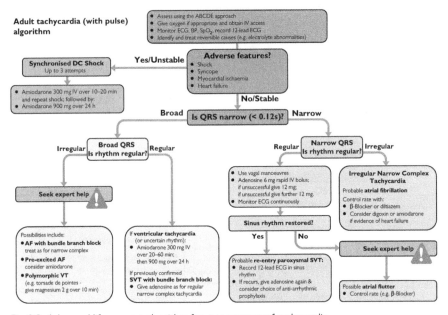

Fig. 2.9 Advanced life-support algorithm for management of tachycardia.

Reproduced with the kind permission of the Resuscitation Council (UK).

4.4 Anti-arrhythmic drugs

4.4.1 Classification

- Anti-arrhythmic drugs are classically presented in the Vaughn–Williams classification (Table 2.21); however, many commonly used drugs fall outwith this classification.
- An alternative system is to classify by the type of arrhythmia the drug is used to manage (Table 2.22).
- Mechanism of action of non-Vaughn–Williams classified drugs is outlined in Table 2.23.

4.4.2 Mechanism of action

Table 2.21 Vaughn–Williams classification of anti-arrhythmic drugs

Class	Mechanism	Examples
1a	Sodium channel blockade (prolongation of action potential)	Quinidine, procainamide, disopyramide
1b	Sodium channel blockade (shortened action potential)	Lidocaine, phenytoin
1c	Sodium channel blockade (unchanged length of action potential)	Flecainide, propafenone
2	Beta-adrenergic receptor blockade	Atenolol, bisoprolol, metoprolol
3	Potassium channel blockade	Amiodarone, sotalol
4	Calcium channel blockade	Verapamil, diltazem

Adapted from *British Journal of Pharmacology*, Singh BN, and Vaughan Williams M., 'The effect of amiodarone, a new anti-anginal drug, on cardiac Muscle'. Copyright (2012) with permission from John Wiley and Sons

Table 2.22 Alternative classification of anti-arrhythmic drugs

Drugs for supraventricular tachyarrhythmia	Digoxin, adenosine, verapamil, beta blockers, quinidine, magnesium
Drugs for ventricular tachyarrhythmia	Lidocaine
Drugs for both supraventricular and ventricular tachyarrhythmia	Amiodarone, flecainide, procainamide, disopyridamide, sotalol

Table 2.23 Commonly used anti-arrhythmics not contained in the Vaughn–Williams classification

Digoxin	Muscarinic agonist acting primarily on AVN. Slows conduction of action potential from atria to ventricles. Na^+/K^+ pump inhibition, increases availability of Ca^{2+} in cell leading to positive inotropic effect.
Adenosine	A naturally occurring purine nucleoside, which acts upon A1 receptors on the SA and AV nodes. A1 activation opens K^+ channels, the cell is hyperpolarized and conduction through the node is temporarily stopped. The half-life is less than 10 seconds and activity is brief. Adenosine may precipitate VF if used in the context of the combination of Wolf–Parkinson–White and atrial fibrillation. It causes bronchospasm in susceptible individuals.
Magnesium sulphate	Magnesium acts to slow calcium influx, thereby decreasing the rate of electrical conduction and increasing the refractory period. It appears as effective as amiodarone in the rate control and cardioversion of atrial fibrillation and has a specific role in the management of torsades de pointes.

4.4.3 Bradycardia

Drugs used in the management of bradycardia are described in Table 2.24.

Table 2.24 Drugs used for bradycardia

Beta adrenergic agonists	Adrenaline, isoprenaline, dobutamine.
Muscarinic antagonists	Atropine, glycopyrronium
Others	Glucagon (beta blocker od), insulin (Ca^{2+} channel blocker od)

4.5 Pacing

Pacing involves artificial initiation of the cardiac action potential.

4.5.1 Routes of pacing

- The initiating electrical energy may be delivered by a number of routes (Table 2.25).

Table 2.25 Routes of pacing

Route	Description	Advantages and disadvantages
Transcutaneous	Energy delivered through thoracic wall via pads attached to skin.	Can be initiated quickly and requires minimal expertise. Skeletal muscle contraction causes discomfort, often requiring sedation, and practical only as a holding measure pending arrival of expert assistance.
Transvenous	Temporary wire inserted via central venous sheath and advanced (via fluoroscopy or balloon) until in contact with endocardium. May be atrial and/or ventricular.	Relatively rapid insertion in trained hands. Avoids the discomfort of transcutaneous pacing. The risk of infection, the limitation it places on patient mobility and the tendency for wires to displace limit duration of use to a few days pending recovery or definitive pacing system.
Epicardial	Temporary wire attached to epicardium during cardiac surgical access. Wires brought out through wound. May be atrial and/or ventricular.	The high incidence of both tachy- and bradyarrhythmia following cardiac surgery (particularly valve surgery) justifies insertion of epicardial pacing wires in many surgeons' opinion. Risk of infection and displacement limit duration of use to a few days.
Permanent	Pacing wires inserted via central vein (usually subclavian). Permanent pacing box inserted into subcutaneous pocket. May be atrial and/or ventricular. Some devices incorporate third wire to allow ventricular synchronization and improved cardiac function. May have defibrillation function.	Require relatively prolonged procedure for insertion. Usually avoided at times of systemic infection as infected permanent pacing system is a significant problem. 'Externalized' system occasionally used as a compromise whereby permanent system inserted but pacing box left external, pending subcutaneous insertion following resolution of sepsis.

4.5.2 Modes of pacing

- All routes of pacing, with the exception of transcutaneous, are capable of a variety of modes.
- Mode is denoted by a four-letter code (Table 2.26).
- The most basic pacemaker mode is V00 in which a single, ventricular pacing wire delivers a pacing impulse at the set rate, regardless of underlying intrinsic activity.
- Whilst this provides a reliable rate and may be useful in an emergency, it does not produce optimal electromechanical coupling or cardiac output.
- Optimal cardiac function is achieved by an intrinsically generated sinus rhythm: atrial contraction assists ventricular filling; ventricular depolarization beginning at the AVN and travelling through the Bundle of His provides far more efficient contraction than depolarization arising elsewhere in the ventricle (as is the case with a ventricular pacing wire).

Table 2.26 Pacemaker codes

Letter			
I	Chamber paced	A = atria, V = ventricle, D = dual (A + V)	The chamber to which the pacing impulse is delivered.
II	Chamber sensed	A = atria, V = ventricle, D = dual (A + V) 0 = none	The chamber in which the pacing system searches for intrinsic electrical activity.
III	Response	T = triggered, I = inhibited, D = dual, 0 = none	The response of the pacemaker to the presence of intrinsic electrical activity.
IV	Rate modulation	R = rate modulation, 0 = none	Automatic rate response to exercise.

- In the absence of normal sinus rhythm, cardiac function is best served by a DDD mode of pacing.
- In DDD mode, the pacemaker will begin each cardiac cycle by searching for atrial depolarization.
- In the absence of atrial activity, or if atrial activity is not occurring at a sufficient rate, it will deliver a pacing impulse to the atrium, precipitating atrial contraction; the DDD pacing system will then await evidence of ventricular electrical activity.
- If, after a user-determined period of time, there is no electrical activity detected in the ventricle, a pacing impulse will be delivered via the ventricular wire.

Table 2.27 Pacemaker parameters

Heart rate (bpm)	The minimum heart rate the pacemaker will allow
Output (mA)	The current delivered by the pacing system
Sensing (mV)	The minimum voltage that the pacing system will regard as intrinsic electrical activity
AV delay (ms)	The maximum time the pacing system will allow for conduction of impulse from atria to ventricle (DDD mode)

4.5.3 Setting parameters on the temporary pacemaker

Pacemaker setup requires the user to establish several variables (Table 2.27). One approach is outlined below:
- Begin by determining the underlying intrinsic heart rhythm. Reduce the pacemaker rate to 40 bpm. Observe the ECG monitor. If no intrinsic rhythm is apparent, then no meaningful underlying rhythm exists. Return pacemaker to desired rate.
- Determine the capture threshold (mA)—the minimum output that will result in cardiac activity evident on the ECG monitor. Increase the pacemaker *rate* above the intrinsic heart rate until a pacemaker spike precedes every QRS complex. Reduce the *output* until pacing output fails to initiate a QRS complex. This is the capture threshold. For a margin of safety, increase the output to double the capture threshold. Excessively high outputs result in scarring of cardiac tissue, which in turn leads to increased electrical resistance and risk of pacemaker failure. The output should, therefore, be maintained at the lowest acceptable level.
- Determine the sensing threshold (mV)—the minimum electrical activity that the device accepts as representing intrinsic cardiac impulse. The lower the value of the sensitivity, the more

sensitive the system (i.e. a pacemaker system with a sensitivity of 2 mV is more sensitive than one of 4 mV). Threshold determination requires the pacemaker rate to be reduced below the intrinsic heart rate. Sensitivity should be increased to the maximum value (i.e. least sensitive) and gradually decreased until the indicator on the pacing box demonstrates recognition of every intrinsic beat. For a margin of safety, the threshold level should be halved (thereby doubling the sensitivity). If the pacemaker is too sensitive, it may incorrectly interpret non-cardiac electrical activity as a cardiac impulse and fail to pace when required; if not sensitive enough it will fail to recognize intrinsic cardiac rhythm and deliver unnecessary pacing spikes.

4.5.4 Indications

Indications for temporary pacing are listed in Table 2.28.

Table 2.28 Indications for temporary pacing

In context of acute myocardial infarction	• Asystole • 2nd or 3rd degree AV Block *with* symptoms (in patients with infarction of any territory) • 2nd or 3rd degree AV block *without* symptoms (in patients with *anterior infarction*) • New trifasicular block
Outwith acute myocardial infarction	• Asystole • 2nd or 3rd degree AV block with symptoms • Sinus or junctional bradycardia with symptoms • Tachyarrhythmia secondary to bradycardia

Perioperative prophylaxis	• Non-cardiac surgery
	    ▪ Sinus node disease *with* symptoms
	    ▪ Bifasicular or trifasicular block *with* symptoms
	    ▪ 2nd or 3rd degree AV block *without* symptoms
	• Cardiac surgery
	    ▪ Particularly valvular surgery and VSD closure
	    ▪ Some surgeons may use in non-valvular surgery

Tachyarrhythmias	• Overdrive pacing for treatment of ventricular tachycardia

FURTHER READING

Reade MC. Temporary epicardial pacing after cardiac surgery: a practical review: part 1: general considerations in the management of epicardial pacing. *Anaesthesia* 2007; 62(3): 264–71.

Reade MC. Temporary epicardial pacing after cardiac surgery: a practical review. Part 2: Selection of epicardial pacing modes and troubleshooting. *Anaesthesia* 2007; 62(4): 364–73.

5 Myocardial infarction and the acute coronary syndromes

5.1 General

5.1.1 Pathophysiology

• Loss of the blood supply to the myocardium leads to myocyte damage and death.
• The extent of the damage to the myocardium and the clinical picture observed are dependent upon the degree of occlusion, the size of the vessel involved, and the period of time over which the occlusion has developed.

- The classical sequence of events resulting in myocardial infarction is:
  - Rupture of an atheromatous plaque within a coronary artery.
  - Activated macrophages are attracted to the exposed collagen initiating an inflammatory response.
  - Platelet aggregation, via glycoprotein IIb/IIIa receptors, initiates the clotting cascade, resulting in thrombus formation.

5.2 ST elevation myocardial infarction

5.2.1 Pathophysiology

- If the occlusion is complete, and no collateral blood supply exists, the myocardium in the territory supplied by the occluded vessel infarcts.
- This manifests clinically as the classic central crushing chest pain radiating into the left arm (although it may present 'silently' in patients with diabetes), electrocardiographically as ST segment elevation in the leads related to the infarcting territory, and echocardiographically as a regional wall motion abnormality in the myocardial segments supplied by the occluded vessel.

5.2.2 Reperfusion therapy

- Such ST elevation myocardial infarction (STEMI) are time-critical emergencies. Early reperfusion is required and this may be mechanical or pharmacological in nature.
- Mechanical reperfusion is by means of percutaneous coronary intervention (PCI) to dilate the occluded segment and simultaneous insertion of a stent to maintain vessel patency. This is the preferred means of reperfusion, as it has a higher likelihood of success and a lower rate of complications than pharmacological techniques.
- PCI requires, however, the expertise of an interventional cardiologist and the availability of an angiography suite. Given the time-critical nature of STEMI, current guidance dictates that, if PCI can be achieved within 90 minutes of presentation to health services (so-called door-to-balloon time), this is the treatment of choice. If not, systemic pharmacological thrombolysis with a fibrinolytic agent should be administered at the earliest opportunity.
- In reality, all people living in urban and suburban regions of developed nations can access PCI within 90 minutes, particularly since most ambulance services will transport patients suspected of STEMI directly to a cardiac centre, bypassing the local hospital.
- Only those in remote areas are likely to require pharmacological reperfusion. Furthermore, there are a group of patients unable to achieve PCI within 90 minutes in whom PCI is still preferable to thrombolysis:
  - Those with contra-indications to thrombolysis (Table 2.29)
  - Cardiogenic shock
  - Previous coronary bypass grafts
  - Extensive anterior infarcts

Table 2.29 Contra-indications to thrombolysis

Absolute Contra-indications	Relative Contra-indications
<ul><li>Intracranial bleed at any time</li><li>Ischaemic stroke less than 6 months</li><li>Closed head trauma within 3 months</li><li>Suspected aortic dissection</li><li>Uncontrolled hypertension (>180/100 mmHg)</li><li>Known structural vascular lesion</li><li>Intracranial tumour</li></ul>	<ul><li>Current anticoagulant use</li><li>Surgery in last 2 weeks</li><li>Prolonged CPR (>10 min)</li><li>Pregnancy</li><li>Retinopathy</li><li>Peptic ulcer disease</li></ul>

5.3 Non-ST elevation acute coronary syndromes

5.3.1 Pathophysiology

- If occlusion of the coronary vessel is incomplete, or if a collateral blood supply exists, thrombus formation within the coronary artery may lead to myocyte ischaemia but not infarction.
- This pathology manifests as a similar clinical presentation to a STEMI but without ST segment elevation on the ECG. It is referred to as a non-ST elevation acute coronary syndrome (NSTEACS).
- Within NSTEACS lies a spectrum of severity:
  - Those with the most significant reduction in myocardial blood supply will exhibit acute changes on the ECG (ST segment depression, T wave inversion) and large rises in the biochemical markers of myocardial injury (namely troponin).
  - Those with less marked ischaemia may demonstrate no ECG changes with myocardial ischaemia only recognizable by rise in troponin.

5.3.2 Management

- NSTEACS does not require immediate reperfusion therapy; early management is based upon impeding thrombus propagation:
  - Aspirin, cyclooxygenase inhibitor
  - Clopidogrel or prausgrel, ADP receptor antagonists; or ticagrelor
  - Low molecular weight heparin
  - Glycoprotein IIb/IIIa inhibitorin high risk cases
- In addition:
  - Coronary artery flow may be improved by the coronary vasodilator glycerol tri-nitrate.
  - Myocardial oxygen demand may be reduced by the introduction of beta blockers, unless contra-indicated.
  - Oxygen, once a mainstay of treatment in coronary artery disease, is no longer recommended, unless to treat hypoxia: supra-normal oxygen levels are believed to be detrimental in STEMI and NSTEACS.

5.3.3 Complications of acute coronary artery occlusion

- Early complications of acute coronary artery occlusion, in particular of STEMI, include:
  - Arrhythmia
  - Acute mitral regurgitation (secondary to papillary muscle rupture)
  - Myocardial rupture (resulting in VSD or free wall rupture)
  - Cardiogenic shock
  - Pulmonary oedema

FURTHER READING

O'Connor RE, Brady W, Brooks SC, et al. Part 10: acute coronary syndromes 2010 American Heart Association Guidelines for cardiopulmonary resuscitation and emergency cardiovascular care. *Circulation* 2010; 122(18 Suppl 3): S787–817.

Steg PG, James SK, Atar D, et al. ESC Guidelines for the management of acute myocardial infarction in patients presenting with ST-segment elevation. *European Heart Journal* 2012; 33(20): 2569–619.

6 Hypertension in the intensive care unit

6.1 General

6.1.1 Hypertension as a cause for admission

Two groups of patients may require admission to intensive care for management of hypertension:

- Those with hypertension that is so extreme or rapidly progressive that it poses immediate threat to end organs (so-called malignant hypertension or hypertensive crisis).
- Those in whom uncontrolled hypertension risks worsening another primary pathology (e.g. aortic dissection, intracerebral haemorrhage, pre-eclampsia).

6.1.2 Hypertension in the intensive care patient

Furthermore hypertension may arise in any intensive care patient, for reasons outlined in Table 2.30.

Table 2.30 Aetiology of hypertension in the intensive care

Idiopathic/essential hypertension
Pain/agitation
Excessive vasoconstriction (due to vasoconstrictors/cold)
Neurogenic (secondary to rise in intracranial pressure)
Drug-related (cocaine, ecstasy)
Vascular (dissecting aneurysm, vasculitis)
Renal (renal failure, renal artery stenosis)
Endocrine (Cushing's, phaeochromocytoma)
Artefact (incorrectly placed or underdamped transducer)

6.2 Hypertensive crisis

6.2.1 Consequences

- Untreated, severe, or accelerated hypertension can rapidly lead to:
  - Renal dysfunction
  - Cardiac failure
  - Neurological injury (either in the form of encephalopathy or intracerebral bleed)
- Rise in blood pressure in relation to the patient's normal level is more important than the absolute pressure; the diastolic pressure in a hypertensive crisis is, however, usually greater than 120–130 mmHg and the mean greater than 140–150 mmHg.
- The presence of life-threatening complications of extreme hypertension—namely, hypertensive encephalopathy or cardiac failure—warrants ICU admission and urgent intervention.
- Hypertensive encephalopathy is believed to occur when hypertension overwhelms the auto-regulatory mechanism of the cerebral circulation, the resultant hyperaemia causing cerebral oedema.

6.2.2 Management

- General principles of care include:
  - Careful history and examination to elicit the underlying cause.
  - Careful physical examination, including fundoscopy.
  - Routine investigations with focus on ECG, CXR, renal function, and urine dipstick.

- Simultaneously initiated management is aimed at reducing blood pressure by 25% in the first hour, or to 160/100 mmHg, whichever is higher.
- Blood pressure control should be guided by invasive monitoring and achieved by use of rapidly acting, titratable anti-hypertensive agents (Table 2.31); a pragmatic approach is to use the agent most familiar to the practitioners involved.
- Care must be taken as overzealous blood pressure reduction may cause cerebral hypo-perfusion and neurological deterioration.

Table 2.31 Agents for hypertensive emergencies

	Action	Comments
Sodium nitroprusside (SNP)	Acts as prodrug, facilitates nitric oxide production, which in turn increases cGMP levels within vascular smooth muscle. This leads to inhibition of Ca^{2+} influx and increased Ca^{2+} uptake by sarcoplasmic reticulum. Decreased cytoplasmic Ca^{2+} causes both arterial and venous dilation.	Very potent. Very fast acting. Reduces both SVR and preload. Cardiac output maintained by reflex tachycardia. Cyanide is a by-product of SNP metabolism—can accumulate under certain circumstances, therefore be wary of unexplained high lactate. Protection of the infusion from light reduces liberation of cyanide ions.
Glyceryl trinitrate (GTN)	Nitrate within GTN forms nitric oxide which causes vascular relaxation in a similar manner to SNP. Acts on venous circulation to greater extent than the arterial circulation.	Rapid onset. May cause headache secondary to cerebral vasodilation. Tachyphylaxis develops over the first 48 hours.
Labetolol	A combined α and β antagonist. Specific to α_1 but non-specific β blockade. Ratio of $\alpha:\beta$ effect around 1:3 for intravenous preparation. α blockade leads to vasodilation; β blockade inhibits reflex tachycardia and reduces shear force on aorta.	Can be administered orally or intravenously.
Esmolol	Cardioselective β antagonist with rapid onset and offset. Metabolized by red cell esterases and therefore unaffected by liver and kidney function.	Only available in intravenous preparation. Lacks the membrane stabilizing properties of other β antagonists.

6.3 Hypertensive emergencies

6.3.1 Aortic dissection

- A life-threatening emergency (mortality of 1% per hour) characterized by separation of the aortic intimal layer from the media, leading to the creation of a false lumen within the artery.
- Typically presents with severe hypertension and chest or back pain.
- If the dissection flap disrupts the origin of arteries arising from the aorta, a myriad of other complications can occur, including:
  - Myocardial infarction
  - Stroke
  - Ischaemia of the limbs, spinal cord, or viscera
  - Aortic regurgitation and pericardial effusion may also result
- Diagnosis requires a high index of suspicion and can be confirmed by:
  - Aortogram

- Contrast CT of aorta
- Transoesophageal echo
- Aortic dissection is classified into:
  - Type A (if ascending aorta is involved)
  - Type B (if ascending aorta is unaffected)
  - The former typically requires surgical intervention; the latter is often managed success-fully with conservative measures
- Intensive care management is primarily aimed at minimizing propagation of the dissection:
  - Control of the severe hypertension, which is a near universal feature of the condition.
  - Reduction in the shear force applied to the aorta by the cardiac output (dependent upon velocity of blood ejected and the rate of rise of the aortic pressure wave).
  - Combination therapy of beta blocker in conjunction with a vasodilator (or combined alpha–beta blocker) should be initiated with a view reducing blood pressure to the low-est level compatible with organ perfusion within 30 minutes.
  - Anti-hypertensives may be converted to oral agents once control has been achieved.

6.3.2 Cocaine overdose

- Cocaine exerts its cardiovascular effects primarily via α adrenergic receptors.
- Systemic hypertension and coronary artery spasm are common features; angina, myocardial infarction, or sudden death may be the consequence.
- Unopposed β blockade may precipitate heart failure (as cardiac contractility is reduced with-out concurrent reduction in afterload).
- Management should, therefore, begin with α blockade followed, if necessary, with beta block-ers to control tachycardia or arrhythmia.

6.3.3 Hypertension and intracranial events

See Chapter 5, Section 3.

6.3.4 Hypertension of pregnancy

See Chapter 10, Section 4.

7 Acute heart failure

7.1 General

7.1.1 Aetiology and presentation

- Acute heart failure is the sudden onset or rapid progression of heart failure symptoms; there are multiple causes (Table 2.32).
- The symptoms of heart failure are generally related to an increase in filling pressures and sub-sequent back pressure:
  - Left-sided heart failure leads to pulmonary congestion, dyspnoea, orthopnoea, and par-oxysmal nocturnal dyspnoea
  - Right-sided heart failure manifests as peripheral oedema, ascites, and venous congestion of visceral organs.

7.1.2 Mechanism

- Cardiac failure may be divided into:
  - Systolic failure (ventricular contractility is impaired)

- Diastolic failure (ventricular relaxation and filling is impaired)
- Arrhythmia (whereby abnormal electrical activity impairs the contractile function)
- Valvular dysfunction
- Or any combination of the four

Table 2.32 Aetiology of heart failure

Ischaemia	Acute ischaemia Ischaemic cardiomyopathy Mechanical complication of myocardial infarction (e.g. septal rupture)
Hypertensive	Hypertensive crisis Aortic dissection Hypertensive disease of pregnancy
Arrhythmia	Any supraventricular or ventricular arrhythmia. Heart failure more likely at extremes of rate or in conjunction with other cardiac pathology
Valvular	Aortic stenosis—LV pressure overload Mitral stenosis—impaired LV filling Aortic regurgitation—LV volume overload and impaired contractility Mitral regurgitation—LV volume overload and retrograde blood flow
Infective	Infective endocarditis causing acute valvular dysfunction Myocarditis Acute cardiac dysfunction of systemic sepsis
Tamponade	Resulting in impaired LV filling
High output	Septicaemia Thyrotoxicosis Severe anaemia Intra-cardiac shunt

7.2 Management

7.2.1 Initial approach

- Initial aims of treatment are to restore oxygen delivery and to improve organ perfusion.
- The underlying cause should be sought and addressed; ECG, cardiac enzymes, and early echocardiography are required.

7.2.2 Vasodilator—GTN

- Causes dilation of the venous system, thereby reducing preload and potentially optimizing position on the Starling curve (Fig. 2.3).
- Causes arterial dilation, reducing afterload, and therefore cardiac work.
- Dilates the coronary arteries and improves flow to ischaemic myocardium.
- Administered intravenously, GTN is the first-line agent in patients with hypertensive heart failure but is contra-indicated in those in a hypotensive heart failure state.

7.2.3 Determination of volume status

- Despite the majority of heart failure symptoms relating to maldistribution of fluid, many heart failure patients are euvolaemic or even intravascularly deplete.
- Management should, therefore, focus not upon reducing total body volume with diuretics, but rather manipulating cardiovascular indices to optimize cardiac function.

7.2.4 Manipulation of volume status

- If there is clear evidence that the patient is volume overloaded (e.g. excessive iatrogenic fluid administration or omission of regular diuretics), the loop diuretic furosemide may have a role.
- The provocation of diuresis in a euvolaemic or hypovolaemic patient will, however, precipitate reflex vasoconstriction, increasing afterload and potentially exacerbating heart failure.
- The hypovolaemic heart failure patient may indeed require intravenous fluids to maintain cardiac output, particularly when administration of vasodilators causes relaxation of the capacitance vessels.

7.2.5 Non-invasive ventilation (NIV)

- Continuous positive airway pressure (CPAP) or bi-level positive airway pressure (BIPAP) reduces preload, reduces afterload (by means of reduction in transmural pressure), increases cardiac output, reduces work of breathing, and improves oxygenation.
- Evidence relating to NIV in heart failure is somewhat conflicting however meta analysis suggests increase in survival.

7.2.6 Inotropes

- Acute heart failure associated with a low cardiac output state warrants introduction of an inotropic agent.
- Many agents with positive inotropic properties also increase myocardial oxygen demand and incidence of arrhythmia—neither desirable in the context of acute heart failure—the exception being the novel calcium sensitizer, levosimendin.
- The other major advantage of levosimendin, shared by the phosphodiesterase inhibitors, is its property as an ino-dilator.
- Ino-dilators increase contractility, whilst decreasing afterload; hypotension can, however, result.

7.2.7 Mechanical assistance

- Low output acute heart failure unresolved by inotropic agents may require initiation of mechanical support.
- The IABP, ECMO, and cardiac assist devices have all been used in this context, although these are typically temporary measures that act as a bridge to recovery or definitive treatment; cardiac assist devices are likely to become destination therapy in selected cases.

FURTHER READING

Gray A, Goodacre S, Newby DE, et al. Non-invasive ventilation in acute cardiogenic pulmonary edema. *New England Journal of Medicine* 2008; 359(2): 142–51.

NICE. *Acute Heart Failure: Diagnosing and Managing Acute Heart Failure in Adults* [CG187], October 2014. https://www.nice.org.uk/guidance/cg187

---

8 Cardiac arrest

8.1 General

8.1.1 Background

- Cardiac arrest is an event with mortality in excess of 80%.

- Intensive care practitioners are frequently called to manage cardiac arrest and to care for patients in the post-resuscitation period.

8.1.2 Management of cardiac arrest

- Cardiac arrest should be managed as per international consensus guidelines.
- These guidelines, developed by the International Liaison Committee on Resuscitation (ILCOR) and adopted with slight variations by national resuscitation councils, are based upon the principle of the 'chain of survival':
  - Early recognition of cardiac arrest
  - Early CPR
  - Early defibrillation
  - High-quality post-cardiac arrest care
- Knowledge of both basic and advanced life-support protocols is commonly assessed in all exam formats but is frequently an area of poor performance; sound understanding of the appropriate algorithms is, therefore, essential.

8.2 The post-cardiac arrest syndrome

8.2.1 Features

- Survivors of cardiac arrest exhibit a range of physiological abnormalities commonly described as the post-cardiac arrest syndrome:
  - Systemic inflammatory response secondary to global ischaemia and subsequent reperfusion
  - Myocardial dysfunction
  - Adrenal dysfunction
  - Coagulopathy

8.2.2 Approach to management

- The 2010 guidelines of the European Resuscitation Council (ERC) recommend a structured, protocolized approach to survivors of cardiac arrest: there is evidence that agreement and documentation of appropriate physiological goals leads to improved outcome.
- The guidelines emphasize the importance of tight glucose control (<10 mmol.l^{-1}) and the potential detrimental effects of supra-normal oxygen levels (therefore target SpO_2 94–96%).
- Urgent coronary artery angiography is recommended, even in the absence of ischaemia on the ECG, as many victims of cardiac arrest have occult coronary artery disease, resolution of which may reduce the risk of further cardiac arrest and improve outcome.

8.3 Therapeutic hypothermia and targeted temperature management

8.3.1 Theory

- Temperature control in the post-cardiac arrest patient has a number of theoretical advantages:
  - Reduction in oxygen consumption
  - Reduction in glutamate production
  - Reduction in cerebral oedema and intracranial pressure
  - Reduction in free radical formation and reduction in neutrophil migration
  - All of which have been implicated in the neurological injury associated with cardiac arrest

8.3.2 Evidence

Three randomized trials have contributed to the understanding of temperature management in the post-cardiac arrest patient:

- Mild therapeutic hypothermia to improve the neurologic outcome after cardiac arrest
  - European study published in 2002.
  - 136 patients suffering out of hospital VF or VT cardiac arrest were randomized to therapeutic hypothermia (32–34°C) for 24 hours or standard management (who had a mean temperature of greater than 37°C in the first 24 hours post-arrest).
  - The therapeutic hypothermia group had a reduction in mortality and an improvement in neurological outcome.
- Treatment of comatose survivors of out-of-hospital cardiac arrest with induced hypothermia
  - Australian study published in 2002.
  - 77 patients with return of spontaneous circulation post-out of hospital VF arrest were randomized to be cooled to 33°C for 12 hours or standard treatment. The primary outcome was neurological outcome.
  - The hypothermia group demonstrated significantly improved neurological outcomes.
- Targeted temperature management at 33°C vs 36°C after cardiac arrest
  - Australian and European study conducted in 36 centres and published in 2013.
  - 950 unconscious patients with return of spontaneous circulation following out of hospital cardiac arrest with any rhythm. Randomized to targeted temperature management of 33 or 36°C for 28 hours. Primary outcome was mortality; secondary outcome of neurological outcome.
  - No difference in mortality or neurological outcome was found.
- The optimum temperature management strategy remains unclear however hyperthermia seems likely to be harmful.
- The rate of rewarming may impact upon neurological outcomes.

8.3.3 Temperature management techniques

Table 2.33 Techniques for temperature control

Surface cooling	Ice packs in groin and axilla; cold air convection blankets; circulating water cooling blankets; immersion in ice bath (practical in children only); cooling garments (e.g. helmet).
Intravenous cooling	Large volume (30 ml/kg) infusion of cold (4°C) crystalloid fluid over 30 min. Cheap and portable.
Intravascular device	Insertion of specific intravascular cooling device allows close control of body temperature.
Body cavity cooling	Bladder lavage; peritoneal lavage.
Extracorporeal circuits	RRT or ECMO circuits, if required, can be used for rapid cooling.

Options for temperature management are outlined in Table 2.33.

8.3.4 Complications of cooling

Table 2.34 Complications of therapeutic hypothermia

System	Complication	Management
Cardiovascular	Bradycardia Vasoconstriction Arrhythmias	Usually well tolerated—observe Invasive BP monitoring
Haematological	Neutropaenia and increased infection risk Thrombocytopaenia Coagulopathy	Vigilance for infection Monitoring for bleeding and product replacement if required
Gastrointestinal	Decreased gut motility Pancreatitis	Caution with enteral feeds
Renal	Cold diuresis and hypovolaemia Hypokalaemia, hypomagnesaemia	Strict fluid balance, adequate volume, and electrolyte replacement
Metabolic	Hyperglycaemia	Strict glucose control with insulin
Musculoskeletal	Shivering, raising temperature, and causing lactic acidosis	Sedation, muscle relaxants if required. Usually disappears <35°C
Neurological	Non-convulsive status epilepticus	Seizure activity may be masked by muscle relaxant use
Pharmacological	Reduced drug metabolism and clearance	Awareness that sedative agents may exert effect for longer than expected; important for prognostication

- Cooling is not without risk (Table 2.34).

8.4 Prognostication post-anoxic brain injury

8.4.1 Prognostication in the age of temperature management

- Determination of the final neurological outcome of a patient sustaining anoxic brain injury is difficult and is rendered more complex by temperature management, which has unpredictable effects of neurophysiology and the pharmacokinetics of sedative drugs.
- Guidelines relating to prognostication post-cardiac arrest predate active temperature management; data relating to the age of therapeutic hypothermia are sparse.

8.4.2 Prognostic markers

- The factors to consider in determining prognosis are outlined in Table 2.35.
- As a general rule, prognostication should not begin until at least 72 hours post-rewarming.
- No single factor, examination, or test reliably predicts outcome, and assessment should be based upon repeated examination and the use of multiple prognostic tools.
- Potentially reversible conditions contributing to the coma state should be identified and corrected, if possible: namely hypothermia, hypotension, electrolyte disturbance, and seizure activity.

Table 2.35 Prognostic markers following anoxic brain injury

	Poor prognostic markers
History	Prolonged downtime, lack of bystander CPR, initial non-shockable rhythm
Examination	Absence of pupillary and corneal reflexes at >72hours, GCS <5 at 72 hours, vestibule-ocular reflexes absent at >24 hours; myoclonic status within the first 24 hours; motor response of 1 or 2 at 72 hours
Imaging	Extensive cortical and subcortical lesions on MRI Loss of grey-white differentiation on CT
Electrical	EEG: generalized suppression to <20 μV, burst suppression associated with generalized electrical activity, diffuse periodic complexes on a flat background. Evoked potentials: bilateral absence of N20 cortical response to median nerve somato-sensory evoked potential
Biomarkers	Elevated plasma neurone-specific elastase (>33 μg/l) in days 1–3

FURTHER READING

Hypothermia after Cardiac Arrest Study Group. Mild therapeutic hypothermia to improve the neurologic outcome after cardiac arrest. *New England Journal of Medicine* 2002; 346(8): 549–56.

Bernard SA, Gray TW, Buist MD, et al. Treatment of comatose survivors of out-of-hospital cardiac arrest with induced hypothermia. *New England Journal of Medicine* 2002; 346(8): 557–63.

Nielsen N, Wetterslev J, Cronberg T, et al. Targeted temperature management at 33°C versus 36°C after cardiac arrest. *New England Journal of Medicine* 2013; 369(23): 2197–206.

Sandroni C, Cariou A, Cavallaro F et al. Prognostication in comatose survivors of cardiac arrest: an advisory statement from the European Resuscitation Council and the European Society of Intensive Care Medicine. *Intensive Care Medicine* 2014; 40: 1816–31.

CHAPTER 3

Renal and metabolic

CONTENTS

1 Acute kidney injury

1.1 Background

1.1.1 Epidemiology

- The incidence of acute kidney injury (AKI) on the ICU varies depending upon definition and is reported to lie between 5.7% and 35.8%.
- In the UK, AKI is thought to account for approximately 9% of ICU bed days.

1.1.2 Outcomes

- In general ICU patients, the absolute excess 90-day attributable mortality of AKI is substantial (8.6%), and the population attributable risk is nearly 20%.
- A significant proportion of ICU survivors with no evidence of prior chronic kidney disease remain dependent on renal replacement therapy (RRT) in the long term: between 3.5% (Scottish ICU cohort) and 13.8% (BEST kidney cohort).
- The management of AKI in hospital inpatients is frequently suboptimal:
  - Only 50% of AKI patients who died were found to have received 'good' care by the UK National Confidential Enquiry into Patient Outcome and Death (NCEPOD) in 2009.
  - This report prompted the National Institute for Clinical Excellence (NICE) to publish guidelines for the management of patients with AKI.
- Given the outcome and cost implications of AKI, a comprehensive knowledge of methods of preventing, detecting, investigating, and managing it is required for delivering high-quality critical care.

1.2 Definition and consequences

- Consensus on the definition of AKI has only recently been reached.

1.2.1 RIFLE criteria

- The RIFLE criteria were developed by the Acute Dialysis Quality Improvement Group (ADQI) in 2004 (Fig. 3.1).
- The RIFLE criteria are based upon serum creatinine or urine output.

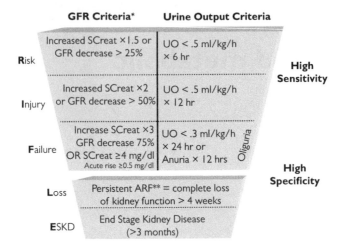

Fig. 3.1 RIFLE criteria.

Reproduced from *Critical Care*, 8, Bellomo R et al., 'Acute renal failure – definition, outcome measures, animal models, fluid therapy and information technology needs: the Second International Consensus Conference of the Acute Dialysis Quality Initiative (ADQI) Group', pp 204–212. Copyright © 2004 Bellomo et al.; licensee BioMed Central Ltd. This figure is from an Open Access article: verbatim copying and redistribution of this article are permitted in all media for any purpose, provided this notice is preserved along with the article's original URL (http://www.ccforum.com/content/8/4/R204)

1.2.2 Kidney Disease Improving Global Outcomes (KDIGO) Group

- KDIGO published further international consensus on AKI management and definition in 2012.
- KDIGO definition of AKI:
  - Increase in serum creatinine by ≥ 26.5 µmol.l^{-1} (≥ 0.3 mg.dl^{-1})
  - Increase in serum creatinine to ≥ 1.5 times baseline within the prior 7 days
  - Urine volume <0.5 ml/kg/hour for 6 hours
- KDIGO stages of AKI (note similarity to RIFLE criteria; RIFLE stages F, L, and E combined into KDIGO stage 3):
  - Stage 1:
    - Serum creatinine: 1–1.5 times baseline OR ≥ 26.5 µmol.l^{-1} (0.3 mg.dl^{-1})
    - Urine output: <0.5 ml/kg/hr for 6–12 hours
  - Stage 2:
    - Serum creatinine: 2–2.9 times baseline
    - Urine output: <0.5 ml/kg/hr for ≥ 12 hours
  - Stage 3:
    - Serum creatinine: 3 times baseline OR increase in serum creatinine to ≥ 353.6 µmol.l^{-1} (≥ 4.0 mg.dl^{-1}) OR initiation of renal replacement therapy OR in patients <18 years old, a decrease in eGFR to <35 ml/min per 1.73 m^2
    - Urine output: <0.3 ml/kg/hr for ≥ 24 hours OR anuria for ≥ 12 h

1.3 Complications

1.3.1 Metabolic

- Metabolic acidosis
- Hyperkalaemia and subsequent cardiac arrhythmia

- Profound electrolyte disturbance
- Uraemic encephalopathy

1.3.2 Fluid-related

- Tissue fluid overload
- Respiratory failure secondary to pulmonary oedema
- Fluid accumulation and prolonged positive fluid balance in critically ill patients is associated with adverse outcomes

1.3.3 Long term

- Survivors of AKI are exposed to increased risk of long-term health issues, such as chronic kidney disease, and a proportion will require long-term RRT.

1.4 Risk factors, aetiology, and pathophysiology

1.4.1 Risk factors

Critical illness is itself a significant risk factor for AKI. The NICE AKI guideline identifies the following as risk factors for AKI in acute illness.
- Chronic kidney disease (CKD)
- Heart failure
- Diabetes
- Liver disease
- Previous AKI
- Any neurological, cognitive, or physical impairment that may compromise the patient's ability to access fluids
- Age 65 or over
- Hypovolaemia
- Sepsis
- Deteriorating early warning score—a simple scoring system based on bedside physiological parameters
- History or symptoms of urological obstruction
- Nephrotoxic drugs
- Iodinated intravenous contrast agents
- Specific perioperative factors in adults:
  - Emergency surgery
  - Intraperitoneal surgery
- Specific factors in paediatrics:
  - Severe diarrhoea
  - Symptoms and signs of nephritis, e.g. haematuria or oedema
  - Haematological malignancy
  - Young age

1.4.2 Aetiology

The large prospective observational 'BEST kidney' study described the aetiological factors for AKI in critically ill patients. AKI in the critically ill patient is usually multifactorial, frequent contributing factors include sepsis, surgical insult, low cardiac output states, hypovolaemia, drugs, contrast, other organ failures/systemic illness, abdominal compartment syndrome, and mechanical obstruction of the renal tract.

- Other causes of AKI to be considered include:
  - Iodinated contrast agents
  - Rhabdomyolysis—following trauma or drug toxicity
  - Haemolytic uraemia syndrome (HUS) e.g. secondary to *E. coli* 0157 infection
  - Tumour lysis syndrome
  - Glomerulonephritis, e.g. post-streptococcal, IgA nephropathy, vasculitis
  - Tubulointerstitial nephritis, e.g. drug hypersensitivity reaction, infection, sarcoidosis, Sjogren's syndrome
- Drugs commonly associated with AKI include:
  - Angiotensin-converting enzyme (ACE) inhibitors
  - Angiotensin 2 receptor blockers (ARBs)
  - Diuretics
  - Aminoglycosides
  - Non-steroidal anti-inflammatory agents

1.4.3 Pathophysiology

- From acute tubular necrosis (ATN) to a more complex model of AKI in critical illness:
  - ATN is an histopathological description of tubular changes believed to be the consequence of hypoperfusion and subsequent ischaemic tubular injury.
  - ATN was previously thought to be the mechanism underlying the majority of AKI in critical illness.
  - Post-mortem examinations have discredited this theory.
  - The mechanism underlying AKI in critical illness is likely to be far more complex involving multiple factors, including immune-mediated dysfunction; may also include a degree of renal 'hibernation' in response to critical illness.

1.5 Prevention and early detection of AKI

1.5.1 Rationale

- AKI is associated with a significant morbidity and mortality and, in many cases, there is little in the way of definitive treatment.
- Prevention or limitation of the progress of early AKI is therefore preferable.

1.5.2 Detection in clinical practice

- Detection of early or developing AKI can be challenging:
  - Significant decreases in glomerular filtration rate (GFR) occur prior to the first rise in serum creatinine (SCr).
  - By the time SCr starts to rise, at least 50% of renal function is lost.

1.5.3 Potential future methods of detection

- Assays with greater sensitivity at the early stages of AKI are used in research settings and may enter clinical practice in the future:
  - During the early stages of AKI pathogenesis, several genes are upregulated and subsequently protein products are released into both the urine and serum. Potential markers include:
    - Neutrophil gelatinase associated lipocalin (NGAL)
    - Kidney injury molecule 1 (KIM 1)

1.5.4 Prevention

- In patients identified as being at risk of AKI:
    - Renal function should be closely monitored (biochemically and clinically)
    - Hydration, perfusion, and oxygen delivery should be optimized
    - Nephrotoxic drugs and agents should be avoided

FURTHER READING

Bellomo R, Ronco C, Kellum JA, Mehta RL, Palevsky P. Acute Dialysis Quality Initiative workgroup. Acute Renal Failure—definition, outcome measures, animal models, fluid therapy, and information technology needs: the second international consensus conference of the Acute Dialysis Quality Initiative (ADQI) Group. *Critical Care* 2004; 8: R204–212.

Chawla LS, Kimmel PL. Acute kidney injury and chronic kidney disease: an integrated clinical syndrome. *Kidney International* 2012; 82(5): 516–24.

Chertow GM, Burdick E, Honour M, et al. Acute kidney injury, mortality, length of stay, and costs in hospitalized patients. *Journal of the American Society of Nephrology* 2005; 16: 3365–70.

KDIGO Group. Kidney Disease: Improving Global Outcomes (KDIGO) Acute Kidney Injury Work Group. KDIGO Clinical Practice Guideline for Acute Kidney Injury. *Kidney Inter* 2012; 2(Suppl): 1–138.

Kolhe NV, Stevens PE, Crowe AV, Lipkin GW, Harrison DA. Case mix, outcome and activity for patients with severe acute kidney injury during the first 24 hours after admission to an adult, general critical care unit: application of predictive models from a secondary analysis of the ICNARC Case Mix Programme Database. *Critical Care* 2008; 12: S2 (doi:10.1186/cc7003).

National Confidential Enquiry into Patient Outcome and Death (NCEPOD). *Acute Kidney Injury: Adding Insult to Injury*, 2008.

Noble JS, MacKirdy FN, Donaldson SI, Howie JC. Renal and respiratory failure in Scottish ICUs. *Anaesthesia* 2001; 56(2): 124–9.

Vaara ST, Pettilä V, Kaukonen K-M., et al. The attributable mortality of acute kidney injury: a sequentially matched analysis. *Critical Care Medicine* 2014; 42(4): 878–85.

1.6 Renal protection in specific situations

The joint ATS/ERS/ESICM/SCCM/SRLF consensus statement recommends the following measures in specific circumstances.

1.6.1 Intravenous iodinated contrast

- Consider risk-to-benefit ratio and withhold contrast if risks>benefit.
- Withhold nephrotoxic drugs.
- Use low- or iso-osmolar contrast agents in low volume, if possible.
- Optimize volume status.
- Infusions of isotonic sodium bicarbonate may be considered but current evidence is not strong.
- Infusion of acetylcysteine may be considered in high-risk patients, however evidence is lacking.

1.6.2 Liver disease

- Albumin resuscitation is recommended in patients with spontaneous bacterial peritonitis and those having large-volume abdominal paracentesis for ascites.

1.6.3 Acute respiratory distress syndrome

- Low tidal volume (6 ml/kg ideal body weight) ventilation is recommended.

1.6.4 Cardiac surgery

- Consider use of 'off pump' coronary bypass grafting in less complex patients.

1.6.5 Patients undergoing cytotoxic therapy at risk of tumour lysis syndrome

- Volume loading with intravenous fluid.
- Sodium bicarbonate infusion not currently recommended.
- Consider prophylaxis with allopurinol or rasburicase.

1.6.6 Rhabdomyolysis

- Occurs as a consequence of skeletal muscle breakdown and subsequent release of muscle components (of which myoglobin is most significant) into the bloodstream.
- Associated with:
  - Trauma (e.g. crush injuries or prolonged immobilization)
  - Exertional muscle breakdown (e.g. endurance activities with inadequate training, seizures, metabolic myopathies)
  - Non-traumatic—non exertional (e.g. drugs and toxins—MDMA intoxication, neuroleptic malignant syndrome, some snake venoms)
- Patients with initial SCr >150 μmol.l^{-1} and creatinine kinase >5,000 U.l^{-1} are at a higher risk of requiring renal replacement therapy and should be monitored closely.
- Large-volume isotonic crystalloid resuscitation with the aim of rehydration and to drive large-volume urine output is recommended.
- Maintain urine pH>6.5—saline resuscitation is usually adequate and bicarbonate is not currently recommended.
- Diuretics should be used with caution; dehydration should be avoided.

1.6.7 Abdominal compartment syndrome

- See Chapter 4, Section 8.

1.7 General approach to assessment and management of critically ill patients with AKI

- AKI can be both a cause and a consequence of critical illness and should be approached in a thorough and systematic manner.
- The following approach is suggested on the basis of NICE and UK Renal Association guidance; consensus ATS/ERS/ESICM/SCCM/SRLF statements; and recent evidence regarding fluid therapy and AKI, in the ICU.

1.7.1 Initial resuscitation

- Ensure that airway is secure and oxygenation is adequate.
- Identify and correct any hypotension:
  - Fluid status assessment

- Cardiovascular support with vasopressors or inotropes following volume optimization
    - Identify and treat sepsis
- Address any immediate life-threatening issues, e.g. hyperkalaemia.

1.7.2 Assessment of fluid status

- Hypovolaemia should be addressed with administration of intravenous fluid:
    - Crystalloids are favoured—there is evidence that hydroxyl-ethyl starch (HES) containing colloids may cause harm (see Chapter 6, Section 5.4.4).
    - Use balanced solutions—observational data suggest that chloride liberal regimes involving mostly 0.9% saline may be associated with increased incidence of AKI and requirement for renal replacement therapy.
- Invasive monitoring and use of cardiac output monitoring (e.g. LiDCO, Doppler CO monitoring) may be useful when assessment of fluid status and fluid responsiveness is difficult, as is often the case in the critical care setting.
- Avoid fluid overload, as high venous pressure (high CVP) decreases renal venous drainage and may cause venous congestion within the kidney.
- Response to fluid therapy should be monitored closely and iatrogenic fluid overload avoided—tissue oedema and salt overload may be detrimental to the kidney and other organ systems.
- Identification of significant oedema or fluid overload is vital:
    - Pulmonary oedema is an indication for urgent renal replacement therapy.
    - A degree of oedema may be remediable with administration of diuretics.
    - Oedema in combination with proteinuria and haematuria can be a sign of glomerulonephritis.

1.7.3 Haemodynamic support

- Haemodynamic support should be initiated, if required to achieve cardiac output and mean arterial pressure (MAP) consistent with adequate oxygen delivery to the kidneys.
- No individual agent has been shown to be superior in patients with AKI.
- Agents should be chosen on the basis of the underlying haemodynamic issue.
- Low-dose dopamine specifically for renal support has *not* been demonstrated to reduce the likelihood of progressive AKI or to reduce the need for RRT.

1.7.4 History and investigation

- Thorough history is essential to ascertain aetiology and direct therapy; specific features may be present:
    - Diarrhoea, vomiting, decreased oral intake make hypovolaemia more likely
    - Bloody diarrhoea raises the possibility of HUS
    - Difficulty passing urine suggests obstructive features and urgent catheterization may be required
    - Haematuria could be suggestive of glomerulonephritis, renal stones, or malignancy
    - Haemoptysis may be suggestive of Wegener's or other of the systemic vasculitides
    - Joint pain or rash may be suggestive of systemic lupus erythematosis (SLE)

1.7.4.1 Past medical history

- Check for risk factors for AKI.

1.7.4.2 Medications
- Review medications and stop potential nephrotoxins.

1.7.4.3 Further clinical examination
- Assess for potential diagnostic features of underlying cause, e.g. vasculitic rash.
- In rhabdomyolysis—check muscle compartments for potential compartment syndrome and seek urgent surgical opinion if compartment syndrome present or suspected.

1.7.4.4 Urinalysis
- May reveal urinary tract infection (UTI) (e.g. protein, blood, leucocytes, nitrites).
- Protein and blood on urinalysis in absence of UTI or traumatic catheterisation may be suggestive of glomerulonephritis.
- Phase contract microscopy enables determination of haematuria source: glomerular (altered RBC morphology) or non-glomerular (intact RBCs).

1.7.4.5 Investigations
- FBC, coagulation, U+E, LFTs, CK (may be indicative of rhabdomyolysis), glucose, Ca^{2+}, PO^{4-}, Mg^{2+} as baseline.
- Further testing directed by clinical suspicion, e.g. blood cultures in sepsis, ANCA in suspected Wegener's or vasculitis, ANA if suspected lupus nephritis, anti-GBM in suspected Goodpasture's syndrome.
- Renal tract ultrasound (US):
  - Not necessary if cause of AKI known
  - Infected and obstructed kidney suspected (i.e. pyonephrosis)—US should be performed within 6 hours of assessment
  - If no obvious cause identified or obstruction suspected—US should be performed within 24 hours of assessment

1.7.5 Criteria for nephrology referral from critical care
- The use of RRT within critical care is well established and not all patients requiring RRT will require renal review whilst in the critical care unit. It is suggested that the critical care team seek nephrology advice in the following situations:
  - AKI with no clear cause
  - Diagnosis suspected or confirmed requiring specialist treatment, e.g. vasculitis, glomerulonephritis
  - Renal transplant patients
  - Established AKI requiring ongoing RRT on or approaching critical care discharge

1.7.6 Criteria for urology referral from critical care
- Urgent urology input may be required for stenting or nephrostomies in patients with AKI thought to be due to an obstructive aetiology. NICE guidelines recommend the following as urology referral criteria:
  - Pyonephrosis
  - Obstructed solitary kidney
  - Bilateral renal tract obstruction
  - Urological obstruction leading to AKI

1.7.7 Renal replacement therapy
- If physiological optimization and supportive therapy are insufficient, then RRT will need to be considered—RRT and its indications are considered in Section 2.

1.7.8 Follow-up

It is recognized that survivors of AKI are at risk of long-term complications and some experts advocate long-term follow-up for such patients; however, such practice is not currently widespread.

1.8 Chronic kidney disease

1.8.1 General

- A significant proportion of patients admitted to the intensive care unit will have a degree of chronic kidney disease; the range will include:
  - Those with mild CKD in whom the acute episode has no significant impact upon renal function.
  - Those with CKD, not normally in need of renal replacement therapy, who have an acute deterioration in renal function requiring temporary or permanent renal support.
  - Those with long-standing renal replacement therapy dependence admitted to the intensive care unit in need of additional physiological support.

1.8.2 Definition and staging

- CKD, by definition, exists for longer than 3 months.
- Classification of CKD is typically based upon glomerular filtration rate (GFR) (GFR in a young adult is around 125ml.min.m^{-2} body surface area):*
  - CKD stage 1—>90 ml/min/1.73 m^2 body surface area
  - CKD stage 2—60–89 ml/min/1.73 m^2 body surface area
  - CKD stage 3—30–59 ml/min/1.73 m^2 body surface area
  - CKD stage 4—15–29 ml/min/1.73 m^2 body surface area
  - CKD stage 5—<15 ml/min/1.73 m^2 body surface area
- The presence and magnitude of proteinuria has prognostic significance.

1.8.3 Implications of CKD in intensive care

- Altered pharmacokinetics:
  - Altered volume of distribution
  - Decreased renal clearance
  - Decreased protein binding
- Fluid and electrolytes:
  - Hyperparathyroidism
  - Hyperphosphataemia
  - Acidosis
  - Risk of fluid overload
- Cardiovascular:
  - Hypertension
  - Increased risk of cardiovascular disease
- Haematological:
  - Anaemia
  - Platelet dysfunction secondary to uraemia

* Adapted from *American Journal of Kidney Diseases*, 39, 'K/DOQI Clinical Practice Guidelines on Chronic Kidney Disease Work Group and Evidence Review Team Membership', pp. S11–S12. Copyright (2002) with permission from Elsevier.

- Neurology:
  - Polyneuropathy
- Impaired immunological function.
- Dialysis access is a consideration.
- In the dialysis-dependent CKD normal intermittent haemodialysis may not be physiologically appropriate or feasible on the intensive care unit.
- Conversion to other modalities of renal replacement therapy may require alternative vascular access

FURTHER READING

Bellomo R, Chapman M, Finfer S, Hickling K, Myburgh J. Low-dose dopamine in patients with early renal dysfunction: a placebo-controlled randomised trial. Australian and New Zealand Intensive Care Society (ANZICS) Clinical Trials Group. *Lancet* 2000; 356(9248): 2139–43.

Brochard L, Abroug F, Brenner M, et al. An official ATS/ERS/ESICM/SCCM/SRLF Statement: prevention and management of acute renal failure in the ICU patient. *American Journal of Respiratory and Critical Care Medicine* 2010; 181(10): 1128–55.

de Geus HR, Betjes MG, Bakker J. Biomarkers for the prediction of acute kidney injury: a narrative review on current status and future challenges. *Clinical Kidney Journal* 2012; 5(2): 102–8.

Lewington A, Kanagasundaram S. Acute Kidney Injury, Clinical Practice Guidelines, UK Renal Association. Nephron Clin Pract 2011;118(suppl 1):c349–c390.

Mehta RL, Kellum JA, Shah SV,et al. Acute Kidney Injury Network: report of an initiative to improve outcomes in acute kidney injury. *Critical Care* 2007; 11: R31.

National Institute for Health and Care Excellence (NICE). *Acute Kidney Injury: Prevention, Detection, and Management of Acute Kidney Injury up to the Point of Renal Replacement Therapy*, Guideline 169, 2013.

National Kidney Association. K/DOQI clinical practice guidelines for chronic kidney disease: evaluation, classification, and stratification. *American Journal of Kidney Diseases: the official journal of the National Kidney Foundation* 2002; 39(2 Suppl 1): S1–266.

Prowle JR, Echeverri JE, Ligabo EV, Ronco C, Bellomo R. Fluid balance and acute kidney injury. *Nature Reviews Nephrology* 2009; 6: 107–15.

Petite CH, Chawla LS. Novel therapeutic targets for prevention and therapy of sepsis associated acute kidney injury. *Current Drug Targets* 2009; 10(12): 1205–11.

Ishikawa K, May CN, Gobe G, Langenberg C, Bellomo R. Pathophysiology of septic acute kidney injury: a different view of tubular injury: cardiorenal syndromes in critical care. *Contributions to Nephrology* 2010; 165: 18–27.

Myburgh JA, Finfer S, Bellomo R et al. Hydroxyethyl starch or saline for fluid resuscitation in intensive care. *New England Journal of Medicine* 2012; 367:901–1911.

Perner A, Haase N, Guttormsen AB et al. Hydroxyethyl starch 130/0.42 versus Ringer's acetate in severe sepsis. *New England Journal of Medicine* 2012; 367: 124–34.

Uchino S, Kellum JA, Bellomo R et al. Acute renal failure in critically ill patients: a multinational, multicentre study. *Journal of the American Medical Association* 2005; 294(7): 813–8.

Wiedemann HP, Wheeler AP, Bernard GR et al. Comparison of two fluid-management strategies in acute lung injury. *New England Journal of Medicine* 2006; 354(24): 2564–75.

Yunos NM[1], Bellomo R, Hegarty C, et al. Association between a chloride-liberal vs chloride restrictive intravenous fluid administration strategy and kidney injury ion critically ill adults. *Journal of the American Medical Association* 2012; 308(15): 1566–72.

2 Renal replacement therapy

2.1 Introduction

2.1.1 Role

- Renal replacement therapy (RRT) describes the support provided to the failing kidneys with the primary objective of fluid and solute removal.
- RRT does not replace the endocrine or cardiovascular functions of the kidney.
- It has been suggested that the term 'renal support therapy' may be more appropriate.

2.1.2 Components

- Modern forms of RRT compatible with current practice in critical care use a veno-venous method of blood circulation/return and consist of:
    - Extracorporeal circuit, including a semi-permeable membrane
    - Blood pumps to generate pressure gradients
    - Pressure sensors and air detectors/traps
    - Vascular access device
    - Anticoagulation to minimize coagulation and subsequent thrombus and circuit failure

2.2 Basic principles

RRT relies on passage of blood through a semi-permeable membrane to achieve solute and fluid removal. This happens, in broad terms, by two standard methods (combinations of these also exist).

2.2.1 Haemofiltration

- Operates on the basis of convection.
- A hydrostatic pressure gradient drives water, across a semi-permeable membrane; *solvent drag* carries low molecular weight solutes (<5,000 Daltons) through the membrane in the same direction as the water; the resultant fluid is described as *ultrafiltrate*.
- The ultrafiltrate is discarded; a buffered, electrolyte fluid is administered post-filter to replace the ultrafiltrate.
- The volume of replaced fluid can be adjusted; the volume of replacement fluid relative to ultrafiltrate determines the net fluid balance.

2.2.2 Haemodialysis

- Operates on the basis of diffusion (i.e. movement of solutes down a concentration gradient).

- Blood and dialysate fluid are separated by a semi-permeable membrane and flow past each other in opposite directions (counter-current flow).
- Dialysate is a fluid containing electrolytes, and a buffer—usually bicarbonate or lactate (bicarbonate is increasingly preferred in critically ill patients).
- Solutes move from blood to dialysate; buffer moves from dialysate to blood.
- Fluid removal can be achieved by ultrafiltration, i.e. by increasing the pressure across the membrane (transmembrane pressure), as described in Section 2.2.1, with fluid moving from the blood to the dialysate compartment. In a pure haemodialysis mode, this filtration component does not contribute significantly to solute removal.

2.2.3 Haemodiafiltration

- Combines the principles of filtration and dialysis.
- Differs from haemodialysis in that the filtration component is increased beyond the point required for fluid removal alone and, therefore, solute drag contributes to solute clearance.
- The dialysis component tends to remove smaller solutes (<500 Daltons; urea, creatinine, electrolytes, and lithium); filtration is more effective in the removal of middle-sized (500–5,000 Daltons; large drugs, e.g. vancomycin) and large (>5,000 Daltons; cytokines, complement) solutes.

2.2.4 RRT membranes

- Membranes are generally either cellulose-based or semi-synthetic:
- Cellulose-based:
  - Low permeability to water, therefore suitable for dialysis
  - Activate inflammatory response
  - Thought to be less suitable for use in critically ill patients
- Semi-synthetic:
  - High permeability to water, allow transfer of solutes <20 kDa, suitable for haemofiltration
  - Less likely to induce inflammatory response
  - Can also be used for both haemodialysis and haemodiafiltration
- Thickness and surface area of the membrane also influence efficiency—thinner membranes and larger surface areas enhance diffusion and convection.

2.2.5 RRT access

- Veno-venous RRT used in modern critical care requires a dual-lumen, wide-bore central venous catheter of at least 11F gauge.
- The internal jugular vein is the preferred site.
- Subclavian lines should be used with caution as they can cause stenosis of the subclavian vein—this is particularly an issue if the patient progresses to needing long-term IHD, as it will interfere with AV fistula formation.
- The femoral route is also suitable; however, it is prone to infection and should be avoided, if possible.
- Patients with chronic kidney disease already on IHD may have a permanent vascular access catheter—if present this can be used in the ICU.
- Patients with AV fistulas may have these cannulated for IHD if local expertise in this method is available.

2.2.6 Indications for RRT

- Historically, RRT was initiated for extreme situations of life-threatening electrolyte disturbance and fluid overload.

- Many practitioners now believe that earlier initiation of RRT (prior to extremes of fluid/ electrolyte imbalance being encountered) and initiation for more relative indications may be advantageous, particularly in the critically ill patient (Table 3.1).

Table 3.1 Indications for renal replacement therapy

Conventional 'rescue' indications	Expanded indications
Urea $\geq$36 mmol.l^{-1}	Volume removal/prevention of overload
Uraemic complications: encephalopathy, pericarditis, bleeding	Immunomodulation in sepsis (potentially)
Hyperkalaemia	Drugs—in overdose, and in drug-induced organ dysfunction
Hypermagnaesaemia	Refractory respiratory acidosis in ARDS
Significant acidosis	Hypercatabolism
Oligo-anuria	Rapidly worsening AKI
Diuretic-resistant fluid overload	To allow adequate nutritional support

Adapted from *Canadian Journal of Anaesthesia*, 57, Bagshaw et al. 'Review article: Renal support in critical illness', copyright (2010) with permission from Springer.

2.3 Modalities of RRT

2.3.1 General

- The modalities of RRT may be grouped as followed:
  - Continuous (CRRT), the most commonly used format on adult critical care.
  - Intermittent, which is limited to haemodialysis (IHD), used in some centres.
  - Hybrid modes, in particular slow low efficiency dialysis (SLED).
  - Peritoneal dialysis, which has limited use in modern adult critical care—due to concerns regarding efficacy and effect on intra-abdominal pressure—but still forms part of paediatric practice, and critical care practice in resource limited settings.
- At present, there is no high-quality evidence from clinical trials suggesting superiority of any of these modalities.
- The advantages and disadvantages of each modality are discussed; each patient's clinical situation should be considered on an individual basis when choosing the appropriate RRT mode and prescription.

2.3.2 Continuous renal replacement therapy (CRRT)

- This is the most widely used RRT modality in modern critical care and includes the following sub-types:
  - Continuous veno-venous haemofiltration (CVVH/CVVHF)
  - Continuous veno-venous haemodialysis (CVVHD)
  - Continuous veno-venous haemodiafiltration (CVVHDF)
- Typically blood flows of 100–200 ml/min are required.
- CVVHDF has the theoretical advantage of increased solute clearance; however, there is no good-quality evidence currently that it improves outcomes in terms of survival.
- The requirement for dialysate provision in CVVHDF may relatively increase costs.

2.3.2.1 Effluent rate (dose) of CRRT

- Current best evidence (RENAL and ATN trials) suggest that effluent rates of 20–25 ml/kg/h should be the target prescription for CRRT.
- Rates above this have no mortality benefit, may cause a degree of harm, and have cost implications.
- It has been suggested that high-volume haemofiltration may be of benefit in severe sepsis; however, at present there is no convincing high-quality evidence to support this.

2.3.2.2 Advantages of CRRT

- Less cardiovascular instability when compared to IHD.
- Compatible with continuous administration of nutrition and drug infusions.
- Potentially associated with better cerebral perfusion in patients with traumatic brain injury or hepatic failure (including therapy for hyperammonaemia).
- Drug dosing/clearance may be more predictable.
- Continuous nature improves solute clearance and limits peak solute concentrations.

2.3.2.3 Disadvantages of CRRT

- Labour-intensive—monitoring; attachment of replacement fluid/dialysate; discarding of ultrafiltrate.
- Expensive in terms of consumables, e.g. replacement fluid/dialysate.
- May impair mobility/rehabilitation of patients in recovery phase of critical care.
- Hypothermia/masking of pyrexia.
- Requirement for anticoagulation.

2.3.3 Intermittent haemodialysis (IHD)

- IHD uses high blood flow rates (e.g. 400 ml/min) against a counter-current flow of dialysate across the membrane—this leads to rapid solute clearance.
- High dialysate flows lead to high filtrate volumes.
- Sessions typically last for 3–5 hours at a time.
- The US ATN study showed no difference in outcome comparing a high-intensity (6 sessions/week) regimen compared to a low-intensity (3 sessions/week) regimen in haemodynamically stable critically ill patients with AKI.

2.3.3.1 Advantages of IHD

- No requirement for replacement fluid.
- Lower costs (once infrastructure in place).
- Rapid solute clearance/increased efficiency.
- Intermittent nature allows mobility and increased rehab potential in recovery phase of critical illness or in context of single organ AKI.
- Less need for anticoagulation than CRRT.

2.3.3.2 Disadvantages of IHD

- Requires established infrastructure to support IHD, e.g. suitable water supply.
- Potential for cardiovascular instability.
- Intermittent nature and gaps between treatments may allow fluid to accumulate (e.g. from nutrition and drugs/infusions) and higher peak solute concentrations to occur.
- Risk of disequilibrium secondary to rapid fluid shifts.
- May increase risk of RRT dependence.

2.3.4 Slow low efficiency dialysis (SLED)

- This newer hybrid mode of RRT combines low blood and dialysate flows over an extended period of 6–12 hours.
- It can be achieved using standard IHD equipment, while having the cardiovascular stability and solute removal advantages of CRRT.
- Its intermittent nature means that patients can be mobile in-between sessions, potentially facilitating investigations and rehab.

2.3.5 Slow continuous ultrafiltration (SCUF)

- Utilizes filtration principle, removing up to 2 litres of fluid per hour.
- No replacement fluid is, however, used making this a simpler, less intensive form of RRT, suitable for patients in whom fluid overload is the only indication.

2.4 Anticoagulation

2.4.1 Rationale

- The continuous nature of CRRT requires the circuit to maintain its integrity for a significant length of time—ideally beyond 24 hours.
- The combination of critical illness and the flow of blood through an extracorporeal circuit may lead to activation of clotting cascades and clotting of the filter or circuit.
- The subsequent circuit 'downtime' significantly affects the dose and efficiency of treatment delivered and may have deleterious effects on outcomes for the patient.

2.4.2 Systemic anticoagulation

- Patients already on systemic anticoagulation for other indications (e.g. venous thrombo-embolism) do not usually require additional treatment.
- It may also be prudent to avoid additional anticoagulation in patients who are coagulopathic or at risk of significant haemorrhage—a clinical decision should be made, taking into account the risks of anticoagulation and the risks of inefficient RRT.
- IHD without anticoagulation may be considered in patients at risk of major haemorrhage.

2.4.3 Unfractionated heparin (UFH):

- Continuous infusion of heparin leading to systemic anticoagulation.
- Commonly used and low associated costs.
- Easily reversible with protamine.
- Relies on availability and interpretation of laboratory indices of clotting.
- Binds primarily to antithrombin (AT)—levels of AT may fall in critical illness leading to decreased efficacy.
- Potentially, increased risk of bleeding when compared to regional citrate anticoagulation.
- Risk of heparin induced thrombocytopaenia.

2.4.4 Low molecular weight heparin (LMWH):

- Once daily subcutaneous injection—systemic anticoagulation.
- Renally excreted and requires monitoring of anti-Xa levels.
- Only partially reversed by protamine.
- Less commonly used than UFH.

2.4.5 Regional citrate anticoagulation

- Administered pre-filter and acts by chelating calcium; subsequent hypocalcaemia impairs thrombin formation; a calcium infusion post filter replaces the chelated calcium which has been filtered into effluent.
- Provides regional filter anticoagulation with no systemic anticoagulation.
- Can cause metabolic alkalosis or acidosis.
- Can lead to systemic electrolyte derangement—hypocalcaemia, hypomagnaesaemia, and hypernatraemia.
- 'Citrate toxicity' manifests as a raised anion gap metabolic acidosis, low ionized calcium, and a high total:ionized calcium ratio. It is more likely in the context of moderate to severe liver dysfunction as citrate cannot be metabolized to bicarbonate.
- May be associated with improved survival and renal recovery in critically ill patients.

2.4.6 Prostaglandins

- Administered as infusion systemically or into the RRT circuit.
- Inhibits platelet function.
- Can lead to systemic vasodilatation—with associated hypotension.

2.5 Discontinuation of RRT

2.5.1 Timing

- There is no compelling evidence as to the correct time to stop RRT.
- Such decisions will be dependent on the individual patient's clinical situation and whether their individual treatment aims have been achieved.
- The BEST KIDNEY study authors found from their international prospective observational multi-centre study that urine output was the most sensitive predictor of successful cessation of CRRT.

2.5.2 Association with outcomes

- Those who required further RRT after planned cessation had a poorer outcome. The authors concluded that patients who passed >400 ml of urine/24 hours, unassisted by diuretics at cessation of CRRT, had an 80% chance of successful CRRT cessation.
- Diuretic use impaired the predictive ability of urine output in this context.

FURTHER READING

Bagshaw SM, Bellomo R, Devarajan P, et al. Review article: renal support in critical illness. *Canadian Journal of Anaesthesia* 2010; 57: 999–1013.

Baker A, Green R. Renal replacement therapy in critical care. World Federation of Societies of Anaesthesiologists—anaesthesia tutorial of the week, 194, 30 August 2010.

Borthwick EM, Hill CJ, Rabindranath KS, et al. High-volume haemofiltration for sepsis. *Cochrane Database of Systematic Reviews* 2013; 1:CD008075. doi: 10.1002/14651858.CD008075.pub2.Jan 21.

Deepa C, Muralidhar K. Renal replacement therapy in ICU. *Journal of Anaesthesiology and Clinical Pharmacology* 2012; 28(3): 386–96.

Brochard L, Abroug F, Brenner M, et al. An official ATS/ERS/ESICM/SCCM/SRLF statement: prevention and management of acute renal failure in the ICU patient. *American Journal of Respiratory and Critical Care Medicine* 2010; 181(10): 1128–55.

Hall NA, Fox AJ. Renal replacement therapies in critical care. *Continuing Education in Anaesthesia, Critical Care, and Pain* 2006; 6(5): 197–202.

Joannes-Boyau O, Honoré PM, Perez P, et al. High-volume versus standard-volume haemofiltration for septic shock patients with acute kidney injury (IVOIRE study): a multicentre randomized controlled trial. *Intensive Care Medicine* 2013; 39(9): 1535–46.

Oudemans-van Straaten HM, Kellum JA, Bellomo R. Clinical review: anticoagulation for continuous renal replacement therapy—heparin or citrate? *Critical Care* 2010; 15: 202.

Oudemans-van Straaten HM, Bosman RJ, Koopmans M, et al. Citrate anticoagulation for continuous venovenous haemofiltration. *Critical Care Medicine* 2009; 37(2): 545–52.

Prowle JR, Schneider A, Bellomo R. Clinical review: optimal dose of continuous renal replacement therapy in acute kidney injury. *Critical Care* 2011; 15: 207.

RENAL Replacement Therapy Study Investigators. Intensity of continuous renal replacement therapy in critically ill patients. *New England Journal of Medicine* 2009; 361: 1627–38.

The VA/NIH Acute Renal Failure Trial Network. Intensity of renal support in critically ill patients with acute kidney injury. *New England Journal of Medicine* 2008; 359: 7–20.

Schneider AG, Bellomo R, Bagshaw SM et al. Choice of renal replacement therapy modality and dialysis dependence after acute kidney injury: a systematic review and meta-analysis. *Intensive Care Medicine* 2013; 39(6): 987–97.

Uchino S[1], Bellomo R, Morimatsu H et al. Discontinuation of continuous renal replacement therapy: a post hoc analysis of a prospective multicenter observational study. *Critical Care Medicine* 2009; 37(9): 2576–82.

Vanholder R, Van Biesen W, Lameire N. What is the renal replacement therapy method of first choice for intensive care patients? *Journal of the American Society of Nephrology* 2001; 12(Suppl 1): S40–43.

3 Electrolyte abnormalities

Electrolyte abnormalities are common in critically ill patients and many are associated with adverse events and outcomes.

3.1 Hyponatraemia

3.1.1 General

- Defined as serum sodium <135 mmol.l^{-1}.
- Present in approximately 15% of ICU patients and associated with adverse outcomes.
- Two mechanisms predominate:
  - Dilution from excess total body water
  - Excess sodium loss—usually gastrointestinal or renal

3.1.2 Clinical features

- Result from fluid shifts and resultant tissue oedema.
- Lethargy, confusion, and nausea may be noted at serum sodium levels <125 mmol.l^{-1}.
- Seizures and depressed conscious level may result from cerebral oedema and raised intracranial pressure—usually occur at serum sodium levels <115 mmol.l^{-1}.

3.1.3 Causes

- Salt and water loss, e.g. diarrhoea, vomiting, or diuretic use:
  - Hypovolaemic state
  - Low urine sodium
- Syndrome of Inappropriate anti-diuretic hormone secretion (SIADH):
  - State of water retention and urinary sodium loss
  - Causes include: paraneoplastic, severe pneumonia, some drugs (e.g. anti-depressants and anti-psychotics)
  - Clinically euvolaemic or mildly oedematous
  - Characterized by inappropriately high urine sodium, may have low serum osmolality, and high urine osmolality
- Drugs (multiple mechanisms)—NSAIDs, ACE inhibitors, diuretics, protein pump inhibitors, anti-depressants, anti-psychotics, carbamazepine, and many others.
- Excess administration of hypotonic fluids.
- Organ failure states leading to fluid retention, e.g. heart failure, MODS, liver failure:
  - Clinically oedematous
- Adrenal insufficiency—hyponatraemia and hypokalaemia may result:
  - Hypovolaemic state
- Severe hypothyroidism.

3.1.4 Clinical assessment

- Particular attention should be paid to fluid status and medications; drugs associated with hyponatraemia should be stopped.
- Measurement of paired serum/urine osmolality and urine sodium can be helpful in the identification of the underlying cause of hyponatraemia; however, critically ill patients will have many confounding factors (e.g. administration of intravenous fluids or diuretic use) and as such the results should be interpreted with caution.

3.1.5 Management

- Management depends on the severity of clinical features, level of hyponatraemia, and underlying aetiology:
  - Salt/water loss—rehydrate with intravenous 0.9% saline.
  - SIADH:
    - Fluid restrict
    - Stop offending drugs
    - Demeclocycline may be considered in severe cases—this induces a state of temporary nephrogenic diabetes insipidus
  - Drug-related:
    - Stop drug
    - Supportive therapy
  - Organ dysfunction/MODS:
    - Treat underlying condition
  - Adrenal insufficiency:
    - Steroids
  - Hypothyroidism:
    - Thyroid hormone replacement

3.1.6 Severe hyponatraemia

- If the patient is comatose or having seizures, infusion of hypertonic saline should be considered.
- The European Society of Endocrinology suggest a pragmatic approach to the initial treatment of severe symptomatic hyponatraemia:
  - Repeated 150-ml boluses of 3% sodium chloride until an increase in serum sodium of 5 mmol/l is achieved
  - Close clinical and biochemical monitoring is recommended to facilitate this, e.g. near patient testing devices
- After the initial rescue treatment, the rate of correction of sodium concentration should remain within 10 mmol.l^{-1}/24 hours for the first 24 hours and then 8 mmol.l^{-1}/24 hours for the following days.

3.1.7 Central pontine myelinolysis

- Rapid correction of plasma sodium can result in central pontine myelinolysis: a catastrophic neurological injury resulting from demyelination of brain stem structures.

3.2 Hypernatraemia

3.2.1 General

- Defined as serum sodium >145 mmol.l^{-1}.
- Found in 5–9% of ICU patients.
- Associated with adverse outcomes.
- Most patients with hypernatraemia in the ICU develop it after ICU admission.

3.2.2 Clinical features

- Usually occur at Na$^+$ >155 mmol.l^{-1}:
  - Agitation and lethargy
  - Coma
- Volume status:
  - Hypovolaemia—in situations of fluid loss, e.g. diuretic use, GI fluid loss
  - Euvolaemia—may be seen in diabetes insipidus
  - Hypervolaemia—administration of hypertonic sodium containing preparations

3.2.3 Causes

- Excess loss of free water:
  - Significant dehydration
  - Diuretics (particularly loop and osmotic diuretics)
  - Nephrogenic diabetes insipidus:
    - Drug-induced, e.g. lithium, amphotericin B, demeclocycline
  - Craniogenic diabetes inspidus:
    - Traumatic brain injury
    - Brain tumour
    - Drug-induced, e.g. phenytoin, ethanol
  - Conn's syndrome
- Excess sodium administration:
  - Use of hypertonic saline solutions, particularly in neurocritical care, as an osmotic agent

3.2.4 Management

- In hypovolaemic states treat underlying cause and replace fluid:
  - Treat shock with fluid resuscitation
  - Once haemodynamically stable, it is recommended that half of the total body water deficit is replaced in the first 24 hours
  - Free water deficit (FWD) can be calculated:

$$\text{FWD (litres)} = 0.6 \times \text{weight (kg)} \times \left(\frac{\text{Current sodium}}{\text{Target sodium}} - 1 \right)$$

  - Target sodium is usually taken to be 140mmol.l^{-1}
  - If Na^+ <160 mmol.l^{-1}—0.9% saline would be an appropriate replacement fluid as it will be relatively hypotonic to the patients plasma
  - If Na+ >160 mmol.l^{-1}—0.45% saline or 5% dextrose can be considered, but used with caution, avoiding rapid changes in sodium concentration
- In hypervolaemic states, hypernatraemia is usually due to iatrogenic hypertonic sodium solutions:
  - Stop offending agent
  - Consider diuresis with loop diuretic
  - Renal replacement therapy offers a rapid means of correction (rate of correction dependent upon the 'dose' used)
- Nephrogenic diabetes insipidus:
  - Stop offending drug
  - Fluid resuscitation, as guided by clinical situation
- Craniogenic diabetes insipidus:
  - Treat underlying cause, if possible
  - Fluid resuscitation, if required
  - Desmopressin or vasopressin administration, if severe
- Conn's syndrome:
  - Spironolactone

3.3 Hypokalaemia

3.3.1 General

- Serum potassium <3.5 mmol.l^{-1}.
- Occurs in over 20% of ICU patients.
- Severe consequences, such as cardiac arrhythmia (including ventricular arrhythmias and cardiac arrest) and muscle weakness, usually occur at serum potassium <2.5 mmol.l^{-1}.

3.3.2 Causes

- Decreased intake:
  - E.g. in eating disorders, chronic disease, or malignancy
- Increased loss:
  - GI losses, e.g. diarrhoea, vomiting
  - Renal loss:
    - Diuretics
    - Excessive mineralocorticoid activity: liquorice toxicity; Conn's syndrome; Cushing's syndrome
    - Renal tubular acidosis, may be drug related, e.g. amphotericin B
    - Osmotic diuresis secondary to uncontrolled hyperglycaemia

- Movement of potassium into cells:
  - Alkalosis
  - Sympathomimetic activity (classically salbutamol)
  - Insulin therapy
  - Refeeding syndrome

3.3.3 Management

- Identify and treat underlying cause.
- Stop culprit medication, if possible (risk:benefit ratio).
- Replace potassium:
  - Mild cases at a rate of 10–20 mmol/hour
  - In cases with unstable cardiac arrhythmia, rate of replacement may be faster; however, administration via a central venous catheter and ECG monitoring are recommended.
- Check serum magnesium and replace, if necessary.
- Continuous ECG monitoring if K^+ <3.0 mmol.l^{-1}.

3.4 Hyperkalaemia

3.4.1 General

- Serum potassium >5 mmol.l^{-1}.
- Occurs in up to 10% of patients in hospital.
- Adverse clinical features generally develop at serum K^+ >6mmol/l:
  - Muscle weakness and paralysis
  - ECG changes—peaked T waves, broadened QRS complexes
  - Rhythm disturbance—ventricular arrhythmia, sine-wave pattern, cardiac arrest

3.4.2 Causes

- AKI and/or CKD.
- Exogenous administration of potassium, e.g. iatrogenic in hospital, bananas.
- Drugs—spironolactone, beta blockers, ace inhibitors, angiotensin 2 receptor blockers, trimethoprim, heparin, suxamethonium, digoxin toxicity.
- Cell lysis—tumour lysis syndrome, rhabdomyolysis, haemolysis, blood transfusion.
- Hypoadrenalism.

3.4.3 Management

- Identify and treat underlying cause.
- Identify and remove precipitants, if possible.
- If asymptomatic, 12 lead ECG shows no acute changes, and serum K^+ <6.0 mmol.l^{-1}—monitor.
- If ECG changes or K^+ >6.0mmol/l:
  - Continuous ECG monitoring
  - 10 ml of 10% calcium gluconate over 2 minutes
  - Nebulized salbutamol
  - 10 units of short-acting insulin (e.g. Actrapid® or Novorapid®) in 50 ml of 50% dextrose over 20 minutes intravenously
  - Consider calcium resonium
- Hyperkalaemia as a consequence of AKI or CKD may require early renal replacement therapy.
- Hyperkalaemia refractory to medical measures will require renal replacement therapy.

3.5 Hypophosphataemia

3.5.1 General

- Serum phosphate <0.8 mmol.l^{-1}.
- Common in ICU.
- Main clinical feature is muscle weakness—doesn't usually occur until serum phosphate <0.3 mmol.l^{-1}.

3.5.2 Causes

- Severe critical illness and its side-effects, e.g. sepsis, polytrauma, malabsorption, alkalosis, hypothermia.
- Drugs—diuretics, aluminium containing antacids, catecholamines.
- Refeeding syndrome.
- Renal replacement therapy.

3.5.3 Management

- Phosphate should be monitored at least daily in critically ill patients and levels should be maintained within the normal range (0.8–1.5 mmol.l^{-1}), being replaced enterally or parenterally, as required.

3.6 Hyperphosphataemia

3.6.1 General

- Serum phosphate >1.6 mmol.l^{-1}
- Uncommon

3.6.2 Causes

- Iatrogenic—excess phosphate administration (IV or enema), vitamin D toxicity.
- Acute Illness—AKI, tumour lysis syndrome, metabolic acidosis, trauma, rhabdomyolysis.
- Endocrine—hypoparathyroidism.

3.6.3 Clinical features

- Hypocalcaemia and its consequences.
- Ectopic calcification.
- AKI.

3.6.4 Management

- Stop exogenous phosphate administration.
- If asymptomatic, may not require treatment.
- Phosphate binders if chronic, e.g. in CKD.
- Hypertonic dextrose may be considered.
- Renal replacement therapy may be required if severe and/or refractory.

3.7 Hypomagnesaemia

3.7.1 General

- Serum magnesium <0.7 mmol.l^{-1}
- Common in the ICU and associated with adverse outcomes.
- Total body magnesium may be depleted despite normal serum magnesium.

3.7.2 Causes

- Critical illness and its consequences—sepsis, trauma, major surgery, burns, malabsorption, starvation.
- Gastrointestinal or renal losses.
- Drugs—diuretics, platinum based cytotoxics, aminoglycosides, cyclosporine, tacrolimus, amphotericin B.

3.7.3 Clinical features

- Cardiac arrhythmia, including torsade de pointes and subsequent cardiac arrest.
- Seizures and coma.
- Hypokalaemia and its consequences.

3.7.4 Management

- Serum magnesium should be monitored at least daily and kept within the normal range in ICU patients.
- Patients with adverse clinical features should have continuous ECG monitoring and should receive 2 g (8 mmol) of magnesium sulphate either by infusion (2 g in 100 ml 0.9% saline over 20–30 minutes); or in the case of unstable arrhythmia/arrest, as a bolus.

3.8 Hypermagnesaemia

3.8.1 General

- Although upper limit of reference range is 1.2 mmol.l^{-1}, clinical features of hypermagnesaemia generally don't occur until serum magnesium >3.5 mmol.l^{-1}, indeed the therapeutic range for magnesium administration in certain conditions, such as eclampsia, is 2.0–3.5 mmol.l^{-1}.
- Uncommon.

3.8.2 Causes

- Generally due to overzealous magnesium administration, especially in the context of renal failure; may be associated with lithium administration.

3.8.3 Clinical features

- Muscle weakness, including respiratory muscles, with potential for respiratory arrest.
- Coma.
- Cardiac conduction defects and cardiac arrest.

3.8.4 Management

- Continuous ECG monitoring.
- Stop magnesium infusion.
- Calcium gluconate for cardiac stabilization.
- Consider renal replacement therapy.

3.9 Hypocalcaemia

3.9.1 General

- Total serum calcium <2.10 mmol.l^{-1}
- Ionized serum calcium <1.15 mmol.l^{-1}
- Total serum calcium is low in nearly all ICU patients.
- Low ionized calcium is present in around 20% of ICU patients.

3.9.2 Causes

- Critical illness and its consequences—sepsis, AKI, CKD, rhabdomyolysis, trauma, pancreatitis.
- Hypoparathyroidism.
- Vitamin D deficiency.
- Hyperphosphataemia and hypomagnesaemia.
- Respiratory alkalosis/hyperventilation.
- Drugs—excess phosphate administration, propofol, edentate containing contrast, heparin, diuretics, fluoride, and oxalate toxicity.
- Citrate toxicity as seen in massive transfusion or in the context of citrate anti-coagulation.

3.9.3 Clinical features

- Tetany.
- Coma and seizures
- Impaired cardiac function
- Coagulation defect

3.9.4 Management

- Identify and treat underlying cause.
- Identify and remove any precipitants, if possible.
- Consider checking vitamin D and PTH levels.
- Asymptomatic individuals may not require any supplementation.
- If adverse features present, then an initial bolus of 10 ml of 10% calcium gluconate should be given over 2 minutes or longer. A subsequent infusion may be required at a rate of 0.7–3.5 mmol/h aiming for serum ionized calcium >0.8 mmol/l. Higher target calcium may be desirable in the context of cardiac dysfunction.

3.10 Hypercalcaemia

3.10.1 General

- Total serum calcium >2.65 mmol.l^{-1}
- Ionized calcium >1.3 mmol.l^{-1}
- Present in up to 15% of critically ill patients.

3.10.2 Causes

- Malignancy
- Hyperparathyroidism
- Renal dysfunction
- Drugs—vitamin D toxicity, thiazide diuretics, lithium, oestrogen, tamoxifen
- Immobility
- Paget's disease of bone
- Sarcoidosis
- Tuberculosis

3.10.3 Clinical features

- Mild toxicity, i.e. total serum calcium 3.0–3.5 mmol.l^{-1}—lethargy, fatigue, abdominal pain, constipation, nephrocalcinosis, pancreatitis.
- Severe toxicity, i.e. total serum calcium >3.5 mmol.l^{-1}—coma, bradycardia.

3.10.4 Management

- Identify and treat underlying cause; check vitamin D and parathyroid levels, if no other obvious explanation.
- Identify and remove any precipitants, if possible.
- Assess fluid status—rehydration alone may be sufficient.
- Bisphosphonates (e.g. pamidronate or zolendronate) may be required if fluids are not sufficient, particularly in the context of hypercalcaemia of malignancy.
- Steroids may be of use in patients with sarcoidosis or vitamin D toxicity.
- Diuretics may promote urinary loss of calcium—this should only be done in the absence of hypovolaemia; concomitant intravenous fluids may be required.

FURTHER READING

Androgue, HJ and Madias NE. Hyponatremia. *New England Journal of Medicine*,2000; 342: 1581–9.

Barker SB, Worthley LI. The essentials of calcium, magnesium, and phosphate metabolism: Part II. Disorders. *Critical Care and Resuscitation* 2002; 4: 307–15.

Buckley MS, Leblanc JM, Cawley MJ. Electrolyte disturbances associated with commonly prescribed medications in the intensive care unit. Critical Care Medicine 2010 Jun; 38(6 Suppl): S253–64.

Evans KJ, Greenberg A. Hyperkalaemia: a review. *Journal of Intensive Care Medicine* 2005; 20: 272–90.

Funk GC, Lindner G, Druml W, et al. Incidence and prognosis of dysnatremias present on ICU admission. *Intensive Care Medicine* 2010; 36(2): 304–11.

Hoorn EJ, Betjes MG, Weigel J, Zietse R. Hypernatraemia in critically ill patients: too little water and too much salt. *Nephrology Dialysis Transplantation* 2007; 23(5): 1562–8.

Lee JW. Fluid and electrolyte disturbances in critically ill patients. *Electrolytes and Blood Pressure* 2010; 8(2): 72–81.

Spasovski G, Vanholder R, Allolio B, et al. Clinical practice guidelines on diagnosis and treatment of hyponatraemia. *European Journal of Endocrinology* 2014; 170: G1–47.

4 Acid–base

4.1 Definitions and relevance

4.1.1 Acid

- An acid is an H^+ donor.
- A strong acid is an H^+ donor that is completely dissociated at physiological pH (e.g. hydrochloric acid).
- A weak acid is an H^+ donor that is incompletely dissociated at physiological pH (e.g. carbonic acid).
- The pH is the reverse logarithmic representation of H^+ activity:
  - The range of pH across which humans can survive (6.8–7.8) represents a ten-fold difference in H^+ concentration.

4.1.2 Base

- A base is an H^+ recipient.
- Base excess is a reflection of the metabolic component of acid–base status:
  - HCO_3^- is a non-linear representation of the metabolic component; it is not measured in blood gas samples but rather derived from pH and $PaCO_2$.
  - (Actual) base excess (ABE) is the amount of acid that must be added to return pH *in vitro* to 7.40 under the standard conditions of 37°C and $PaCO_2$ of 5.33 kPa; it is measured in $mEq.l^{-1}$.
  - Standard base excess (SBE)is the acid required when haemoglobin is 50 $g.l^{-1}$; the reduced buffering capacity of this haemoglobin depleted blood is more representative of extracellular acid–base status.

4.1.3 Changes in pH

- Changes in pH have a number of implications:
  - Impact upon the ionization status of molecules, which may in turn affect the ability of those molecules to cross membranes.
  - Impact upon enzyme systems, with metabolic derangement impacting upon cellular function.

4.2 Acid–base theories

- Metabolic acidosis can be both a cause and a consequence of critical illness. There are two commonly used approaches to acid–base:
  - Siggaard–Anderson approach
  - Stewart approach
- Both methods are acceptable; however, the Stewart approach offers more understanding of the underlying mechanism.

4.2.1 Siggaard–Anderson approach

This approach is based upon:
- The Henderson–Hasselbalch equation:
  - Arises from the dissociation equation for carbonic acid:

$$CO_2 + H_2O \leftrightarrow H^+ + HCO_3^-$$

  - Based upon the premise that HCO_3^- and $PaCO_2$ are the determinants of pH
  - That the relationship between HCO_3^-, $PaCO_2$, and pH may be represented by the equation:

$$pH = 6.1 + \log \frac{HCO_3^-}{0.03 \times P_aCO_2}$$

- Base excess (BE)
- Anion gap (AG)
- A negative BE suggests a metabolic acidosis is contributing to the acid–base state; this may be viewed as the consequence of an excess of negatively charged ions (anions) relative to positively charged ions (cations).

- Identification of a metabolic acidosis should prompt identification of the precipitating bio-chemical abnormality:
  - Anion gap:
    - Calculated as $(Na^+ + K^+) - (Cl^- + HCO_3^-)$ (normal range 14–17)
      - Raised anion gap metabolic acidosis is caused by strong acid accumulation.
      - Normal anion gap metabolic acidosis can be caused by bicarbonate loss, decreased renal excretion of H^+, and infusion/ingestion of acid, e.g. HCl.
- The differential diagnosis of metabolic acidosis according to anion gap is listed in Table 3.2.

Table 3.2 Differential diagnosis of metabolic acidosis according to anion gap

Normal anion gap metabolic acidosis	Raised anion gap metabolic acidosis
Diarrhoea	Lactic acidosis
Ileostomy	Ketoacidosis—in uncontrolled diabetes, starvation, alcohol excess
Renal tubular acidosis	AKI/CKD
Parenteral nutrition	Toxic alcohols, e.g. methanol, ethylene glycol
Dilutional	Chronic paracetamol use—glutathione deficiency
Colonic ureteric implant/diversion	Salicylate poisoning

- This approach has the advantage of being relatively uncomplicated, and it is the standard approach to metabolic acidosis for most clinicians.
- Its main disadvantage is that it doesn't take into account the many unmeasured cations/anions that contribute to acid–base physiology.
- Albumin is the most abundant unmeasured anion in normal physiology; it can be corrected for in the standard anion gap calculation by adjusting for any fall in serum albumin from normal:
  - Serum anion gap (corrected for albumin) = (measured serum anion gap) + (2.5 × (45 – oberved serum albumin g.l^{-1}))

4.2.2 Stewart approach

- Canadian physiologist Peter Stewart developed a mathematical and physiochemical approach to acid–base disturbances in the 1970s.
- It is based on six simultaneous equations and relies on complex mathematics. It involves the following basic concepts:
  - Acids are defined as substances that, relative to hydroxyl ion concentration, increase the H^+ concentration of a solution, and bases are defined as substances that decrease the H^+ concentration.
  - HCO3$^-$ is not independent of pH/H^+, rather it is dependent on it.
  - Acids/bases are said to be 'strong' if they are fully dissociated in plasma and 'weak' if they are only partly dissociated.
  - Importantly, it takes into account the influence of albumin on acid–base disturbances.
- In terms of clinical utility, it identifies three major contributors to acid–base balance:
  - Strong ion difference (SID)
  - Concentration of non-volatile weak acids in plasma (Atot)
  - $PaCO_2$

4.2.2.1 Strong ion difference (SID):

- The SID reflects the difference between the number of strong cations and number of strong anions; a strong ion being an ion which is completely dissociated at physiological pH and temperature:
  - Strong cations: $Na^+ K^+ Ca^{2+} Mg^{2+}$
  - Strong anions: $Cl^- Lactate^-$
- An increase in strong cations relative to strong anions (an increase in the SID) leads to an alkalosis; conversely a decrease in SID leads to acidosis.
- The 'apparent' SID is calculated as:

$$(SIDapp) = ((H^+) + (K^+) + (Ca^{2+}) + (Mg^{2+})) - ((Cl^-) + (lactate^-))$$

- SIDapp is approximately 40 mEq.l^{-1} in normal physiology.
- The SIDapp is referred to as 'apparent' as it only includes those strong ions which are routinely measured.
- The true, or 'effective' strong ion difference (SIDeff) can be calculated using an equation developed by Figge *et al*:

$$SIDeff = 1,000 \times 2.46 \times 10^{-11} \times PCO_2/(10^{-pH}) + [Alb] \times (0.12 \times pH - 0.631)$$
$$+ [PO_3^-] \times (0.309 \times pH - 0.469).$$

- The difference between SIDeff and SIDapp is the strong ion gap (SIG).
- The SIG is similar to the anion gap in that, if it is elevated (>2), this indicates the presence of unmeasured strong cations contributing to acidosis (e.g. ketones, salicylates, paraldehyde).

4.2.2.2 Concentration of non-volatile weak acids in plasma (Atot)

- Albumin and phosphate act as weak acids in plasma.
- An increase in the concentration in either of these weak acids will lead to a reduction in the SIDeff, thereby shifting the equilibrium towards acidosis.
- Hypoalbuminaemia will cause a shift towards alkalosis.
- The inclusion of albumin is one of the major advantages of the Stewart hypothesis over earlier theories.

4.2.2.3 PaCO$_2$

- P_aCO_2 acts as an independent determinant of acid-base status.

FURTHER READING

Chawla G, Drummond D. Water, strong ions, and weak ions. *Continuing Education in Anaesthesia, Critical Care, and Pain* 2008; 8 (3): 108–12.

Corey HE. Stewart and beyond: new models of acid–base balance. *Kidney International* 2003; 64: 777–87.

Emmett M and Szerlip H. *Approach to the Adult with Metabolic Acidosis*. uptodate.com, July 2013.

Figge J, Rossing TH, Fencl V The role of serum proteins in acid–base equilibria. *Journal of Laboratory and Clinical Medicine* 1991; 117(6): 453–67.

Handy JM, Soni N. Physiological effects of hyperchloraemia and acidosis. *British Journal of Anaesthesia* 2008; 101(2), 141–150.

Kitching J, Edge CJ. Acid–base balance: a review of normal physiology. *British Journal of Anaesthesia* CEPD Reviews, 2002; 2 (1): 3–6.

Rastegar A. Clinical utility of Stewart's method in diagnosis and management of acid–base disorders. *Clinical Journal of the American Society of Nephrology* 2004; 4(7): 1267–4.

Rinaldi S, De Gaudio AR. Strong ion difference and strong anion gap: the Stewart approach to acid base disturbances. *Current Anaesthesia and Critical Care* 2005; 16(6): 395–402.

Stewart PA. Modern quantitative acid–base chemistry. *Canadian Journal of Physiology and Pharmacology* 1983; 61: 1444–62.

Story DA et al. Quantitative physical chemistry analysis of acid–base disorders in critically ill patients. *Anaesthesia* 2001; 56(6): 530–3.

Watkinson P. *The Stewart Hypothesis of Acid–Base Balance.* frca.co.uk, February 2009.

5 Glycaemic control

5.1 General

5.1.1 Hyperglycaemia

- Hyperglycaemia occurs in the majority of critically ill patients at some point of their illness and its aetiology is multifactorial:
  - Increased gluconeogenesis
  - Insulin resistance
  - Catecholamines—both endogenous and exogenous
  - Glucose-containing preparations
  - Corticosteroids
- A degree of hyperglycaemia is associated with the physiological response to critical illness; however, uncontrolled hyperglycaemia is associated with excess mortality and increased rates of healthcare associated infection.
- In patients with traumatic brain injury it may be associated with poor neurological outcome.

5.1.2 Hypoglycaemia

- Hypoglycaemia may occur as a result of insulin administration or severe illness, such as septic shock, hepatic failure, or cardiac failure. It is also associated with an excess mortality.
- Systemic effects of hypoglycaemia include:
  - Inflammatory response
  - Neuroglycopaenia
  - Cerebral vasodilatation
  - Autonomic dysfunction
  - Impaired stress response

5.2 Glycaemic control strategies

Glycaemic control in critical illness is a controversial topic.

5.2.1 The Van den Berghe study

- Interest in tight glycaemic control in the ICU was initially stimulated in 2001 by Van den Berghe's single-centre RCT, which demonstrated decreased mortality in surgical ICU patients using intensive insulin therapy (blood glucose target 4.4–6.1 mmol.l^{-1}).

5.2.2 Nice-Sugar

- Subsequent multi-centre NICE-SUGAR RCT found tight glycaemic control achieved by intensive insulin therapy was associated with:
  - Excess mortality
  - Increased rates of hypoglycaemia

5.2.3 Current guidance

- Recent guidelines form the Society of Critical Care Medicine suggest aiming for the more liberal target of blood glucose <10 mmol.l^{-1} and the avoidance of hypoglycaemia.
- It should be acknowledged that point-of-care glucose monitoring systems themselves are not always reliable and accurate—this is likely to be more of an issue when using these devices to maintain blood glucose within a tight control range.
- It has also been postulated that glycaemic variation may be as detrimental as hyperglycaemia itself.

5.3 Diabetic ketoacidosis

5.3.1 Background

- Diabetic ketoacidosis (DKA) occurs in patients with insulin deficiency and is defined metabolically as a triad of ketonaemia, hyperglycaemia, and metabolic acidosis.
- The clinical presentation includes profound dehydration in combination with the biochemical findings.
- It is usually found in type 1 diabetics and may prompt undiagnosed cases of type 1 diabetes mellitus (DM) to present to hospital.
- DKA can occur in patients with type 2 DM who develop insulin deficiency.
- The underlying defect of insulin deficiency and a concurrent increase in counter-regulatory hormones (including glucagon and adrenaline) result in the following pathophysiological response:
  - Decreased utilization of glucose and increased hepatic gluconeogenesis leading to hyperglycaemia
  - Glycosuria and subsequent osmotic diuresis
  - Increased lipolysis in liver mitochondria and subsequent production of acetoacetic acid, acetone, and 3-beta-hydroxybutyrate
- It is a life-threatening condition but is both preventable and treatable; mortality from DKA has fallen from around 8% to less than 1% over the last 20 years.
- The most common causes of death are cerebral oedema (mostly in adolescents and young children), ARDS, hypokalaemia, and co-morbidities.

5.3.2 Precipitants

- DKA is often precipitated by the following events:
  - New onset diabetes
  - Non-compliance with insulin
  - Administration of out-of-date insulin
  - Lipohypertrophy of injection sites due to non-rotation of injection sites and subsequent impaired insulin absorption
  - Intercurrent illness, e.g. infection, gastroenteritis, myocardial infarction

5.3.3 Management

As recommended by the Joint British Diabetes Societies (JBDS) Inpatient Working Group.
- Restore circulating volume with administration of IV fluids.

- Suppress ketogenesis and clear ketonaemia by administration of insulin and fluids.
- Treat hyperglycaemia while avoiding hypoglycaemia.
- Replace potassium and avoid hypokalaemia.
- Identify and treat any precipitating factor.
- Historically, DKA management has been guided by bedside blood glucose measurement and monitoring of bicarbonate and pH as surrogates for ketone clearance.
- The development of bedside meters that reliably measure the most abundant ketone in DKA (3-beta-hydroxybutyrate) has allowed management to focus on directly reversing the underlying pathophysiological process by suppression of ketogenesis and clearance of ketonaemia.
- Until recently there has been wide variation in the management of DKA; the JBDS Inpatient Care Group has therefore produced a DKA management guideline and care pathway. It makes the following recommendations:
  - Use of a fixed rate insulin infusion (0.1 units.kg.h^{-1}):
    - Aimed at suppressing ketogenesis
    - 10% dextrose can be administered to permit insulin administration if required (when blood glucose is <14 mmol.l^{-1})
    - Insulin infusion rate can be increased if the desired rate of ketone clearance is not achieved
  - Administration of 0.9% saline as resuscitation fluid:
    - There is widespread experience of this crystalloid in the treatment of DKA.
    - It is the only appropriate fluid to come pre-mixed with potassium in the UK.
    - It is acknowledged that Hartmann's solution may be used in critical care units, and its use may be associated with less hyperchloraemic acidosis, although there is no evidence that either fluid is superior in terms of outcomes in the management of DKA.
    - Colloids are not recommended.
  - Measurement of blood ketones should guide management:
    - The aim of treatment should be the suppression of ketogenesis and the clearance of ketones.
    - A fall in blood ketones of at least 0.5 mmol.l^{-1} per hour should be targeted—the insulin infusion rate should be increased if this is not being achieved.
    - In the absence of the availability of blood ketone monitoring, a fall in serum glucose by 3.0 mmol.l^{-1} per hour and a rise in serum bicarbonate by 3.0 mmol.l^{-1} per hour should be targeted.
    - Serum bicarbonate may remain low once DKA has resolved due to hyperchloraemia induced by 0.9% saline administration—this further underlines the benefit of ketone measurement.
  - Venous bicarbonate/pH should be used rather than arterial:
    - The difference in pH between arterial and venous samples is not large enough to significantly influence management, it is therefore preferable for patient safety and comfort to use venous samples.
    - Arterial catheters should *not* be inserted routinely for blood sampling; they can be inserted for respiratory or cardiovascular instability, if required.
  - Long-acting subcutaneous insulin should be continued:
    - If the patient is normally on a long-acting insulin analogue such as Levemir® or Lantus® this should continue to be administered.
    - This strategy reduces the risk of rebound hyperglycaemia.

- Patients with markers of severity should be considered for admission to the critical care unit:
  - Most patients with DKA improve with standard therapy and will need Level 2 critical care at most.
  - Patients who present late, have severe co-morbidities, or have a concurrent critical illness (e.g. severe pneumonia) may require Level 3 support.
  - The UK guidelines suggest the following as markers of DKA severity:
    - Blood ketones >6 mmol.l^{-1}
    - Serum bicarbonate <5 mmol.l^{-1}
    - Venous or arterial pH <7.0
    - Potassium <3.5 mmol.l^{-1} on admission
    - GCS <12
    - SaO2 <92% on room air
    - Heart rate <60 or >100
    - Anion gap >16
- Guidance around stopping IV insulin infusion and re-starting subcutaneous insulin regime:
  - The diabetes specialist team should be involved in this transition.
  - The subcutaneous regime can be restarted when the patient is able to take sufficient diet and fluids; and blood ketones are <0.6 mmol/l and serum pH is >7.3.
  - Subcutaneous regime should be restarted with a meal and the IV insulin infusion stopped 30–60 minutes after the subcutaneous dose.
- Administration of phosphate is discouraged in most cases:
  - There is no evidence that supplementation improves outcome.
  - Should be reserved for those cases with respiratory or skeletal muscle weakness.
- Intravenous bicarbonate is not recommended:
  - It is associated with cerebrospinal fluid acidosis and is implicated in cerebral oedema in children.
- Sodium correction in hyperglycaemia:
  - The osmotic effect of plasma glucose draws water into the intravascular compartment, diluting ionic concentrations, most significantly sodium.
  - Correction of sodium concentration for hyperglycaemia more accurately reflects sodium and allows sodium to be tracked as hyperglycaemia resolves.
  - Tracking of corrected sodium is particularly important in children and adolescents who are at greater risk of cerebral oedema as the DKA resolves: it is the fall in corrected sodium that is the primary precipitant of the cerebral oedema.
  - Corrected sodium in the context of hyperglycaemia:

  Corrected sodium = Measured sodium + (0.3(plasma glucose − 5.5))

5.4 Hyperosmolar hyperglycaemic state

5.4.1 Background

- Hyperosmolar hyperglycaemic state (HHS) typically presents in older patients and tends to develop over several days; however, with changes in the demographic of diabetes, it can be seen in younger patients.
- It is usually associated with type 2 diabetes and has a high mortality (15–20%), although it is relatively uncommon.

- There is no standard diagnostic definition for HHS, however, JBDS Inpatient Working Group states that it is characterized by the following features:
  - Marked hypovolaemia
  - Blood glucose >30 mmol.l^{-1} in the absence of significant hyperketonaemia (<3.0 mmol.l^{-1}) or significant acidosis (pH >7.3, serum bicarbonate >15 mmol.l^{-1})
  - Serum osmolality >320 mosmol.kg^{-1}
- The pathogenesis of HHS is unclear.
- A degree of insulin deficiency occurs; however, it is not significant enough to promote lipolysis and the marked ketosis that is seen in DKA.
- Osmotic diuresis does, however, lead to profound dehydration (fluid deficit estimated at 100–220 ml/kg) and electrolyte disturbance.
- Until recently HHS was known as hyperosmolar non-ketotic coma (HONK); however, as a mild degree of ketosis can be found and most patients are not comatose, this term has been superseded by HHS.
- Patients with HHS frequently experience vascular complications, such as arterial/venous thrombosis and foot ulceration, and less frequently complications of fluid/electrolyte shifts, such as cerebral oedema and central pontine myelinosis.

5.4.2 Management

- As with DKA, the JBDS Inpatient Working Group has produced HHS management guidelines.
- The goals of management are to replace fluid and electrolytes and to normalize osmolality and blood glucose, whilst preventing potential complications.
- The guidelines recommend treating any underlying cause (e.g. infection or MI) and using the following approach to management:
  - Osmolality should be monitored frequently:
    - Should be measured or calculated frequently to guide therapy
    - Ideally results should be plotted on a graph to evaluate rate of change
    - If laboratory measurement of osmolality is not readily available, it should be calculated using the formula:

    $$osmolality = 2 [Na] + [glucose] + [urea].$$

  - Fluid and potassium replacement:
    - 0.9% saline should be the resuscitation fluid of choice.
    - 50% of the estimated fluid deficit (see Section 3.2.4 to calculate fluid deficit) should be replaced in the first 12 hours of management.
    - Fluid resuscitation should lower blood glucose and subsequently serum osmolality—this should be gradual with a rate of fall in blood glucose no more than 5 mmol.l^{-1} per hour optimal.
    - Rapid changes in osmolality result in large fluid shifts and their potential deleterious effects.
    - Serum sodium may rise; however, this should only be of clinical concern if the serum osmolality is not falling and 0.45% saline should only be considered if osmolality is not falling and blood glucose is not falling adequately with adequate 0.9% saline administration (see corrected sodium in Section 5.3.3).
    - Potassium should be monitored and replaced; however, some patients will present with hyperkalaemia secondary to AKI and this should be considered.
    - Fluid and electrolyte abnormalities may take up to 72 hours to normalize.

- Insulin administration when necessary:
  - Insulin therapy should only be started in the initial phase if significant ketosis is present, i.e. blood ketones >1 mmol.l^{-1} or urine ketones >2+. Otherwise blood glucose should fall with fluid administration.
  - When blood glucose ceases to fall with fluids, then insulin administration can be considered.
  - When insulin is required acutely, fixed rate IV insulin is recommended with a starting dose of 0.05 units/kg/h. Target blood glucose is 10–15 mmol.l^{-1}.
- Monitoring and prevention of complications:
  - Monitoring for complications of treatment (such as fluid overload or cerebral oedema) should take place every 1–2 hours.
  - Feet are particularly vulnerable to pressure sores and should be examined daily and heel protectors considered.
- Anticoagulation:
  - Unless contraindicated, prophylactic dose low molecular weight heparin (LMWH) should be administered.
  - Prolonged administration of LMWH for up to 3 months post-discharge should be considered in high-risk patients.
  - Some centres advocate the use of full-dose LMWH given the high risk of thrombotic complications—the national guidelines state that there is no robust evidence for this approach, and indeed patients may be exposed to an unacceptable bleeding risk if this approach is employed.
- Specialist advice:
  - Should be sought as soon as practically possible.
  - Most patients will require subcutaneous insulin regimes after the acute phase.
- Critical care—admission to the critical care unit and invasive monitoring should be considered for patients with the following markers of severity:
  - Osmolality >350 mosmol.kg^{-1}
  - Na^+ >160 mmol.l^{-1}
  - Venous/arterial pH>7.1
  - K^+ <3.5 mmol.l^{-1} or >6 mmol.l^{-1} on presentation
  - GCS <12
  - SaO_2 <92% on room air
  - Systolic BP <90 mmHg
  - Heart rate <60 or >100 bpm
  - Urine output <0.5 ml.kg^{-1} per hour
  - Serum creatinine >200 μmol.l^{-1}
  - Hypothermia
  - Acute macrovascular event
  - Significant co-morbidities

FURTHER READING

Egi M, Finfer S, Bellomo R. Glycaemic control in the ICU. *Chest* 2011; 140(1): 212–20.

Jacobi J, Bircher N, Krinsley J, et al. Guidelines for the use of an insulin infusion for the management of hyperglycaemia in critically ill patients. *Critical Care Medicine* 2012; 40(12): 3251–76.

Kitabchi AE, Umpierrez GE, Miles JM, Fisher JN. Hyperglycemic crises in adult patients with diabetes. *Diabetes Care* 2009; 32(7): 1335–43.

Mahler SA, Conrad SA, Wang H, Arnold TC. Resuscitation with balanced electrolyte solution prevents hyperchloraemic acidosis in patients with diabetic ketoacidosis. *American Journal of Emergency Medicine* 2011; 29(6): 670–4.

NICE-SUGAR. Study Investigators Intensive versus conventional glucose control in critically ill patients. *New England Journal of Medicine* 2009; 36013: 1283–97.

Rudd B, Patel K, Levy N, Dhatariya K. A survey of the implementation of the NHS diabetes guidelines for management of diabetic ketoacidosis in the intensive care units of the East of England. *Journal of the Intensive Care Society* 2013; 14(1): 60–4.

Savage M.W., Dhatariya K.K., Kilvert A., et al., *Joint British Diabetes Societies guideline for the management of diabetic ketoacidosis.* Diabetic Medicine 2011; 28(5): p. 508–515.

Scott A.R., *Management of hyperosmolar hyperglycaemic state in adults with diabetes.* Diabetic Medicine, 2015; 32(6): p. 714–24.

van den Berghe G, Wouters P, Weekers F, Verwaest C, et al. Intensive insulin therapy in the critically ill patients. *New England Journal of Medicine* 2001; 34519: 1359–67.

Van Zyl DG, Rheeder P, Delport E. Fluid management in diabetic-acidosis—ringer's lactate versus normal saline: a randomized controlled trial. *QJM* 2012; 105(4): 337–43.

6 Thyroid axis

Acute illness results in multiple changes in the hypothalamic–pituitary–thyroid (HPT) axis. Although some changes are part of the physiological response to acute illness and may be advantageous, others are the result of prolonged critical illness.

6.1 Thyroid changes in acute illness

6.1.1 Early changes

- Circulating total T3 and free T3 levels decrease
- Circulating levels of the inactive reverse T3 (rT3) increase
- Circulating T4 levels may increase transiently, however, in severe illness they will fall and may be low at presentation
- TSH levels may rise transiently in very early acute illness

6.1.2 Subsequent changes

- Depression of the HPT axis compounds the earlier changes
- Decreased circulating T4 levels
- Decrease in thyroid-binding globulin (TBG) levels—this may return to normal in prolonged illness
- TSH levels fall

6.1.3 Drugs

- Commonly used drugs in critical care can also have effects of the HPT axis (Table 3.3).

Table 3.3 Drugs affecting the thyroid axis

Drug	Mechanism of interference with HPT axis
Glucocorticoids	TSH suppression and inhibition of peripheral conversion
Iodinated contrast agents and dressings	Inhibition of hormone synthesis and secretion in thyroid
Propranolol	Inhibition of peripheral conversion
Amiodarone	Inhibition of peripheral conversion
Barbiturates	Increased T4 clearance
Dopamine	TSH suppression
Opiates	TSH suppression
Benzodiazepines	Inhibition of peripheral conversion
Sulfonamides	Inhibition of hormone synthesis
Somatostatin	TSH Suppression
Furosemide	Interaction with binding proteins

Reproduced from *Best Practice and Research Clinical Endocrinology and Metabolism*, 25, Mebis L et al. 'Thyroid axis function and dysfunction in critical illness', pp. 745–757. Copyright (2011) with permission from Elsevier.

- The changes in thyroid function that occur during acute illness are known by a number of terms, including:
  - Low T3 syndrome
  - Non thyroid illness
  - Sick euthyroid state
- Routine serum thyroid function tests (TFTs) show low levels of circulating T3 and T4, and inappropriately low TSH (i.e. low or within reference range TSH—this is still low in the context of low T3/T4).
- The prognostic significance of these changes is unclear and there is currently no evidence to support the use of supplementary thyroid hormones is this situation.

6.2 Thyroid storm

6.2.1 Background

Thyroid storm is an exaggerated response to hyperthyroidism; its exact pathophysiology is poorly understood. It can result from any thyrotoxic state but is seen most frequently in Graves' disease. It is a rare condition that is associated with a high mortality rate (10–30%). The pathophysiology of thyroid storm is poorly understood; however, it is generally characterized by:

- Hypermetabolic state
- Increased sympathetic activity and excess circulating catecholamines
- Increased oxygen consumption

6.2.2 Precipitants

Thyroid storm is usually precipitated by another condition or insult such as:

- Infective illness
- Vascular/thrombotic, e.g. myocardial infarction, stroke, pulmonary embolism
- Perioperative—thyroid surgery, non-thyroid surgery, and anaesthesia
- Metabolic upset
- Burns or trauma
- Pregnancy

- Therapeutic—iodinated contrast, amiodarone, pseudoephedrine, interferon, acute excess thyroid hormone ingestion, non-compliance with, or cessation of, treatment for thyrotoxicosis
- Thyroiditis
- Diabetic ketoacidosis

6.2.3 Diagnosis

Diagnosis is made on the basis of clinical suspicion and recognition of key clinical features—this requires a high index of suspicion. TFTs are usually no different from those found in established thyrotoxicosis. Clinical features include:

- Pyrexia—most common feature
- Profuse sweating
- Tachyarrhythmia
- Organ dysfunction—cardiac, hepatic, CNS, renal
- Elderly patients may present atypically with lethargy or cardiac failure

6.2.4 Management

Management of thyroid storm includes the following general measures:

- Invasive organ support in ICU if clinical situation merits, including nutritional support
- Fluid resuscitation
- Cooling measures and antipyretics (avoid salicylates as can displace T4 from TBG)
- Sedation if required for agitation (may also decrease oxygen consumption in this situation)
- Identification and treatment of precipitating cause

Thyroid specific therapy should be introduced after consultation with endocrine services.

6.3 Myxoedema coma

6.3.1 Background

- Myxoedema coma is the clinical manifestation of profound hypothyroidism.
- The widespread availability of thyroid function testing and oral levothyroxine have made it a relatively rare occurrence.
- Despite the name, patients are not necessarily comatose.

6.3.2 Features

Clinical features include:

- Cardiovascular instability—due to myocardial depression and vasodilatation
- Hypothermia
- Confusion or decreased conscious level—as a result of decreased cerebral blood flow and metabolism
- Hypercapnia—secondary to impaired respiratory centre response to hypoxia
- Macroglossia, myxoedema of larynx, and typical hypothyroid features may occur (e.g. dry, coarse skin and eye/periorbital changes)—macroglossia/laryngeal oedema may be particularly relevant if considering intubation
- Decreased gut motility
- Renal failure
- Biochemistry—raised TSH, low T3/T4, raised CK, raised LDH, hypoglycaemia

TFTs reveal raised TSH and low T3 and T4; however, the actual values may be no different to those found in hypothyroid patients who are clinically stable—a high index of suspicion is therefore required to make the diagnosis. Mortality rates are quoted from 20% to 65%—this underlines the importance of recognition and commencement of definitive therapy.

Myxoedema is more common in elderly females. Those with previous thyroid surgery or radio-active iodine treatment are particularly at risk.

6.3.3 Precipitants

Precipitating factors include:
- Systemic infection
- Hypothermia
- Trauma
- Anaesthesia

6.3.4 Management

- Due to the rarity of this condition, there is little good evidence regarding therapy.
- Supportive care in the ICU should be provided.
- Precipitants should be identified and treated.
- Adrenal insufficiency can co-exist and as such IV steroid therapy is recommended until this can be excluded.
- Intravenous thyroid hormone should be administered as definitive therapy until stability and normal gut motility has been obtained, at which point oral therapy can be commenced.
- Both T3 and T4 monotherapy and combination regimes have been described—this should be guided by advice from local endocrinologists.

FURTHER READING

Beynon J, Akhtar S, Kearney T. Predictors of outcome in myxoedema coma. *Critical Care* 2008; 12: 111.

Burch HB, Wartofsky L. Life-threatening thyrotoxicosis. Thyroid storm. *Endocrinology Metabolism Clinics North America* 1993; 22(2): 263–77.

Carroll R, Matfin G. Endocrine and metabolic emergencies: thyroid storm. *Therapeutic Advances in Endocrinology and Metabolism* 2010; 1(3): 139–45.

Chiha M, Samarasinghe S, Kabaker AS. Thyroid storm: an updated review. *Journal of Intensive Care Medicine* 2013. 30(3):131–40.

Dutta P, Bhansali A, Masoodi SR, et al. Predictors of outcome in myxoedema coma: a study from a tertiary care centre. *Critical Care* 2008; 12: R1.

Kwaku MP, Burman KD. Myxoedema coma. *Journal of Intensive Care Medicine* 2007; 22(4): 224–31.

Mebis L, Van den Berghe G. Thyroid axis function and dysfunction in critical illness. *Best Practice and Research Clinical Endocrinology and Metabolism* 2011; 25: 745–57.

7 Adrenal response to critical illness

7.1 The hypothalamic–pituitary–adrenal axis (HPA)

7.1.1 The stress response

- The stress response to critical illness includes activation of the HPA axis and the sympatho-adrenal system:
  - Hypothalamus secretes corticotrophin-releasing hormone (CRH)

- CRH stimulates the anterior pituitary to release adrenocorticotrophic hormone (ACTH)
- ACTH stimulates the adrenal cortex to produce cortisol
- Adrenal medulla secretes increased amounts of adrenaline and noradrenaline
- During health the majority of cortisol is bound to corticosteroid-binding globulin (CBG), however in critical illness the amount of CBG falls therefore increasing the amount of active cortisol.

7.2 Critical illness-related corticosteroid insufficiency (CIRCI)

7.2.1 Background

- In addition to the stress response described earlier, some patients with severe critical illness may display an inadequate corticosteroid response to their degree of critical illness—this is known as critical illness-related corticosteroid insufficiency (CIRCI) (sometimes also termed relative adrenal insufficiency, RAI) and it is thought to arise for the following reasons:
  - Suppression/failure of the HPA axis and adrenals
    - Aetiology is multifactorial and includes some drugs used in the ICU, e.g. corticosteroids, etomidate, rifampicin, and phenytoin
    - Typically seen in patients with marked systemic inflammation and may be due to effects of TNF α and Interleukin 1
  - Corticosteroid resistance
    - Thought to be a consequence of systemic inflammation and inflammatory mediators, including TNF α
- Unlike patients who present with chronic forms of adrenal failure (e.g. Addison's disease), patients with CIRCI do not typically present with hyponatraemia and hyperkalaemia.
- CIRCI should be considered in critically ill patients with fluid refractory cardiovascular instability requiring inotropes or vasopressors, and patients with progressive ARDS.

7.2.2 Definition and diagnosis

- Traditional diagnosis of adrenal insufficiency is based upon measurement of baseline cortisol and ACTH levels, and dynamic testing by measuring the change in serum cortisol produced by administering 250 μg of synthetic ACTH (the 'short Synacthen test').
- This may be inaccurate in the critically ill patient for a number of reasons:
  - The majority of commercially available assays measure total serum cortisol—critical illness decreases the amount of CBG, therefore free cortisol levels may increase making total cortisol measurements difficult to interpret.
  - Elimination of cortisol may be impaired, therefore complicating the interpretation of dynamic tests.
  - Serum cortisol levels may vary from hour to hour making random measurements unhelpful.
- The American College of Critical Care Medicine recommends the following as diagnostic parameters of adrenal insufficiency in critical illness; however, as described these criteria have significant limitations:
  - Random serum cortisol <10 μg.dl^{-1}
  - Change in serum cortisol (delta cortisol) <9 μg.dl^{-1} following administration of 250 μg of synthetic ACTH

7.2.3 Administration of steroids to patient with CIRCI

- The use of steroids in critical illness is an area of debate:
  - Administration of supraphysiological doses of corticosteroid may be associated with harm.

- Recent research has focused on the use of physiological stress-dose steroid (in the range of 200 mg of hydrocortisone per 24 hours) in critical illness.
- The work of a French group led by Annane led to the widespread use of stress-dose steroid in septic shock, dependant on the patient's baseline cortisol and response to synthetic ACTH.
- Subsequently the multi-centre randomized controlled trial CORTICUS failed to show any outcome benefit in the administration of stress-dose steroids to patients with septic shock—regardless of their response to synthetic ACTH. Although there was no clear mortality benefit of steroids in the CORTICUS study, patients who received steroid did have a faster reversal of their shock state.
- Subsequent meta-analyses have consistently shown that steroids improve shock but provide conflicting results regarding mortality. Subgroup analysis suggests that patients with higher illness severity scores are more likely to have mortality benefit with steroids.

7.3 The role of exogenous steroids in critical illness

- In the light of the difficulties in diagnosing CIRCI and identifying patients likely to benefit from steroid administration, the American College of Critical Care Medicine has made the following recommendations:
  - Steroid administration should be considered in vasopressor dependent septic shock—hydrocortisone 200 mg per 24 hours for at least 7 days
  - Response to synthetic ACTH administration should not be used to determine who should receive steroids in the above groups.
  - Steroids should be weaned rather than stopped abruptly.
- See Section 1.6.3 for a discussion of steroids in ARDS and Section 1.10.3 for the use of steroids in community acquired pneumonia.

FURTHER READING

Annane D, Sébille V, Charpentier C, et al. Effect of treatment with low doses of hydrocortisone and fludrocortisone on mortality in patients with septic shock. *Journal of the American Medical Association* 2002; 288(7): 862–71.

Boonen E, Vervenne H, Meersseman P, et al. Reduced cortisol metabolism during critical illness. *New England Journal of Medicine* 2013; 368: 1477–88.

Davies M. Anaesthesia and adrenocortical disease. *Continuing Education in Anaesthesia, Critical Care and Pain* 2005; 5(4): 122–6.

Gomez-Sanchez, CE. Adrenal dysfunction in critically ill patients. *New England Journal of Medicine* 2013; 368: 1547–9.

Marik PE, Pastores SM, Annane D, et al. Recommendations for the diagnosis and management of corticosteroid insufficiency in critically ill adult patients: consensus statements from an international task force by the American College of Critical Care Medicine. *Critical Care Medicine* 2008; 36(6): 1937–49.

Marik PE. Critical illness-related corticosteroid insufficiency. *Chest* 2009; 135(1): 181–93.

Sprung CL[1], Annane D, Keh D, et al. Hydrocortisone therapy for patients with septic shock. *New England Journal of Medicine* 2008; 358: 111–24.

CHAPTER 4

Gastroenterology and hepatology

CONTENTS

1 Liver failure syndromes

Patients with both acute (fulminant) liver failure and acute-on-chronic liver failure may require support on the ICU. These two groups of patients typically have differing underlying disease processes, present different problems, and require different approaches to management.

1.1 Comparison of acute and acute-on-chronic liver failure

1.1.1 Aetiology

- Whilst there is a degree of crossover between the aetiologies of acute and chronic liver failure, certain pathologies are more commonly associated with one or the other (Table 4.1).

Table 4.1 Aetiology of acute and chronic liver failure (described in further detail in Sections 2.2 and 3.2, respectively)

Acute liver failure	Chronic liver failure/cirrhosis
<ul><li>Paracetamol overdose</li><li>Drug-induced liver injury</li><li>Viral hepatitis (A, B, and E)</li><li>Ischaemic hepatitis and Budd–Chiari syndrome</li><li>Wilson's disease</li><li>Mushroom (Amanita phalloides) poisoning</li><li>Post-surgical resection</li><li>Post-orthotopic liver transplantation</li></ul>	<ul><li>Viral hepatitis (B and C)</li><li>Alcoholic liver disease</li><li>Non-alcoholic steatohepatitis (NASH)</li><li>Haemochromatosis</li><li>Autoimmune processes<ul><li>Autoimmune hepatitis</li><li>Primary sclerosing cholangitis</li><li>Primary biliary sclerosis</li></ul></li><li>Right-sided heart failure</li><li>Veno-occlusive disease</li></ul>

1.1.2 Management issues

- Although acute and chronic liver failure share some features, they are two distinct clinical entities (Table 4.2).

Table 4.2 Defining features of acute and chronic liver failure

Acute liver failure	Chronic liver failure/cirrhosis
• Coagulopathy • Encephalopathy associated with raised intracranial pressure • Hyperbilirubinaemia	• Hyperbilirubinaemia • Ascites and spontaneous bacterial peritonitis • Variceal disease • Encephalopathy *without* raised intracranial pressure • Increased risk of hepatocellular carcinoma • Hepatorenal syndrome

2 Acute (fulminant) liver failure

2.1 Background

2.1.1 General

- Acute liver failure (ALF) (also described as fulminant liver failure) is a rare, life-threatening disease with a high risk of progression to multi-organ failure and death.
- ALF is a different entity from acute-on-chronic liver failure, which describes deterioration, or decompensation of chronic, cirrhotic, liver disease.

2.1.2 Definition

- Definition of ALF requires:
  - Absence of chronic liver disease
  - Hepatic insult leading to the triad:
    - Encephalopathy (this is the most important clinical defining event)
    - Coagulopathy
    - Jaundice

2.1.3 Timing

- Subcategorized depending upon time from onset of jaundice to encephalopathy:
  - Hyperacute: <7 days
  - Acute: 7–28 days
  - Sub-acute: 5–12 weeks

2.2 Aetiology

2.2.1 Drug-induced

- The commonest cause of ALF is that secondary to drug-induced liver injury:
  - Paracetamol overdose (POD) is the leading drug-induced liver injury in Europe and the USA.

- Changes to the packaging of paracetamol (acetaminophen in the USA and Canada) have reduced the incidence and severity of POD ALF significantly.
- Less common causes of drug-induced liver injury are:
  - Antibiotics
  - Anti-epileptics (particularly valproate)
  - Anti-tuberculosis medication (particularly isoniazid)
  - Recreational drugs (ecstasy, methamphetamine)

2.2.2 Non-drug-induced

- Non-drug-related causes of ALF include:
  - Viral hepatitis (hepatitis A, B and E)
  - Non-hepatitic viruses (Ebstein–Barr Virus (EBV), Cytomegalovirus (CMV), Herpes Simplex Virus (HSV))
  - Non-drug poisoning (e.g. *Amanita phalloides* mushroom poisoning).
  - Wilson's disease is a special case in that the liver failure generated by copper deposition is commonly associated with fibrotic changes in the liver, including cirrhosis.

2.3 Clinical manifestations

Acute liver failure is typically a rapidly progressive process.

2.3.1 Haemodynamic instability

- High cardiac output vasodilatory shock

2.3.2 Acute kidney injury

- May be the consequence of the underlying disease process (e.g. POD), concurrent sepsis, or due to the haemodynamic changes associated with acute liver failure.

2.3.3 Coagulopathy

- A defining feature of ALF, but risk of spontaneous bleeding is low: this is because of reduced production of both pro- and anti-coagulant factors.

2.3.4 Encephalopathy and coma

- Ammonia is generated in the gut from breakdown of amino acids and is normally detoxified in the healthy liver to ammonium, which is renally excreted.
- During ALF, and in cases of portosystemic bypass, plasma ammonia levels rise and freely cross the blood–brain barrier.
- Within the brain, ammonia is converted to glutamine by glutamate dehydrogenase.
- Glutamine is a powerful intracellular oncotic in its own right. In addition, it causes increased peri-mitochondrial hyperammonaemia and mitochondrial dysfunction: this 'Trojan horse hypothesis' results in failure of water homeostasis in the astrocyte due to reduced ATP production.
- Whilst the precise pathophysiological mechanism remains the subject of debate, the end result is accepted to be astrocyte swelling with resultant cerebral oedema and raised intracellular pressure.
- The higher the serum level of ammonia, the greater the rise in intracranial pressure and risk of death.

- - Ammonia levels >100 μmol.l⁻¹ are strongly associated with severe encephalopathy
  - Ammonia levels >200 μmol.l⁻¹ are associated with intracranial hypertension
- Hepatic encephalopathy is graded using the West Haven scale (Table 4.3).

2.3.5 Infection

- A state of functional immunosuppression evolves and the risk of infection is high.
- Sepsis may contribute to vasodilatory shock.

Table 4.3 West Haven grading of hepatic encephalopathy

Grade	Features
I	Trivial lack of awareness
	Euphoria or anxiety
	Shortened attention span
	Impaired performance of addition
II	Lethargy or apathy
	Minimal disorientation for time or place
	Subtle personality change
	Inappropriate behaviour
	Impaired performance of subtraction
III	Somnolence to semi-stupor, but responsive to verbal stimuli
	Confusion
	Gross disorientation
IV	Coma (unresponsive to verbal or noxious stimuli)

Reprinted from *Gastroenterology*, 72, Conn HO et al., 'Comparison of Lactulose and Neomycin in the Treatment of Chronic Portal-Systemic Encephalopathy', pp.573–583. Copyright (1977) American Gastroenterological Association. Published by Elsevier Inc.

2.4 Management

2.4.1 Specialist input

- Early discussion and transfer to a specialist hepatic centre is important.
- Low threshold for endotracheal intubation prior to transfer, as encephalopathy can rapidly progress to coma.

2.4.2 Specific therapies

- Remove the hepatic insult and consider specific antidotes (e.g. N-acetylcysteine for paracetamol overdose; see Chapter 9, Section 3.1).

2.4.3 Supportive management

- Airway protection in comatose patients
- Invasive haemodynamic monitoring and vasopressors for shock
- Renal replacement therapy for acute kidney injury (concerns that RRT may mask creatinine as a marker of severity of ALF should not delay initiation of therapy)

2.4.4 Encephalopathy and raised intracranial pressure

- Can rapidly progress to death and therefore early and aggressive management is warranted.
- Removal of ammonia:
  - Renal replacement therapy ('high-dose' haemodiafiltration)
  - Pharmacological (e.g. lactulose, L-ornithine L-arginine (LOLA), rifaximin), although none have demonstrated a survival benefit in ALF
- Management of cerebral oedema:
  - Similar management as employed in other forms of cerebral oedema (see Chapter 5, Section 3.4):
    - Temperature management
    - High-normal plasma sodium
    - Sedation
    - Head up nursing
    - Optimization of cerebral perfusion pressure
- Some centres use invasive intracranial pressure monitoring, particularly in high-risk groups (young age, high ammonia); this is of unclear benefit and carries a risk of bleeding.

2.4.5 Coagulopathy

- Careful use of pro-coagulant blood products (e.g. fresh frozen plasma, platelets, and fibrinogen):
  - Routine correction of coagulopathy is *not* recommended, as modulating PT could affect transplant decisions.
  - Therefore only used to cover procedures with high risk of bleeding or in which consequences of bleeding are catastrophic, e.g.:
    - Intracranial pressure monitor insertion
    - Prior to liver transplant
    - Not typically for arterial or central venous catheters
- Vitamin K replacement is suggested to remove any nutritional cause of coagulopathy; whilst nutritional deficiency is relatively common in chronic liver disease it is unlikely in the early stages of ALF.

2.4.6 Emergency liver transplantation

- Decision-making based on the King's College Hospital criteria (KCC) (Table 4.4):
  - Developed in 1989 by O'Grady et al. and remain the benchmark for listing decision.
  - Criteria differ for POD and non-POD cases of ALF.
  - The criteria have been the subject of several meta-analyses confirming excellent specificity but poor sensitivity in determining mortality with or without liver transplantation.
  - The acute liver failure early dynamic (ALFED) model is an alternative scoring system that is based upon the trajectory of liver markers and has been proposed as a more specific prognostic tool; use is, however, not widespread.
- Contra-indications to emergency liver transplantation include:
  - Severe cerebral oedema
  - Rising vasopressor requirements
  - Uncontrolled sepsis
  - Major psychiatric co-morbidity

Table 4.4 The King's College criteria for emergency liver transplant in acute liver failure

Acute liver failure secondary to paracetamol overdose	Acute liver failure secondary to aetiology other than paracetamol overdose
pH <7.3 24 hours post-admission following fluid resuscitation	PT >100 s (INR >6.5)
Or	Or
Combination of: • Hepatic encephalopathy grade 3 or 4 • PT >100 s (INR >6.5) • Creatinine >300 µmol.l⁻¹ or Arterial lactate >3.5 mmol.l⁻¹ at 4 hours or Arterial lactate >3 mmol.l⁻¹ at 12 hours (after fluid resuscitation)	Any three of: • PT >50 s (INR >3.5) • Non-hepatitis A/B aetiology • Age <10 or >40 • Bilirubin>300 µmol.l⁻¹ • Duration of jaundice prior to hepatic encephalopathy onset > 7 days

Adapted from *Gastroenterology*, 97, O'Grady et al., 'Early indicators of prognosis in fulminant hepatic failure', pp. 439–445. Copyright (1989) with permission from Elsevier. INR, International Normalised Ratio; PT, Prothrombin Time.

FURTHER READING

Bernal W, Wendon J. Acute liver failure. *New England Journal of Medicine* 2013; 369: 2525–34.

Kumar R, Sharma H, Goyal R, et al. Prospective derivation and validation of early dynamic model for predicting outcome in patients with acute liver failure. *Gut* 2012; 61: 1068–75.

O'Grady JG, Alexander G, Hayllar KM, et al. Early indicators of prognosis in fulminant hepatic failure. *Gastroenterology* 1989; 97: 439–45.

3 Chronic liver failure and cirrhosis

The incidence of cirrhosis in the general population is rising due to increasing numbers of cases of alcohol-related liver disease, non-alcoholic steatohepatitis, and viral hepatitis. These three main causes dominate incidence rates and liver transplant activity, and will become a significant burden on intensive care services.

• There are multiple reasons for ICU admission of the cirrhotic patient:
  ▪ Variceal haemorrhage
  ▪ Hepatic encephalopathy
  ▪ Renal or metabolic dysfunction, including ascites and hepatorenal syndrome
  ▪ Standard extra-hepatic reasons for admission (septic shock, respiratory failure)

3.1 Cardiovascular changes in cirrhosis

• A number of cardiovascular abnormalities are associated with chronic liver disease. A number of vasoactive substances are involved.

3.1.1 Hyperdynamic circulation

• Decreased peripheral vascular resistance

- Increased cardiac output
- Decreased blood pressure

3.1.2 Cirrhotic cardiomyopathy (despite an increased cardiac output at rest)

- Blunted response to catecholamines (either intrinsic or extrinsic)
- Diastolic dysfunction

3.1.3 Alterations in hepatic and splanchnic flow

- Increased intra-hepatic resistance leads to portal venous congestion and varices
- Formation of collateral circulation and subsequent porto-systemic shunt
- Splanchnic vasodilation

3.1.4 Vascular changes within other organs

- Inappropriate vasodilation within the pulmonary circulation may lead to ventilation-perfusion mismatch—the hepato-pulmonary syndrome, which manifests as hypoxaemia.
- Splanchnic vasodilation may lead to neuro-humorally mediated renal vasoconstriction, which may contribute to the hepatorenal syndrome.

3.2 Mortality of cirrhotic patients in intensive care

3.2.1 General

- Patients with cirrhosis are functionally immunocompromised, frequently deconditioned, and often have pre-existing liver failure and dysfunction of other organs.
- There exist many reports demonstrating the poor survival rates of these patients in intensive care units compared with patients without liver disease.
- Predicting survival in these patients can be difficult and there exist several schemas from both the hepatology and intensive care communities designed to assist prognostication.
- Studies reporting survival of critically ill patients with cirrhosis in ICU suggest overall mortality to range between 40% and 80%, with a progressive increase in mortality with the number of organ systems failing.
- The reason for ICU admission must also be considered as underlying aetiology impacts upon mortality: cirrhotic patients admitted with variceal haemorrhage demonstrate relatively high survival; those admitted with undifferentiated sepsis, however, have poorer outcomes.

3.2.2 Mortality scoring systems specific to cirrhosis

- Mortality prediction scores exist, some of which are specific to cirrhosis:
    - Child–Pugh–Turcotte score:
        - Scores outlined in Table 4.5
        - On addition of the individual score, patients are stratified into Child–Pugh A (5–6), B (7–9), or C (>9)
        - Mortality post-operatively and in the outpatient setting increases with rising score
    - Model for end-stage liver disease (MELD) score:
        - Calculation outlined in Box 4.1
        - Range 1–40
        - 3-month mortality increases with rising score
        - Patients with MELD >15 are suitable for transplant assessment/listing
        - In the United Kingdom, this has been modified to the UKELD (United Kingdom end-stage liver disease score) by inclusion of serum sodium into the model.

Table 4.5 Child–Pugh scoring for patients with cirrhosis

	1 point	2 points	3 points
Total bilirubin, μmol.l^{-1}	<34	34–50	>50
Serum albumin, g.l^{-1}	>35	28–35	<28
INR	<1.7	1.71–2.30	> 2.30
Ascites	None	Mild	Moderate to severe
Hepatic encephalopathy	None	Grade I–II (or suppressed with medication)	Grade III–IV (or refractory)

Adapted from *British Journal of Surgery*, 60, Pugh et al., 'Transection of the oesophagus for bleeding oesophageal varices', pp.646–9. Copyright (1973) with permission from John Wiley and Sons.

Box 4.1 Model for end-stage liver disease (MELD) score (ln—natural logarithm)

MELD Score $= 10$ $((0.957\ ln(Creatinine/88.4)) + (0.378\ ln(Bilirubin/17.1)) + (1.12\ ln(INR)) + 6.43$

Adapted from *Hepatology*, 31, Malinchoc et al, 'A model to predict poor survival in patients undergoing transjugular intrahepatic portosystemic shunts', pp.864–71. Copyright (2000) with permission from John Wiley and Sons

3.2.3 General intensive care scoring systems in cirrhosis

- Chapter 12, Section 3 explores scoring systems in the intensive care.
- In patients who require support of one or more extra-hepatic organs, intensive care organ failure scoring systems are often used in preference to MELD.
- In critically ill patients with cirrhosis, SOFA has been shown to be better than APACHE II or other ICU systems in predicting intensive care unit survival.
- Recently a major initiative to define acute-on-chronic liver failure generated a chronic liver failure-specific modification of the SOFA score (CLIF-SOFA) from a mainly ward-based cohort of patients; it is postulated to have a still higher accuracy for patients with cirrhosis.
- The CLIF-SOFA accommodates INR instead of platelets as a coagulation score, raises the threshold for bilirubin to be graded as organ failure and uses grades of hepatic encephalopathy as opposed to GCS for neurological failure.
- In summary, prognostication in chronic liver disease patients who require admission to intensive care is difficult. Intensive care admission of the cirrhotic patient is not however universally futile and patients should not be denied admission on the basis of their liver disease alone. Early liaison with specialist hepatology and transplant centres is beneficial.

FURTHER READING

Arabi Y, Ahmed QA, Haddad S, et al. Outcome predictors of cirrhosis patients admitted to the intensive care unit. *European Journal of Gastroenterology and Hepatology* 2004; 16: 333–9.

Cholongitas E, Senzolo M, Patch D, et al. Risk factors, sequential organ failure assessment and model for end-stage liver disease scores for predicting short term mortality in cirrhotic patients admitted to intensive care unit. *Alimentary Pharmacology and Therapies* 2006; 23: 883–93.

Das V, Boelle PY, Galbois A, et al. Cirrhotic patients in the medical intensive care unit: early prognosis and long-term survival. *Critical Care Medicine* 2010; 38: 2108–16.

Kamath PS, Wiesner RH, Malinchoc M, et al. A model to predict survival in patients with end-stage liver disease. Hepatology 2001; 33: 464–70.

Kamath PS, Kim WR, Advanced Liver Disease Study G. The model for end-stage liver disease (MELD). *Hepatology* 2007; 45: 797–805.

Levesque E, Hoti E, Azoulay D, et al. Prospective evaluation of the prognostic scores for cirrhotic patients admitted to an intensive care unit. *Journal of Hepatology* 2012; 56: 95–102.

Malinchoc M, Kamath PS, Gordon FD, et al. A model to predict poor survival in patients undergoing transjugular intrahepatic portosystemic shunts. *Hepatology* 2000; 31: 864–71.

Pugh RN, Murray-Lyon IM, Dawson JL, et al. Transection of the oesophagus for bleeding oesophageal varices. *British Journal of Surgery* 1973; 60: 646–9.

3.3 Renal dysfunction

- Renal dysfunction is common in patients with cirrhosis.

3.3.1 Contributors to renal dysfunction in the cirrhotic population

- Hypovolaemia:
    - Loop diuretics and aldosterone antagonists are frequently used for control of ascites
    - Osmotic laxatives (e.g. lactulose) are used to manage encephalopathy
    - Blood loss from the GI tract
- Sepsis:
    - Spontaneous bacterial peritonitis
    - Higher incidence of extra-abdominal sepsis in the presence of cirrhosis
- Nephrotoxic agents:
    - Diuretics
- Hepatorenal syndrome (HRS):
    - Loss of renal function related to chronic hepatic failure (although has been described with severe acute alcoholic hepatitis)
    - Believed to be related to inappropriate splanchnic vasodilation and associated reduction in renal perfusion
    - Associated with poorly controlled ascites
    - The renal injury in HRS is rapid in onset (rapid rise in creatinine and onset of oligo-anuria)
    - Is associated with a high mortality
    - It occurs in two forms:
        - Type I—two-fold increase in serum creatinine (to a peak of greater than 221 $\mu mol.l^{-1}$) in less than 2 weeks.
        - Type II—hepatorenal syndrome, which does not fulfil the above criteria; often manifests as ascites refractory to diuretic therapy.
        - Type I is associated with the highest early (90-day) mortality.
    - Essentially a diagnosis of exclusion:
    - Diagnostic guidelines issued by the International Ascites Club (Box 4.2).

Box 4.2 International Ascites Club definition for hepatorenal syndrome

- Cirrhosis with ascites
- Serum creatinine >133 μmol.l^{-1}
- No improvement in serum creatinine after at least 2 days with diuretic withdrawal and volume expansion with albumin.
  - The recommended dose of albumin is 1 g.kg^{-1} of body weight per day up to a maximum of 100 g.day^{-1}
- Absence of shock
- No current or recent treatment with nephrotoxic drugs
- Absence of parenchymal kidney disease
  - As indicated by proteinuria 4,500 mg/day, microhaematuria and/or abnormal renal ultrasonography

3.3.2 Management

The approach to renal dysfunction in the general intensive care patient is discussed in Chapter 3, Section 1. In the cirrhotic population, in whom inappropriate splanchnic vasodilation may be the primary, or at least a contributing, cause, certain variations to practice exist.

3.3.2.1 Volume replacement—the role of albumin

- In contrast to the sepsis literature, human albumin solution is the primary colloid of choice in this group.
- Doses of 1 g.kg^{-1} as a loading dose, then 20–40 g.day^{-1} are required, although the evidence is based on comparison with hydroxyethyl starches.
- The theoretical beneficial functional aspects of albumin are its ability to bind nitric oxide and inflammatory cytokines.
- In cases where sepsis predominates, the diagnosis of hepatorenal syndrome is less likely and the benefit of HAS therefore less proven. In these cases crystalloid resuscitation should not be delayed.

3.3.2.2 Vasoconstriction—the role of terlipressin

- Terlipressin (a synthetic vasopressin analogue) is the vasoconstrictor of choice amongst hepatologists in cases of HRS.
- Terlipressin is primarily (but not exclusively) a splanchnic vasoconstrictor: renal perfusion and the effective blood volume are increased.
- Common side-effects are hypertension, bradycardia, and ischaemic complications in the heart, gut, and periphery.
- It should be avoided with concomitant use of high-dose noradrenaline.
- A typical starting dose is 1 mg IV bolus every 4–6 hours, although up to 12 mg can be used daily in refractory cases.
- Terlipressin—unlike other vasoactive agents—may be given in specialized liver units outwith the critical care area; this has logistical advantages.

- Approximately 50% of patients with HRS will respond to this treatment. The most appropriate management strategy for non-responders is debated:
  - For those already wait-listed for liver transplantation or who can be safely assessed as transplant candidates, then renal replacement therapy for standard indications may be used as a bridge to transplant.
  - In patients who have been declined or are not eligible for LT, then RRT can be considered but is not associated with long-term normalization of renal function.
  - Despite at least three randomized control trials regarding this matter, there are no liver support devices yet licensed for the treatment of HRS.

3.4 Ascites

3.4.1 Aetiology

- Ascites may be the consequence of:
  - Portal hypertension (e.g. cirrhosis, heart failure, Budd–Chiari syndrome)
  - Hypoalbuminaemia (e.g. malnutrition, nephrotic syndrome)
  - Peritoneal disease (e.g. ovarian cancer, mesothelioma, peritoneal infection)

3.4.2 Sequelae

- Consequences of ascites include:
  - Pressure effects:
    - May contribute to an abdominal compartment syndrome
    - Compromise of respiratory mechanics
  - Potential for spontaneous bacterial peritonitis
  - Hepatic hydrothorax
  - Contribute to hepatorenal syndrome
  - Discomfort

3.4.3 Management

3.4.3.1 Medical management

- Sodium restriction
- Diuretics:
  - Typically a combination of furosemide and spironolactone

3.4.3.2 Paracentesis

- The benefits and risks of paracentesis are outlined in Table 4.6.

Table 4.6 Benefits and risks of paracentesis

Benefits	Risks
• Reduction in intra-abdominal hypertension • Improved renal, splanchnic and hepatic blood flow • Improved lung compliance • Patient comfort	• Cutaneous or intra-abdominal infection • Haemodynamic collapse • Renal dysfunction from hypotension • Variceal haemorrhage from abdominal wall varices • Perforation of abdominal viscous

- Paracentesis may be classified into:
  - Total abdominal paracentesis (TAP):
    - Attempted removal of entirety of ascites in pre-defined time-frame
  - Limited abdominal paracentesis (LAP):
    - Removal of ascites to a predefined endpoint (e.g. intra-abdominal pressure of <20 mmHg).

A variety of drains are available; none are licensed for this use in the UK. Most utilize a catheter-over-needle approach (Box 4.3).

Box 4.3 Technique of drain insertion for paracentesis

- Verbal or written consent
- Assessment of bleeding risk from FBC and coagulation profile +/− functional assays
- Identification of insertion site by clinical examination or abdominal ultrasound (with Doppler US if abdominal wall varices suspected)
- Preparation of sterile pack
- Skin decontamination
- Infiltration of local anaesthesia
- Insertion of 21G needle into ascites and aspiration of 20 ml for diagnostic investigation—fluid protein, albumin, LDH, amylase, microscopy & culture, +/− cytology
- Superficial laceration (approximately 5 mm) to intended insertion site
- Insertion of catheter-over-needle until flange sits on skin
- Temporarily secure flange with adherent dressing
- Documentation and plan for drainage

- No drain should be left in for more than 6 hours for infection-prevention reasons.
- It is common practice to administer 100 ml of 20% Human Albumin Solution intravenously for every 1–2 litres of ascites drained, to avoid haemodynamic instability.
- In cases of spontaneous bacterial peritonitis, the risk of haemodynamic instability may be increased and paracentesis may be deferred until the sepsis and shock are under control.

3.5 Hepatic encephalopathy

3.5.1 Classification

- The International Society for Hepatic Encephalopathy and Nitrogen metabolism (ISHEN) guidelines divide hepatic encephalopathy (HE) into:
  - Type A—related to acute liver failure
  - Type B—related to porto-systemic bypass
  - Type C—related to cirrhosis
- Hepatic encephalopathy (HE) in patients with cirrhosis occurs for different reasons than in acute liver failure and without a significant risk of life-threatening intracranial hypertension.
- Circulating ammonia levels correlate less well with the severity of HE compared with patients with ALF, especially at low West Haven grades.

3.5.2 Precipitants

- Common precipitants for HE in patients with cirrhosis include:
  - Constipation
  - Sepsis

- Electrolyte disturbance
- Gastrointestinal haemorrhage
- Medication, including:
  - Benzodiazepines (commonly used to treat delirium tremens)
  - Propanolol (commonly used to control portal hypertension)

3.5.3 Management

- Ammonia-lowering strategies include:
  - Lactulose
  - Phosphate enemas
  - L-ornithine L-aspartate
  - Branch chain amino acids
  - Renal replacement therapy (RRT):
    - Capable of significant reduction in ammonia levels
    - Indicated in hyperammonaemia, even in absence of renal indications for RRT
- Gut decontamination strategies include:
  - Rifaximin
  - Patients with portosystemic bypass, such as TIPSS, may be particularly challenging; in such cases, if refractory to conventional management, the calibre of the TIPSS can be reduced or even occluded.

3.5.3.1 Nutrition and encephalopathy

- Enteral nutrition in patients with CLD and HE should be provided by standard formulary feed.
- Branched chain amino acid enriched solutions should only be used when HE is refractory to the above measures and is not recommended for all patients.
- Low-protein dietary intake does not prevent HE, precipitates sarcopaenia, and may delay liberation from the ventilator.
- All liver patients in intensive care require specialist input from dieticians and high-protein EN, if possible.

FURTHER READING

Nadim MK, Kellum JA, Davenport A, et al. Hepatorenal syndrome: the 8th International Consensus Conference of the Acute Dialysis Quality Initiative (ADQI) Group. *Critical Care* 2012; 16: R23.

---

4 Liver transplantation

4.1 General

4.1.1 Indications

- Acute liver failure
- Hepatocellular carcinoma
- Decompensated chronic liver disease
- Congenital and acquired biliary diseases
- Miscellaneous metabolic syndromes

4.2 Peri-transplant care

4.2.1 Phases of transplant procedure

- Resection phase
- Anhepatic phase
- Reperfusion phase

4.2.2 Factors to consider post-transplant on the ICU

- Indication for transplant
- Complications of liver failure pre-transplant.
- Extra-hepatic pre-transplant complications
- Nature of the graft
- Blood group of donor and recipient
- Blood loss
- CMV status of graft and recipient
- Organ support required following reperfusion

4.2.3 Monitoring

- Plasma lactate should be monitored; this would be expected to normalize over the first 6 hours post-operatively.
- Normalization of coagulation and return of gluconeogenesis (as evidenced by rising plasma glucose) are also indicators of hepatic function.

4.2.4 General

- In the absence of complications, early extubation and early enteral feed are advocated.
- A short course of intravenous antibiotics and enteral anti-fungal are common.

4.2.5 Immunosuppression

- Intravenous hydrocortisone/low-dose methylprednisolone is typically administered perioperatively.
- If gut function is intact, enteral immunosuppression is commenced early; options include:
    - Tacrolimus
    - Cyclosporin
    - Azathioprine
- High-dose methylprednisolone is typically reserved for those with evidence of inadequate immunosuppression.
- In patients with pre-existing or acquired renal dysfunction, nephrotoxic immunosuppressants (e.g. tacrolimus) are given in low dose with alternative immunosuppressants added (e.g. basilixumab).

4.3 Post-transplant complications

4.3.1 Primary non-function of the graft

- Defined as the failure of the graft to start normal hepatic enzymatic processes; it is indistinguishable from acute liver failure.
- Occurs in 1–2% of all liver transplants and more likely in patients transplanted for acute liver failure.
- Diagnosis is based on failure of transaminases to normalize and/or rebound severe transaminitis, hyperbilirubinaemia, and coagulopathy.
- Isolated rise in transaminases may be amenable to management with supportive management; however, if a fulminant picture develops, urgent relisting is the only available therapy.

4.3.2 Hepatic artery thrombosis

- Diagnosed on Doppler ultrasound from 24 hours post-transplant.
- Weak or absent Doppler signal is an indication for triple-phase CT of the liver where patency of the new vasculature can be assessed.
- Urgent revascularization may salvage the transplant however for most relisting is the only treatment option.

4.3.3 Venous thrombosis

- Thrombosis of the portal or hepatic vein complicates a small proportion of transplants.
- Anticoagulation and/or radiological stenting may offer a solution.

4.3.4 Biliary complications

- Include bile leak and obstruction to biliary flow.
- Rising bilirubin and alkaline phosphatase may indicate obstruction to biliary flow; investigation by cholangiography; endoscopic insertion of a stent or percutaneous insertion of t-tube can relieve obstruction.
- Biliary leak may arise from a defect in the biliary tree or from the cut edge of a 'split' graft (many high-quality donor organs are split between two recipients); this may result in biliary peritonitis; management includes peritoneal drain and interventions to repair the biliary system.

4.3.5 Sepsis

- Transplant recipients are often colonized with resistant organisms.
- Immunosuppression is required for the graft; intensive care interventions carry an inherent risk of infection.
- Liver transplant recipients are therefore at risk of sepsis.
- Careful observation for evidence of infection, strict infection control, and early use of appropriate antibiotics are important.

5 Gastrointestinal haemorrhage

5.1 Non-variceal upper GI haemorrhage

5.1.1 General

- Upper gastrointestinal (GI) haemorrhage is defined as that which occurs between the pharynx and ligament of Treitz.
- Non-variceal upper GI haemorrhage accounts for 80% of cases of bleeding admitted acutely to hospital or occurring during hospital stay for other reasons.
- Although the incidence of *Helicobacter pylori* infection in the general population is falling, the use of non-steroidal anti-inflammatory drugs remains high and bleeding from peptic ulcer disease is still a common reason for admission to hospital.
- Despite modern therapies, such as continuous proton pump inhibitor infusions and a variety of endotherapy options, mortality rates remain high at 10–20%.
- The presentation of bleeding is usually with melaena, 'coffee ground vomiting' and/or anaemia.
- Frank haematemesis is a poor prognostic sign and indicative of significant ongoing blood loss requiring prompt haemostasis via urgent upper GI endoscopy.
- Isolated tachycardia alone is worrisome, even without postural or overt hypotension, and requires discussion with endoscopy providers.
- 15% of patients with bright red PR blood loss have a source in the upper GI tract.

5.1.2 Pre-endoscopic management

- 'ABCDE' approach
- Early, 'aggressive' resuscitation is associated with a reduction in mortality
- Correction of coagulopathy (see Chapter 7, Section 4)
- Transfusion to maintain adequate but not normal haemoglobin concentrations:
  - A 'restrictive' transfusion target of 70 g.l^{-1} has been demonstrated to reduce mortality when compared with a target of 90 g.l^{-1}
- Risk stratification by Glasgow–Blatchford scale (Table 4.7) or Rockall score (Table 4.8)
- Proton pump inhibition:
  - Administered on the basis that increase in gastric pH reduces the risk of clot auto-digestion
  - Meta-analysis, however, demonstrates no reduction in mortality or re-bleed rate.

Table 4.7 Glasgow Blatchford Score

Admission risk marker	Score component value
Blood urea	
≥6·5 <8·0	2
≥8·0 <10·0	3
≥10·0 <25·0	4
≥25	6
Haemoglobin (g/l) for men	
≥12.0 <13.0	1
≥10.0 <12.0	3
<10.0	6
Haemoglobin (g/l) for women	
≥10.0 <12.0	1
<10.0	6
Systolic blood pressure (mmHg)	
100–109	1
90–99	2
<90	3
Other markers	
Pulse ≥100 (per min)	1
Presentation with melaena	1
Presentation with syncope	2
Hepatic disease	2
Cardiac failure	2

In a validation cohort patients with a score of 0 could be treated as an outpatient and of those with a score of >6, 50% needed an intervention.

Adapted from *The Lancet*, 356, Blatchford O et al., 'A risk score to predict need for treatment for upper-gastrointestinal haemorrhage', pp.1318–21. Copyright (2000) with permission from Elsevier.

Table 4.8 Rockall score (upper GI endoscopy is required to complete the score)

Variable	Score 0	Score 1	Score 2	Score 3
Age	<60	60–79	>80	
Shock	No shock	Pulse >100 BP >100 Systolic	Systolic BP<100	
Co-morbidity	Nil major		CHF, IHD, major morbidity	Renal failure, liver failure, metastatic cancer
Diagnosis	Mallory-Weiss tear	All other diagnoses	GI malignancy	
Evidence of bleeding	None		Blood, adherent clot, spurting vessel	

Adapted from *Gut*, 38, Rockall TA et al., 'Risk assessment after acute upper gastrointestinal haemorrhage', pp. 316–321. Copyright (1996) with permission from BMJ Publishing Group Ltd.

- These scores are of most benefit during assessment in the emergency department to assess timing of endoscopy and are not validated in the ICU population.
- The post-endoscopy Rockall score has the most predictive accuracy.

5.1.3 Gastroscopy and non-variceal upper GI haemorrhage

- Complete gastroscopy must include intubation to D2 and retroflexion in the fundus.
- This provides diagnosis in the majority of cases of suspected upper GI haemorrhage
- The most common pathological finding in the non-ICU patient is peptic ulceration. Alternative, non-variceal causes include:
  - Nasogastric tube trauma
  - Erosive tumours
  - Vascular ectasia
  - Angiodysplasia
  - Mallory–Weiss tear
  - Dieulafoy lesions (mucosal vascular lesions)
- Risk stratification:
  - Based upon the presence of 'major-stigmata' of recent haemorrhage
  - Assists in choice of therapy
  - Allows analysis of risk of rebleeding that can prompt admission to higher acuity areas of the hospital, a decision for early repeat endoscopy, or pre-emptive plans for non-endoscopic management of major re-bleed (interventional radiology or surgery).
- Endotherapy:
  - Small well-covered ulcers with no signs of recent bleeding do not require endotherapy, as the risk of complications of endotherapy outweighs the benefits.
  - Major stigmata of haemorrhage requiring endotherapy:
    - Deep ulcers with visible or spurting vessels
    - Adherent clot
    - Blood in the lumen

5.1.4 Endotherapy options

- Three main options are available to the endoscopist—two of the three should be deployed to minimize chance of rebleed:
    - *Submucosal injection of adrenaline* 1:10,000 via a retractable needle passed through the biopsy channel of the endoscope; 10–15 ml provides reduced re-bleed rates compared to lower amounts.
    - Bipolar diathermy via dedicated diathermy lines.
    - Aluminium clips—tendency to fall off within days or hours; more than one clip is required to reduce risk of rebleeding.
- Several emerging new modalities, such as Doppler endoscopic ultrasound to assess underlying vessels depth from the submucosa and risk of bleeding and haemostatic spray, are not yet part of standard practice but may be encountered in specialist centres.
- Following endoscopy a clear escalation plan should be documented and handed over to the treating team; this may include interventional radiology or surgical techniques.

FURTHER READING

Baradarian R, Ramdhaney S, Chapalamadugu R, et al. Early intensive resuscitation of patients with upper gastrointestinal bleeding decreases mortality. *American Journal of Gastroenterology* 2004; 99: 619–22.

Blatchford O, Murray WR, Blatchford M. A risk score to predict need for treatment for upper-gastrointestinal haemorrhage. *Lancet* 2000; 356: 1318–21.

Rockall TA, Logan RF, Devlin HB, et al. Risk assessment after acute upper gastrointestinal haemorrhage. *Gut* 1996; 38: 316–21.

Sreedharan A, Martin J, Leontiadis GI, et al. Proton pump inhibitor treatment initiated prior to endoscopic diagnosis in upper gastrointestinal bleeding. *The Cochrane Library* 2010; (7): CD005415.

Villanueva C, Colomo A, Bosch A, et al. Transfusion strategies for acute upper gastrointestinal bleeding. *New England Journal of Medicine* 2013; 368: 11–21.

5.2 Stress ulceration

5.2.1 General

- Stress ulceration represents a special case of non-variceal upper gastrointestinal haemorrhage.
- First described in the 1970s by Lucas, then Skilmen and Sulen.
- May be defined as superficial ulceration of the gastric mucosa in patients undergoing invasive ventilation for sepsis, resulting in overt gastrointestinal blood loss.
- Pre-gastric protection-era reports suggested an incidence of stress ulceration as high as 25% of ventilated patients; modern studies show only 1% to 4% of such patients have clinically important stress ulceration.

5.2.2 Pathophysiological mechanism

- Believed to be related to reduced splanchnic blood flow and loss of mucosal protective measures.
- Unlike peptic ulceration, stress ulceration is more likely to occur in the gastric fundus and be associated with diffuse mucosal oozing.
- Deeper ulceration leading to overt haemorrhage can occur.

- The following factors are associated with an increased risk of stress ulceration:
  - Mechanical ventilation for more than 48 hours (15.6x risk)
  - Coagulopathy (either thrombocytopaenia or INR/APTTr >1.5) (4.3x risk)
  - Multiple organ failure
  - History of GI bleeding
  - Major trauma or severe burns
  - Steroids
  - Renal failure

5.2.3 Stress ulcer prophylaxis

- Establishing enteral feeding is protective and has the added, theoretical benefits of improving splanchnic blood flow and stimulating gut associated lymphoid tissue.
- In patients at low risk of stress ulceration, established enteral feeding is generally accepted to offer sufficient protection and no further prophylaxis required; in those with multiple risk factors, there is a need for pharmacological prophylaxis.
- Pharmacological options include:
  - Proton pump inhibitors (PPI)—acid suppression
  - H_2 receptor antagonists (H_2RA)—acid suppression
  - Sucralfate—mucosal protection
- Meta-analysis of over 1,700 patients in trials comparing PPI and H_2RA has demonstrated superiority of PPI for reducing overt or clinically important GI haemorrhage with no difference in rates of pneumonia during ventilation.
- Sucralfate is not as effective as PPI and H_2RA and should be regarded as a second-line measure when PPI are only partially effective.
- No ICU stay or mortality benefit associated with the use of PPI or H_2RA.
- Potential adverse effects of pharmacological prophylaxis:
  - Drug interaction:
    - Sucralfate inhibits absorption of digoxin, warfarin, phenytoin, fluoroquinolones
    - Modern H_2RA agents have minimal interaction
    - PPI may interact with anti-platelet agents
  - Pneumonia:
    - It is postulated that acid suppression increases the risk of nosocomial pneumonia, presumably due to increased bacterial colonization of the stomach and duodenum with increased gastric pH. The results of studies attempting to demonstrate this association have however been conflicting.
  - Clostridium difficile:
    - There is an epidemiological association between acid suppression and Clostridium difficile. The significance in the critically ill population is unclear.

FURTHER READING

Alhazzani W, Alenezi F, Jaeschke RZ, et al. Proton pump inhibitors versus histamine 2 receptor antagonists for stress ulcer prophylaxis in critically ill patients: a systematic review and meta-analysis. Critical Care Medicine 2013; 41: 693–705.

Cook DJ, Fuller HD, Guyatt GH, et al. Risk factors for gastrointestinal bleeding in critically ill patients. New England Journal of Medicine 1994; 330: 377–81.

5.3 Variceal haemorrhage

5.3.1 General

- Variceal haemorrhage (VH) is associated with portal hypertension, usually as a consequence of cirrhosis.
- VH should be managed on the ICU if haemostasis is not confirmed or in the presence of concomitant organ failure.
- The main reason for varices forming and rupturing is sudden worsening of chronic portal hypertension.
- Portal pressures are normally lower than 5 mmHg in the non-cirrhotic splanchnic circulation.
- Portal pressures above 5 mmHg represent portal hypertension; varices and variceal haemorrhage occur with portal pressures greater than 10mmHg.
- Varices can form at any part of the GI tract but are more common in the:
  - Oesophagus
    - Most common
    - Occur secondary to retrograde filling of splenic or long gastric vein
    - Generate columns of varices where blood flows from the distal oesophagus and gastro-oesophageal junction proximally
    - Endoscopically graded as 1, 2 or 3 (Table 4.9)
  - Gastric fundus
  - Rectum
  - Bare area of the liver
  - Retroperitoneum
  - Abdominal wall

Table 4.9 Grading of oesophageal varices by endoscopic appearance—the risk of bleeding increases with grade and correlates with portal pressures

Grade of oesophageal varices	Endoscopic appearance
1	Small, well epithelialized, disappear on insufflation of the oesophagus
2	Between grade 1 and 3
3	Large varices which occlude the lumen

Adapted from *Gut*, 46, Jalan R and Hayes P, 'UK guidelines on the management of variceal haemorrhage in cirrhotic patients. Copyright (2000) with permission from BMJ Publishing Group Ltd.

- The approach to variceal bleeding differs from other forms of upper GI bleed, as outlined in Table 4.10.

5.3.2 Medical management of variceal bleeding

- Antibiotics
  - Secondary infection (urinary, respiratory or spontaneous bacterial peritonitis) is common in cirrhotic patients presenting with haemorrhage; it is associated with an increase in mortality.
  - Prophylactic antibiotics have been demonstrated to reduce mortality, length of hospital stay, and rebleeding rate.

- ■ Choice of antibiotic should be guided by local policy; ciprofloxacin and ceftriaxone are commonly employed agents.
- Vasoactive medications
  - ■ Pharmacological reduction in portal blood flow may be achieved with vasopressin or somatostatin analogues; this is associated with a reduction in rebleeding rate and mortality.
  - ■ The vasopressin analogue terlipressin constricts mesenteric arterioles thus reducing blood flow and pressure in the portal system; it has a stronger evidence-base than other vasoactive agents.
  - ■ Terlipressin may be administered as intermittent injections of 0.5–2 mg 4-hourly.

5.3.3 Sengstaken–Blakemore tube

- Temporary haemostasis can be achieved using the Sengstaken–Blakemore tube (SBT).
- Consists of:
  - ■ Essentially two modified Foley catheters joined along their length
  - ■ Two balloons, which can take up to 500 ml of fluid/air
    - ▪ One gastric balloon
    - ▪ One oesophageal balloon
  - ■ Two suction ports
- Typically the gastric balloon alone is inflated: oesophageal varices fill from distal oesophagus/gastro-oesophageal junction upwards, therefore gastric balloon inflation and SBT traction is normally sufficient; inflation of the oesophageal balloon inflation is associated with a high risk of necrosis and perforation.
- Insertion is described in Box 4.4.

Box 4.4 Insertion of Sengstaken–Blakemore tube

- Airway protection by endotracheal intubation and invasive ventilation preferred
- Intubate the oesophagus per oral and pass the tip of the tube to the stomach
- 250 m of air/water/contrast is used to inflate the *gastric* balloon (contrast allows confirmation of placement on chest radiograph but do not delay insertion waiting for contrast)
- The entire catheter should be pulled back until engaged at the gastroesophageal junction
- Secure against the face with strong tape
- Urgent arrangements for definitive haemostasis must then be made
- Do not leave the SBT *in situ* for >12 hours to prevent oesophageal necrosis

- A plan for removal of the SBT and expertise to manage problems pending definitive haemostasis are required for successful continued haemostasis.
- Nevertheless in cases of refractory VH, where endoscopy is not available or has failed, use of the SBT can be life-saving.

5.3.4 Endoscopic management of varices

- Grade 1 varices require no therapy.
- Grade 2 and 3 are at higher risk of spontaneous haemorrhage and the patient should have portal pressure reduction by non-selective beta blockade +/− endoscopic band ligation.
- Endoscopic band ligation(EBL) is the preferred form of endoscopic variceal eradication, both electively and in the case of acute VH.

- Placement of bands from a dedicated cap placed at the end of the gastroscope starting at the gastro-oesophageal junction immediately reduces pressure proximally and a single banding session commonly achieves haemostasis in acute VH.
- As bands spontaneously detach, varices can reform, so further endoscopic surveillance over the following days to weeks is necessary.
- Increased risk of rebleed is associated with:
  - High Child–Pugh grade
  - Increasing portal pressure
  - High risk features at endoscopy
- Rebleeding can be treated with further endoscopy and EBL.

5.3.5 Transjugular intrahepatic porto-systemic shunt (TIPSS)

- Refractory variceal haemorrhage is one of the main indications for TIPSS; other indications include:
  - Refractory or recurrent ascites
  - Hepatorenal syndrome
  - Hepatopulmonary syndrome
  - Hepatic hydrothorax
- Recent evidence supports the earlier use of TIPSS in patients with rebleed or high risk of re-bleed following the index admission.
- Work up for TIPSS includes:
  - Doppler study of portal vein and biliary system (as portal vein patency is (mostly) required; biliary obstruction must be relieved prior to TIPSS)
  - Echocardiogram (to assess right heart function; TIPSS leads to significant rise in right ventricular preload; severe tricuspid regurgitation, severe pulmonary hypertension, and congestive cardiac failure are absolute contra-indications)
  - EEG (as TIPSS can provoke HE)—in practice in the high-risk bleeding patient the risk of HE is accepted and EEG not performed.
- TIPSS services are centralized to centres with liver transplant experience or high-volume interventional radiology.
- The TIPSS procedure involves:
  - Venous access is obtained (usually via the right internal jugular vein) and a catheter advanced down the vena cava into the hepatic vein.
  - The portal vein is identified and a needle directed from the hepatic vein to the portal vein.
  - A guidewire is passed through the needle, balloon dilation of the tract undertaken, and finally a stent deployed.
  - Portal venography and pressure measurements may be undertaken and the calibre of the stent altered if decompression is insufficient.
- Complications of TIPSS include:
  - Access-related:
    - Liver capsule puncture with potential for intraperitoneal haemorrhage
    - Biliary puncture and fistula formation
    - Hepatic infarction
  - Stent-related:
    - Stent thrombosis
    - Stent migration
  - Shunt-related:
    - Hepatic encephalopathy

Table 4.10 Differences in management of variceal and non-variceal upper GI haemorrhage

	Non-variceal haemorrhage	Variceal haemorrhage
Pre-endoscopic management	Intravenous proton pump inhibitor	Terlipressin
		Broad spectrum IV antibiotics
Endoscopic management	Sub-mucosal injection of adrenaline 1:10,000	Endoscopic band ligation
	Bipolar diathermy	Sclerotherapy
	Endo-clip mechanical haemostasis	
Rescue haemostasis	Repeat endoscopy	Repeat endoscopy
	Mesenteric angiography & embolization	Sengstaken–Blakemore tube insertion
	Surgery	Dani stent
		TIPSS
		Liver transplantation

5.4 Small or large bowel gastrointestinal haemorrhage

5.4.1 General

- The majority of cases of bleeding presenting as an emergency are proximal to the ligament of Trietze and defined as upper GI tract bleeds.
- If gastroscopy does not demonstrate the site of bleeding, then the patient should be investigated for lower GI bleeding distal to this landmark.
- Potential causes of small or large bowel bleeding include:
  - Ulcers
  - Polyps
  - Tumours
  - Colitis/enteritis
  - Ulcerative colitis/Crohn's disease
  - Haemorrhoids
  - Aortoenteric fistulae
  - Angiodysplasia

5.4.2 Investigation

- Potential investigations for lower GI bleeding are:
  - Flexible sigmoidoscopy
  - Colonoscopy
  - Capsule endoscopy
  - Push or balloon enteroscopy
  - CT angiogram abdomen/pelvis
  - Mesenteric angiography
- While endoscopic examination of the lower GI tract provides the opportunity to provide therapy, the view during acute bleeding is often obscured.
- Determination of a bleeding point by CT angiogram is often preferable to guide endoscopic, radiological, or surgical intervention.

5.4.3 Management

- Interventional methods to treat lower GI bleeding include:
  - Endotherapy—adrenaline injection, bipolar coagulation, endoclips
  - Interventional radiological embolization and coil placement
  - Surgical resection—limited resection or colectomy

FURTHER READING

Jalan R, Hayes P. UK guidelines on the management of variceal haemorrhage in cirrhotic patients. *Gut* 2000; 46: iii1.

Patidar KR, Sydnor M, Sanyal AJ. Transjugular intrahepatic portosystemic shunt. *Clinics in Liver Disease* 2014; 18: 853–76.

---

6 Diarrhoea

6.1 General and mechanisms

- The World Health Organization defines diarrhoea as three or more loose or watery stools per day.
- Diarrhoea occurs as a consequence of an imbalance in water or solute transport.
- Diarrhoea may occur secondary to a number of mechanisms.

6.1.1 Osmotic diarrhoea

- Failure of the gut to absorb osmotically active solutes:
  - Magnesium
  - Bile salts
  - Osmotic laxatives (e.g. lactulose)
  - Malabsorption (chronic pancreatitis, coeliac disease)
- Typically moderate in volume
- Stops with starvation

6.1.2 Secretory diarrhoea

- Occurs due to either increase in secretion from bowel mucosa or decrease in absorption of luminal contents.
- Mechanism underlying some infective diarrhoea (e.g. cholera, which stimulates the secretion of chloride ions into the lumen).
- Typically large in volume (>1,000ml/24-hour period).
- Does not improve with starvation.

6.1.3 Inflammatory diarrhoea

- Inflammatory process leads to loss of mucosal integrity.
- Often bloody in nature.
- May be the consequence of an autoimmune inflammatory bowel disease (e.g. Crohn's disease or ulcerative colitis) or infection (e.g. *E. coli*, *Shigella*, *Salmonella*).

6.2 Infective diarrhoea

6.2.1 Clostridium difficile

- The most common infective cause of diarrhoea in intensive care units in Europe, Australasia, and North America.
- *C. difficile*:
  - A Gram-positive bacterium
  - Many carriers in the community: present in the intestinal flora of 3% of the population but 20% of patients receiving antibiotics
  - Infection manifests profuse watery diarrhoea and abdominal pain; associated fever is suggestive of severe infection
  - Risk factors for infection:
    - Antibiotics, in particular:
      - Penicillins
      - Cephalosporins
      - Clindamycin
      - Fluroquinolones
    - Long-standing inflammatory bowel disease
    - Recent intestinal surgery
    - Proton pump inhibitor use
- Diagnosis:
  - Polymerase chain reaction (PCR) positivity for *C. difficile* represents colonization (carriers).
  - Presence of *C. difficile* toxin(CDT) in stool indicates active infection.
  - Colonoscopy may demonstrate pseudomembranes (pseudomembranous colitis).
- Complications of C. difficile colitis:
  - Fulminant colitis:
    - Represents around 3% of cases and associated with a mortality between 30% and 80%
    - Severe abdominal pain
    - Hypovolaemia
    - Lactic acidosis
    - Fever
    - Markedly elevated white cell count
  - Toxic megacolon
    - Fulminant colitis, as described above, with radiological evidence of severe colonic dilation (>7 cm)
  - Bowel perforation
- Treatment:
  - Metronidazole (oral or intravenous)
  - Vancomycin (enteral route only as it does not cross from blood to gut)
  - Fidaxomicin:
    - New class of macrolide antibiotic licensed for treatment of *C. difficile* infection
    - Demonstrated to be non-inferior to oral vancomycin with similar side effect profile
    - May be associated with lower rate of recurrence and is some centres is now first line for severe infection
  - Faecal transplant may be considered for resistant cases
  - Surgical
    - Severe cases of *C. difficile* infection may require emergency colectomy

6.2.2 Other infective causes of diarrhoea

- First-line anti-microbial agent shown in parenthesis.
- Bacterial
  - Inflammatory:
    - *Escherichia coli* (generally avoid)
    - *Shigella* (ciprofloxacin, ceftriaxone)
    - *Campylobacter* (ciprofloxacin)
    - *Salmonella* (ciprofloxacin)
  - Secretory:
    - *Cholera* (doxycycline, ciprofloxacin).
- Viral
  - Norovirus (N/A)
  - Rotavirus (N/A)
  - Adenovirus (N/A)
  - Cytomegalovirus (ganciclovir)
- Parasitic
- *Giardia* (metronidazole)
- *Entamoeba* (metronidazole)
- *Cryptosporidium* (nitazoxanide)

6.2.3 Management of infective diarrhoea

- Supportive therapy (in particular fluid management)
- Appropriate antimicrobial therapy
- Investigation including HIV testing (infective diarrhoea may be the initial presentation of HIV disease)
- Liaison with relevant public health authorities

6.3 Non-infective diarrhoea

6.3.1 Drugs

- Antibiotics
  - Decrease intestinal bacterial load, thereby increasing luminal carbohydrate concentration resulting in an osmotic diarrhoea.
- Laxatives
- Magnesium-containing agents

6.3.2 Enteral feed

- High osmotic content of enteral feed is a common cause of diarrhoea in the intensive care unit.
- Continuous feed is associated with lower rates of diarrhoea than intermittent feed.
- No apparent difference between nasogastric and nasojejunal feeding.
- Changing feed to soluble fibre containing or small peptide suspensions, or decreasing the rate of feed may be beneficial.

6.3.3 Other non-infective causes

- Inflammatory bowel disease (ulcerative colitis/Crohn's disease)
- Ischaemic colitis
- Malabsorption (coeliac disease, pancreatitis, pancreatic insufficiency, post-operative)

7 Acute pancreatitis

7.1 General
7.1.1 Background
- Acute pancreatitis (AP) is an acute inflammatory process affecting the pancreas.
- The cardinal symptom is severe epigastric pain.
- The incidence is estimated to be between 320 and 440 per million of population.
- There is a wide range of severity, with between 10% and 20% categorized as severe.

7.1.2 Aetiology
- Common causes of AP:
  - Gallstones
  - Alcohol
  - Post-endoscopic retrograde cholangiopancreatography (ERCP) and sphincterotomy
  - Trauma
  - Pharmacological (5-ASAs, azathioprine/mercaptopurine, diuretics, steroids)
  - Metabolic (hyperlipidaemia, hypercalcaemia)
  - Infections (*cytomegalovirus*, mumps, ascaris, *mycoplasma pneumoniae*)

7.2 Diagnosis and investigation
7.2.1 Criteria
- Based upon two of three of:
  - Abdominal pain
  - Serum amylase or lipase >3 times the upper range of normal
  - Characteristic CT findings

7.2.2 Imaging
- Abdominal ultrasound is the preferred early modality: may provide ultrasonographic evidence of pancreatitis and identify gallstones.
- Early CT (within the first few days) of the abdomen is not recommended, as may under-estimate severity; CT should be performed if no improvement in first 72 hours.
- The primary radiological findings in AP are interstitial oedema of the pancreatic parenchyma in 85% of cases; necrosis (defined radiologically as absence of intravenous contrast) is seen in around 15%.

7.3 Risk stratification and prognostication
7.3.1 Atlanta criteria
- The Atlanta criteria categorize AP as:
  - Mild—no organ failure or local/systemic complication
  - Moderate—transient (<48 hours) of organ failure or local/systemic complication
  - Severe—persistent organ failure or complication (>48 hours)

7.3.2 Determinant-based classification of acute pancreatitis severity
- Concerns regarding the subjectivity and over-simplicity of the Atlanta criteria led to the development of a determinant-based classification system by consensus of experts.
- Severity is based upon a number of 'determinants'; these determinants are divided into 'local' and 'systemic':

- Local determinants:
  - Relates to the severity of necrosis in the pancreas or peri-pancreatic tissue.
  - The identification of necrosis and assessment of severity are based upon CT imaging and, if appropriate, fine needle aspiration to assess for the presence of infection.
- Systemic determinants:
  - Based upon the presence and persistence of organ failure.
  - Organ failure is defined as a SOFA score of 2 or more (see Chapter 12, Section 3.2).
  - Transient organ failure is defined as a SOFA score of 2 or more for less than 48 hours; persistent organ failure is defined as greater than 48 hours.
- Definitions:
  - *Mild acute pancreatitis*: characterized by the absence of both pancreatic necrosis and organ failure.
  - *Moderate acute pancreatitis*: characterized by the presence of sterile pancreatic necrosis and/or transient organ failure.
  - *Severe acute pancreatitis*: characterized by the presence of either infected pancreatic necrosis or persistent organ failure.
  - *Critical acute pancreatitis*: characterized by the presence of infected pancreatic necrosis and persistent organ failure.
- The persistence of organ failure appears to be the most important single determinant of outcome.

7.3.3 Ranson score

- The Ranson score provides risk stratification and prediction of mortality.
- Half of the criteria are scored based on admission; the remainder scored at 24 hours.
- The Ranson score is outlined in Table 4.11.
- A Ranson score of greater than 3 is considered to represent severe pancreatitis; associated mortality is outlined in Table 4.12.
- The Ranson score was developed for alcohol induced pancreatitis; variations for other aetiology are available.

Table 4.11 The Ranson score—one point is allocated for each positive criterion

Scored on admission	Scored at 24 hours
Age >55 years	Fall in haematocrit >10%
AST >250 IU.l^{-1}	P_aO_2 <8 kPa
Glucose >11.2 mmol.l^{-1}	Base deficit >4 mEq.l^{-1}
White cell count > 16,000 cells.mm^{-3}	Fluid sequestration >6 litres
LDH >350 IU.l^{-1}	Rise in urea >1.8 mmol.l^{-1}

Adapted from *Journal of the American College of Surgeons*, 139, 1974, Ranson JH et al., 'Prognostic signs and the role of operative management in acute pancreatitis', pp. 69-81. Reprinted with permission from the *Journal of the American College of Surgeons*, formerly Surgery, Gynecology & Obstetrics.

Table 4.12 Ranson score and mortality

Score	Predicted mortality
0–2	2%
3–4	15%
5–6	40%
7–8	100%

Local complications include acute necrosis, walled off necrosis, pancreatic pseudocyst, and acute pancreatic fluid collection.

7.3.4 Alternative scoring systems

- The Glasgow–Imrie score
  - An alternative prognostic score for both alcohol-induced and gallstone pancreatitis
  - Eight criteria (oxygenation, age, white cell count, calcium, urea, LDH, albumin, and glucose), which are assessed at the time of admission
  - A score of 3 or more should prompt admission to a critical care area
- APACHE score (see Chapter 12, Section 3.2)
  - General severity score for critical illness
  - Has been demonstrated to be a robust predictor of outcome in AP

7.4 Complications of pancreatitis

7.4.1 Local

- Necrosis (see Section 7.6)
- Pseudocyst:
  - Encapsulated bodies of fluid within the pancreas
  - Typically occur late (>4 weeks)
- Peri-pancreatic collection:
  - Develop early and usually resolve spontaneously
- Mesenteric vein thrombosis
- Pseudoaneurysm

7.4.2 Systemic

- Defined in the Atlanta criteria as an exacerbation of pre-existing disease, e.g. coronary artery disease.

7.4.3 Organ failure

- Pancreatitis may provoke a systemic inflammatory response, which can result in failure of distant organ systems.
- Organ failure commonly associated with AP include:
  - ARDS, pleural effusions, atelectasis
  - Shock
  - AKI
  - Ileus, metabolic derangement, abdominal compartment syndrome
- These should be managed with standard supportive therapy.

7.5 Management

7.5.1 General management of acute severe pancreatitis

- Admission to critical care unit if Ranson score >3 or other organ failure.

- Supportive management:
  - Fluid replacement
    - The type, volume, and rate of fluid replacement are a matter of debate (see editorial by Wu 2011)
  - Adequate analgesia
  - Organ support, as required

7.5.2 Nutrition

- Historically, gut rest was prescribed in acute pancreatitis as a means of reducing pancreatic excrine activity and ameliorating the clinical course of AP; this is no longer practiced.
- Patients with mild AP can continue to eat and drink as tolerated.
- For patients with severe AP, enteral nutrition via the nasogastric route is safe and generally well tolerated.
- Nasojejunal feeding is reserved for those who do not tolerate the nasogastric route and parenteral nutrition reserved for those who fail the enteral route entirely.
- PYTHON is a randomized controlled trial which is currently recruiting and seeks to determine whether very early or delayed nutrition is most appropriate in AP.
- Present guidance is that early (<48 hours) enteral nutrition is preferred.

7.5.3 Antibiotics

- The routine use of prophylactic antibiotics is not recommended.
- Antibiotics should be reserved for cases of infected necrosis, ideally confirmed by positive microbiological sample via fine-needle aspiration of the necrosis.
- Probiotics have no role in the treatment of acute pancreatitis; the results of the placebo controlled PROPATRIA trial demonstrated increased rates of bowel ischaemia and mortality in the probiotic arm.

7.5.4 Endoscopic retrograde cholangiopancreatography (ERCP)

- Specific questions often arise around the role of early ERCP in gallstone pancreatitis.
- Gallstone pancreatitis is suggested by:
  - Presence of gallstones on abdominal ultrasound
  - ALT >150 IU.l^{-1}
  - Confirmation on gold standard modalities of magnetic retrograde cholangiopancreatography (MRCP) or endoscopic ultrasound (EUS) (although these modalities are often unsuitable for the critically ill)
- Urgent ERCP is considered in the following cases of acute pancreatitis:
  - In the presence of cholangitis (strong indication)
  - Cholestasis
  - Predicted severe gallstone pancreatitis (in some centres)
- For predicted mild pancreatitis, ERCP is not required, as the risk of inducing pancreatitis with sphincterotomy outweighs the benefits of pancreatic/biliary duct decompression.

7.6 Necrotic pancreatitis

- Necrosis of the pancreas is due to severe AP can be sterile or infected.
- Infected necrosis is defined by:
  - Positive bacterial/fungal microscopy/culture on fine needle aspiration
  - Presence of gas in the pancreatic bed on imaging

- The treatment of infected necrosis involves:
  - Intravenous broad-spectrum antibiotics (typically a carbapenem)
  - Delayed intervention (4 weeks) to allow collections to become walled off
  - Percutaneous or endoscopic drainage as the preferred route
  - Minimally invasive surgical necrosectomy if no other feasible options
- At present the 'Transluminal endoscopic step-up approach versus minimally invasive surgical step-up approach in patients with infected pancreatic necrosis' (TENSION) study is recruiting to guide the best approach to dealing with infected necrosis.

FURTHER READING

Dellinger EP, Forsmark CE, Layer P, et al. Determinant-based classification of acute pancreatitis severity: an international multidisciplinary consultation. *Annals of Surgery* 2012; 256: 875–80.

Ranson JH, Rifkind KM, Roses DF, et al. Prognostic signs and the role of operative management in acute pancreatitis. *Surgery Gynecology and Obstetrics* 1974; 139: 69–81.

Schepers NJ, Besselink MG, van Santvoort HC, et al. Early management of acute pancreatitis. *Best Practice and Research in Clinical Gastroenterology* 2013; 27: 727–43.

Tenner S, Baillie J, DeWitt J, et al. American College of Gastroenterology guideline: management of acute pancreatitis. *The American Journal of Gastroenterology* 2013; 108: 1400–15.

Wu BU. Editorial: fluid resuscitation in acute pancreatitis: striking the right balance. *The American Journal of Gastroenterology* 2011; 106: 1851–2.

8 Abdominal compartment syndrome

8.1 Definitions

8.1.1 Definition

- Normal intra-abdominal pressure (IAP) is 5–7 mmHg.
- As the volume of intra-abdominal contents increases, the abdominal wall will expand to a point, but when the extent of elasticity is reached, further increase in volume will generate an increase in intra-abdominal pressure.
- Intra-abdominal pressure may be measured:
  - Directly—laparoscopy
  - Indirectly—by means of a balloon tipped catheter in either the stomach or the bladder
- Abdominal perfusion pressure (APP) is defined as

$$\text{Mean Arterial Pressure} - \text{Intraabdominal pressure}$$

8.1.2 Intra-abdominal hypertension

- Intra-abdominal hypertension (IAH) is graded as:
  - Grade I—12–15 mmHg
  - Grade II—16–20 mmHg
  - Grade III—21–25 mmHg
  - Grade IV—>25 mmHg

8.1.3 Abdominal compartment syndrome

- Abdominal compartment syndrome (ACS) is defined as IAP >20 mmHg (or APP <50 mmHg) with associated organ failure.

8.2 Aetiology and consequences

8.2.1 Aetiology

- The causes of raised IAP are outlined in Table 4.13. Multiple factors may contribute.

Table 4.13 Aetiology of intra-abdominal hypertension

Surgical	Intra-abdominal haemorrhage
	Reduction of large hernia
	Closure of abdominal wound under excess tension
	Ileus
	Prolonged pneumoperitoneum
Medical	Peritoneal dialysis
	Ascites
	Intra-abdominal infection
	Pancreatitis
	Generalized intestinal oedema
Post-traumatic	Haemorrhage
	Fluid resuscitation
Burns	Restriction of abdominal wall
	Fluid resuscitation

8.2.2 Consequences

- The consequences of raised IAP are outlined in Table 4.14.

Table 4.14 Consequences of intra-abdominal hypertension

Respiratory	Diaphragmatic splinting reduces compliance, increased risk of atelectasis, decrease in functional residual capacity, results in hypoxaemia and propensity to infection.
Cardiovascular	Reduced venous return may reduce stroke volume and cardiac output.
Renal	Renal perfusion is reduced at IAP >15 mmHg; anuria is typical at IAP >30 mmHg.
Gastrointestinal	Hepatic and splanchnic blood flow is impaired, liver dysfunction ensues, gut function is further impaired with potential loss of mucosal barrier.
Nervous system	Increase in IAP may lead to rise in intracranial pressure.

8.3 Management

- The 2013 World Society of Abdominal Compartment Syndrome made a series of recommendations on the identification and management of IAH and ACS:
  - There is no routine clinical examination finding that accurately replaces the need for measuring IAP.
  - The simple, cheap, and reproducible transurethral route is preferred.
  - In patients at risk of IAH (Table 4.13), measurements should be made every 4 hours until the risk is deemed low.
  - In patients with IAP short of ACS (12–20 mmHg), the preferred treatment is medical.
- Optimization of blood pressure and abdominal perfusion pressure.

- Medical methods to reduce intra-abdominal pressure include:
  - Total body water removal and negative fluid balance (diuretics or renal replacement therapy)
  - Gastric aspiration
  - Prokinetic agents
  - Laxatives
  - Reduction in abdominal wall tone:
    - Analgesia
    - Sedation
    - Neuromuscular blockade
- When IAP exceeds 20 mmHg with organ failure, then medical methods and measurement should be intensified.
- If these are unsuccessful or the IAP increases to >30 mmHg, then surgical decompression may be necessary (laparostomy).
- Surgical decompression of ACS will inevitably lead to the patient being left with an open abdomen.
- This presents considerable technical and physiological challenges, as well as psychological stress on aware patients.

FURTHER READING

Bjorck M, Wanhainen A. Management of abdominal compartment syndrome and the open abdomen. *European Journal of Vascular and Endovascular Surgery* 2014; 47: 279–87.

Kirkpatrick AW, Roberts DJ, De Waele J, et al. Intra-abdominal hypertension and the abdominal compartment syndrome: updated consensus definitions and clinical practice guidelines from the World Society of the Abdominal Compartment Syndrome. *Intensive Care Medicine* 2013; 39: 1190–206.

---

9 Nutrition

9.1 General

9.1.1 Importance

- A key aspect of critical care but an area with limited high-level evidence.
- Nutrition is of particular importance at times of critical illness due to:
  - Increase in resting energy expenditure.
  - Failure to meet energy requirements may lead to:
    - Catabolism with associated detrimental effect on wound healing, immune function, coagulation, muscle strength, and respiratory function
    - Hypoglycaemia
    - Loss of mean body mass
    - Hypoalbuminaemia
  - Malnutrition may be associated with worse outcomes.
  - Overfeeding may also have detrimental effects.

9.1.2 Assessment

- Biochemical markers of nutrition (e.g. albumin, pre-albumin, transferrin) are of little use in critical illness due to their acute phase nature.
- The involvement of a critical care dietician is imperative in clinical practice.

9.2 Nutritional need

- It is difficult to estimate the nutritional requirements of critically ill patients.

9.2.1 Energy requirements

- Methods of estimating energy requirements include:
  - Indirect calorimetry:
    - The gold standard
    - Calorific requirements calculated on the basis of oxygen consumption
    - Not readily available on the majority of units
  - Measurement of CO_2 production:
    - Provides a reasonable estimate of energy requirement under stable conditions; however, overfeeding will lead to an over-estimate of energy expenditure.
  - Estimation:
    - For the majority of units, energy requirements are based upon population derived calculations +/− correction for underlying disease (e.g. Schofield formula); as a general rule these are:
      - Age under 65 years: 25 kilocalories per kg per day
      - Age over 65 years: 20 kilocalories per kg per day
- Some patient groups present particular problems in determining the energy requirements:
  - Obese
  - Malnourished
  - Patients with particularly hypermetabolic states (e.g. major trauma, severe burns)
- It was postulated that patients with ARDS may benefit from a lower calorific intake at the beginning of their admission; this however was not borne out in the recent EDEN study.

9.2.2 Daily requirements

- Standard daily requirements for various nutritional components are outlined in Table 4.15.

Table 4.15 Daily nutritional requirements

	Requirement (/kg/day)
Energy	● Under 65 years—25 kilocalories ● Over 65 years—20 kilocalories
Carbohydrates	● Should provide ~ 60% of non-protein calories ● 3–4 g
Protein	● Normally 1–1.5 g ● Increased to 1.5–2 g for burns, major trauma and other hypercatabolic states ● Comprised of a mixture of essential and non-essential amino acids
Lipid	● Should provide ~ 40% of non-protein calories ● 0.7–1.5 g
Electrolytes	● Water 30 ml ● Sodium 1–2 mmol ● Potassium 0.7–1 mmol ● Calcium 0.1 mmol ● Magnesium 0.1 mmol ● Phosphate 0.4 mmol
Trace elements	● Role unclear ● Selenium may have a mortality benefit

9.3 Route of nutrition

- If volitional intake can be maintained, this is the preferred option.
- Patients unable to meet nutritional requirements will require enteral nutrition (EN) or parenteral nutrition (PN).

9.3.1 Enteral nutrition

- Administered via an enteral tube, which is either gastric or jejunal:
  - Jejunal feeding tubes are more expensive and are more difficult to site.
  - The suggestion that the use of jejunal tubes would increase energy delivery or decrease the rate of ventilator associated pneumonia has not been borne out in trials.
  - Jejunal tubes are therefore reserved primarily for those patients who are not tolerating gastric feed.
- Suggested advantages over PN include:
  - Cheaper
  - Easier to administer
  - Lower risk of infection
  - More 'gut protective'
- Disadvantages compared to PN:
  - Requires gastrointestinal function
  - Potential increased risk of ventilator associated pneumonia
  - Less reliable delivery of energy
- Bowel sounds or passage of flatus/stool are a poor indicator of readiness for EN in the ICU.
- Measuring the volume aspirated from the feeding tube every 4 hours is typically used to assess tolerance of enteral feeding.
  - Aspirates of >500 ml are generally accepted to be an indication of hold enteral feed.
  - High aspirates should prompt search for a cause of gut failure (e.g. constipation; obstruction; acute abdomen; ACS).
  - Prokinetics may have a role in improving tolerance.
  - Avoidance of opiates and other agents which reduce gut motility should be considered.
  - Jejunal feeding and PN offer alternatives.

9.3.2 Parenteral nutrition

- In patients in whom the enteral route is not available, or who fail to tolerate enteral feed, PN is indicated.
- Complications of PN include:
  - Access-related
    - Central venous line insertion
  - Liver-related
    - Hepatic steatosis
    - Cholestasis
    - In rare cases, liver failure
  - Increased risk of sepsis with PN
  - Increased risk of hyperglycaemia

9.3.3 Enteral versus parenteral (CALORIES trial)

- A large pragmatic multi-centre trial, which compared early PN with EN, found no difference in mortality at 30 days; EN was associated with a higher risk of vomiting and hypoglycaemia.

- The authors conclude that 'Early nutritional support through the parenteral route is neither more harmful nor more beneficial than such support through the enteral route'.
- Of note, neither group achieved energy requirements in the trial and there was no significant difference in energy delivered between groups; this challenges the assertion that PN is more effective at delivering energy requirements.

9.4 Timing of nutrition

9.4.1 Early versus late

- Timing of nutritional intervention (either EN or PN) is generally divided into 'early' or 'late'.
- Whilst there is no absolute consensus on the timings these terms represent, early is generally taken to represent less than 48 hours after ICU admission and late greater than 7 days.

9.4.2 Evidence and practice

- Whilst high-grade evidence is lacking, there is general consensus that, where possible, EN should be initiated early—this may improve mortality.
- If the enteral route is not available, early initiation of PN is slightly more controversial, although this is not borne out by the CALORIES study.
- In patients with pre-existing malnutrition, the need for early nutrition is probably greater.

9.5 Immune-enhancing nutrition

- A number of fractional nutrients are believed to augment the immune system or modulate the inflammatory response.

9.5.1 Glutamine

- The most abundant circulating amino acid.
- The preferred energy source for leukocytes and enterocytes.
- Evidence that it has a beneficial role in the inflammatory response, oxidative stress, and gut integrity.
- Outcome benefit has been demonstrated in trauma and burns patients.

9.5.2 L-arginine

- Essential during metabolic stress.
- Up-regulates macrophage activity.
- High-dose supplementation has been demonstrated to enhance wound healing and to reduce infection in the elective surgical population; may increase mortality in other groups.

9.5.3 Omega 3

- Exhibits potent immune-modulatory activity via arachadonic acid inhibition.
- Some evidence of improved outcomes in ARDS.

9.6 Refeeding syndrome

9.6.1 Definition and aetiology

- Refeeding syndrome develops when a carbohydrate load is delivered following prolonged fast.
- Hypo-insulinaemia is common during fast and the sudden increase in circulating insulin provokes the intracellular movement of potassium, magnesium, phosphate, and/or calcium.
- The electrolyte disturbance can provoke cardiac failure and circulatory collapse, as well as symptoms of particular electrolyte losses.

9.6.2 Avoidance and management

- All patients at risk of refeeding syndrome should have prophylactic thiamine replacement, normalization of electrolytes prior to enteral feeding commencement and daily measurement of electrolytes as EN is established (first 24–72 hours).
- Feeding should be commenced at lower rates (10 kcal per kg per day).

FURTHER READING

Harvey SE, Parrott F, Harrison DA, et al. Trial of the route of early nutritional support in critically ill adults. *New England Journal of Medicine* 2014; 371: 1673–84.

Kreymann K, Berger M, Deutz Ne, et al. ESPEN guidelines on enteral nutrition: intensive care. *Clinical Nutrition* 2006; 25: 210–23.

Martindale RG, McClave SA, Vanek VW, et al. Guidelines for the provision and assessment of nutrition support therapy in the adult critically ill patient: Society of Critical Care Medicine and American Society for Parenteral and Enteral Nutrition: Executive Summary. *Critical Care Med* 2009; 37: 1757–61.

Rice TW, Wheeler AP, Thompson BT, et al. Initial trophic vs full enteral feeding in patients with acute lung injury: the EDEN randomized trial. *Journal of the American Medical Association* 2012; 307: 795–803.

Singer P, Berger MM, Van den Berghe G, et al. ESPEN guidelines on parenteral nutrition: intensive care. *Clinical Nutrition* 2009; 28: 387–400.

CHAPTER 5

Neurosciences

CONTENTS

1 Sedation and analgesia

1.1 General

1.1.1 Role of sedation

- Airway—placement and tolerance of endotracheal tube
- Breathing—facilitate compliance with mechanical ventilation
- Circulation—reduce oxygen consumption
- Disability—maintain comfort; augment analgesia; manage neurological disturbance (anxiety, agitation, delirium); control raised intracranial pressure

1.1.2 Adverse effects

- Prolongation of mechanical ventilation
- Prolongation of intensive care stay
- Difficulty in assessment of underlying neurological function
- Side-effects of the drugs (delirium, hypotension)

1.1.3 Sedation holds

- There is a general consensus that minimizing administered sedation is preferable.
- Many advocate the daily interruption of sedation (often described as a 'sedation hold').
- Sedation holds have been suggested to:
  - Decrease ventilator time
  - Decrease length of stay
  - Decrease post-traumatic stress disorder and other psychological sequelae
  - Decrease use of vasoactive drugs
  - Decrease hospital mortality
  - Increase likelihood of successful extubation

- ▪ Decrease the likelihood of tracheostomy
- ▪ It does, however, increase likelihood of unplanned self-extubation and increases nursing workload.
- ● These positive findings are not, however, consistent; some studies have failed to demonstrate advantages to daily sedation holds.

1.1.4 Sedation scoring systems

- ● Degree of sedation should be regularly assessed and recorded.
- ● The most commonly used system is the ten-point Richmond agitation–sedation score (RASS).
- ● In RASS:
  - ▪ Negative scores denote sedation, positive scores denote hyperarousal, and a patient with a neutral score is calm and spontaneously interacts with staff.
  - ▪ RASS –1 is often regarded as the ideal target for the intubated patient.
  - ▪ Precise definitions for the RASS score can be found in the original paper by Sessler et al. (2002).

1.2 Sedative agents

1.2.1 Mechanism of action of sedative agents

- ● Sedative agents exert their effects by one of several mechanisms:
  - ▪ As an agonist at inhibitory neurotransmitter receptors (namely GABA (Gamma-aminobutyric acid) A and glycine):
    - ▫ GABA A and glycine are chloride ion gated receptors, activation of which results in influx of chloride, hyperpolarization of the neuronal membrane and therefore inhibition of neuronal activity.
  - ▪ As an antagonist of excitatory neurotransmitter pathways:
    - ▫ Antagonism of the NMDA (N-methyl D-Aspartate)receptor prevents binding of glutamate, thereby inhibiting neuronal activity.
  - ▪ As an agonist at $\alpha 2$ receptors:
    - ▫ Agonism of pre-ganglionic receptors reduces central sympathetic outflow; stimulation of post-ganglionic receptors within the central nervous system leads to the sedative effect.

1.2.2 The 'ideal' agent

- ● The properties of the 'ideal' sedative agent are outlined in Table 5.1.

Table 5.1 The ideal sedative agent

Physical	● Long shelf-life at room temperature ● Water soluble (to facilitate storage) ● No physical interactions ● High lipid solubility (to facilitate passage across membranes) ● No pain on injection or extravasation
Pharmacokinetics	● Rapid onset and offset ● No accumulation ● Not altered by renal or hepatic failure ● No effect on the handling of other drugs
Pharmacodynamics	● Analgesic properties ● Anxiolytic properties ● No effect on cardiovascular, respiratory, or gastrointestinal systems ● Amnesic effect may be beneficial

1.2.3 Commonly used sedative agents

- The perfect sedative agent does not exist.
- Commonly used sedatives in the intensive care unit are described in Table 5.2.

Table 5.2 Commonly used sedative agents

Agent	Mechanism	Comments
Propofol	GABA A agonist (Glycine agonist)	Presented as a lipid/water emulsion in 1% or 2% preparations. Rapid onset and offset: popular choice as both induction agent and for maintenance of sedation. Use is curtailed by dose-dependent hypotension (reduces both SVR and contractility); respiratory depression to point of apnoea; propofol infusion syndrome (see Chapter 9, Section 3.14); and its high calorie load.
Benzodiazepines (midazolam, lorazepam, diazepam)	GABA A agonist	Slower onset and offset than propofol. Have anxiolytic, anti-convulsant, amnesic, and muscle-relaxing properties. Relatively cardiostable therefore often preferred in shocked patients. Useful in alcohol and drug withdrawal. Tend to accumulate, particularly in renal and hepatic failure. Associated with increased incidence of ICU delirium.
α2 receptor agonists (clonidine, dexmedetomidine)	α2 agonist	Provide a degree of sedation and anxiolysis with no effect on respiratory function. Analgesic. Useful in alcohol and drug withdrawal. Use limited by dose-dependent bradycardia and hypotension.
Thiopental	GABA A agonist (Glycine agonist)	Primarily used as an induction agent it has a more predictable onset and less haemodynamic disturbance than propofol. Use in maintenance of sedation is reserved for management of refractory seizures and refractory intracranial hypertension; accumulation of drug in this context leads to prolonged half-life and slow recovery of consciousness.
Etomidate	GABA A agonist	An imidazole derivative that induces anaesthesia with no haemodynamic compromise. Inhibition of 17α hydroxylase and 11β hydroxylase impairs steroid synthesis and even single-dose use of etomidate has been linked to increased mortality in the critically ill. Consequently it is not available in Australasia and has fallen out of favour in Europe.
Ketamine	NMDA antagonist	A phencyclidine derivative; a centrally acting stimulant of the sympathetic nervous system. Induction of anaesthesia is accompanied by increase in cardiac output and blood pressure (but at the expense of increased intracranial pressure and myocardial oxygen demand). It is currently the induction agent of choice in the haemodynamically unstable patient, although traditionally contra-indicated in those with head injuries. It has bronchodilator properties and consequently has a role in induction and maintenance in asthma.

- In recent years there has been significant interest in the potential of dexmedetomidine as a sedative agent in intensive care:
  - Dexmedetomidine has been demonstrated not to be inferior to propofol or midazolam in terms of achieving sedative goals.
  - It is associated with a shorter period of mechanical ventilation and less delirium than midazolam, and better patient interaction than propofol.
  - It is, however, associated with the theoretical risks of hypotension and bradycardia (although these do not appear to have been major issues in the clinical trials).

1.3 Analgesic agents

1.3.1 Role

- Management of pain
- Adjunct to sedation

1.3.2 Agents

- Commonly used analgesic agents are described in Table 5.3.

Table 5.3 Commonly used analgesic agents

Agent	Mechanism	Comments
Opiates (morphine, fentanyl, alfentanil, remifentanil)	Provide analgesia primarily by action on Mu receptors (inhibitory G-protein-linked receptors), located throughout the central nervous system. Sedative effects occur via Kappa receptors.	Side-effects include respiratory depression, hypotension, pruritus, decreased gut motility, and constipation, urinary retention. Opiates differ in their pharmacokinetic properties.
Non-steroidal anti-inflammatory drugs (NSAIDS)	Inhibit cyclo-oxygenase at the site of inflammation, thereby reducing production of pro-inflammatory prostaglandins and thromboxanes.	Potential side-effects include gastric irritation, worsening of asthma, worsening of renal function, and worsening of platelet function.
Paracetamol	Believed to inhibit cyclo-oxygenase-3 within the central nervous system providing analgesic and anti-pyretic effects.	Safe in therapeutic doses. Caution in patients with low weight.
Neuropathic agents (gabapentin, pregabalin, amitriptyline)	Gabapentin and pregabalin act on calcium channels within the central nervous system, reducing excitatory neutrotransmitter release. Amitriptyline has multiple mechanisms of action, including the inhibition of noradrenaline and serotonin reuptake and antagonism of muscarinic and histaminergic receptors.	Commonly used as an adjunct in the management of neuropathic pain. Some sedative properties.
Ketamine	See Table 5.2	

FURTHER READING

Girard TD, Kress JP, Fuchs BD, et al. Efficacy and safety of a paired sedation and ventilator weaning protocol for mechanically ventilated patients in intensive care (Awakening and Breathing Controlled trial): a randomised controlled trial. *Lancet* 2008; 371(9607): 126–34.

Jackson D, Proudfoot C, Cann K, Walsh T. A systematic review of the impact of sedation practice in the ICU on resource use, costs and patient safety. *Critical Care* 2010; 14(2): R59.

Jakob S, Ruokonen E, Grounds R, et al. Dexmedetomidine for Long-Term Sedation Investigators: dexmedetomidine vs midazolam or propofol for sedation during prolonged mechanical ventilation: Two randomized controlled trials. *JAMA: the Journal of the American Medical Association* 2012; 307(11): 1151–60.

Kress JP, Pohlman AS, O'Connor MF, Hall JB. Daily interruption of sedative infusions in critically ill patients undergoing mechanical ventilation. *New England Journal of Medicine* 2000; 342(20): 1471–7.

Mehta S, Burry L, Cook D, et al. Daily sedation interruption in mechanically ventilated critically ill patients cared for with a sedation protocol: a randomized controlled trial. *Journal of the American Medical Association* 2012; 308(19): 1985–92.

Riker R, Shehabi Y, Bokesch P, et al. SEDCOM (Safety and Efficacy of Dexmedetomidine Compared With Midazolam) Study Group. Dexmedetomidine vs midazolam for sedation of critically ill patients: a randomized trial. *JAMA: the Journal of the American Medical Association* 2009; 301(5): 489–99.

Sessler CN, Gosnell MS, Grap MJ, et al. The Richmond Agitation–Sedation Scale: validity and reliability in adult intensive care unit patients. *American Journal of Respiratory and Critical Care Medicine* 2002; 166(10): 1338–44.

Strøm T, Martinussen T, Toft P. A protocol of no sedation for critically ill patients receiving mechanical ventilation: a randomised trial. *Lancet* 2010; 375(9713): 475.

2 Coma

2.1 Coma on the intensive care

2.1.1 General

- Investigation of unexplained coma may be required either:
    - On admission to intensive care (in the unconscious patient with unclear diagnosis)
    - Or at a later stage in stay (in the patient failing to regain consciousness from iatrogenic coma)

2.1.2 Aetiology and investigation

- The causes are many and extensive work up is often required (Table 5.4).

Table 5.4 Causes of coma

System	Pathologies	Investigations
Neurological	Seizure	CT brain
	CNS infection (meningitis, encephalitis)	MRI brain
	Intracranial mass lesion (tumour, haemorrhage, abscess)	EEG
		Lumbar puncture
	Cerebrovascular event	
Cardiovascular	Low cardiac output state	ECG, echo
Respiratory	Hypoxia	ABG
	Hypercapnia	
	Carbon monoxide	
Metabolic	Uraemia	U&E
	Hepatic encephalopathy	LFT
	Hypoglycaemia	Ammonia
	Hypo-/hypernatraemia	Blood glucose
	Hypothyroidism	TFT
	Hypothermia	
	Hypo-/hyper-osmolar state	
Pharmacological	Opiates	Urine or plasma toxicology if appropriate
	Benzodiazepines	
	Barbituates	
	Tricyclic anti-depressants	
	Alcohol	

U&E, urea and electrolytes; LFT, liver function tests; TFT, thyroid function tests; ABG, arterial blood gas; EEG, electroencephalogram.

2.1.3 Coma-like states

- Coma may be confused with one of the coma-like states (Table 5.5).

Table 5.5 Coma-like states

Locked-in syndrome	Occurs due to bilateral pontine lesion transecting descending pathways; ascending and reticular activating system pathways unaffected. Cortex intact.
	Alert and aware. Blinking and vertical eye movement intact but no other voluntary movement. EEG is normal.
Persistent vegetative state	Secondary to bilateral cortical damage but preservation of brainstem.
	Spontaneous but non-purposeful limb movements occur, as does yawning. There is no speech. Patient is unaware. EEG is abnormal. Definition of persistent requires >4 weeks.
Akinetic mutism	Due to bilateral frontal lobe damage, hydrocephalus or third ventricular mass lesion.
	Partially or fully awake but immobile and silent. Diffuse slowing on EEG.

Catatonia	A condition of psychiatric origin.
	Awake but mute and decreased motor activity. May have fixed posture. EEG non-specific.
Minimally conscious state	Secondary to global neuronal damage.
	Globally impaired responsiveness but with evidence of partial preservation of self and environmental awareness. Theta and alpha waves on EEG.

3 Traumatic brain injury

3.1 Background

3.1.1 Significance

- Traumatic brain injury (TBI) is a major cause of morbidity and mortality, and is frequently associated with major trauma.

3.1.2 Classification

- Initial assessment is by means of the Glasgow coma score (GCS) (Table 5.6).
- TBI is classified as:
  - Mild (GCS 13–15)
  - Moderate (GCS 8–12)
  - Severe (GCS <8)
- TBI is, by definition, the result of external force; however, many of the physiological, pathological, and management principles also apply to other, non-traumatic forms of brain injury.

Table 5.6 Glasgow coma score

Eyes	4—Open spontaneously
	3—Open to voice
	2—Open to painful stimulus
	1—No response
Voice	5—Orientated
	4—Confused
	3—Inappropriate words
	2—Incomprehensible sounds
	1—No response
Motor	6—Obeys commands
	5—Localises to painful stimulus
	4—Withdraws from painful stimulus
	3—Abnormal flexion to painful stimulus
	2—Extension to painful stimulus
	1—No response

Adapted from The Lancet, 304, Teasdale G. et al., 'Assessment of coma and impaired consciousness-a practical scale', pp. 81–84. Copyright (1974) with permission from Elsevier.

3.2 Mechanisms and physiology

The mechanisms of TBI are divided into primary and secondary injury.

3.2.1 Primary brain injury

- Occurs at the time of injury, and is the result of axial loading and shearing forces causing in a diffuse axonal injury.
- Presents radiologically as diffuse swelling, loss of grey-white differentiation, and is often associated with contusions (both at point of impact and at the opposite side of the brain—the *contrecoup* injury).
- There may be associated vascular injury resulting in extradural haematoma (commonly due to middle meningeal artery injury), subdural haematoma (due to bridging vein injury), or intra-parenchymal bleeding.
- Primary brain injury is immediate and can only be avoided by accident prevention.

3.2.2 Secondary brain injury

- Arises when cerebral oxygen consumption ($CMRO_2$) exceeds cerebral oxygen delivery (Table 5.7). This may be a result of:
  - Increase in $CMRO_2$ (e.g. seizures, pyrexia)
  - Inadequate systemic delivery of oxygen (e.g. hypotension, hypoxaemia)
  - Rise in intracranial pressure impeding blood flow to the brain (the cerebral perfusion pressure, CPP). CPP is dependent upon systemic blood pressure and intracranial pressure (ICP):

$$CPP = MAP - ICP$$

Table 5.7 Causes of secondary brain injury

	Mechanisms of secondary brain injury
Intracranial	Seizures ($\uparrow CMRO_2$)
	Haematoma ($\uparrow$ ICP)
	Hydrocephalus ($\uparrow$ ICP)
	Infection ($\uparrow$ ICP; $\uparrow CMRO_2$)
Systemic	Hypoxia ($\downarrow O_2$ delivery; $\uparrow$ ICP)
	Hypercarbia ($\uparrow$ ICP)
	Hypocarbia ($\downarrow O_2$ delivery)
	Pyrexia ($\uparrow CMRO_2$)
	Hyponatraemia ($\uparrow$ ICP)
	Hypoglycaemia (impaired cerebral metabolism)

3.2.3 Determinants of intracranial pressure

- ICP is governed by the Monro–Kellie doctrine: a relationship based upon the fact that the skull is a rigid box.
- Increase in volume of the contents of the box (e.g. from bleeding or oedematous brain parenchyma) can be compensated to a degree by displacement of CSF.

- When compensatory mechanisms are overwhelmed, however, large pressure rises occur in response to small increases in the volume of intracranial contents (Fig. 5.1).
- The volume of parenchyma (and hence ICP) is sensitive to plasma osmotic pressure:
  - Reduction in plasma osmolality causes fluid shift from plasma into neuronal cells resulting in cerebral oedema and raised intracranial pressure.
  - The most significant osmotically active particle is sodium; in the brain-injured patient, even a small drop in plasma sodium can precipitate a clinically significant rise in ICP.

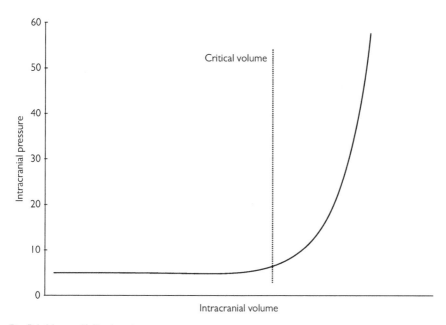

Fig. 5.1 Monro–Kellie doctrine.

3.2.4 Determinants of cerebral perfusion

- Cerebral perfusion is governed by a number of physiological variables.
- The healthy brain autoregulates blood flow and this allows maintenance of a steady cerebral blood flow throughout a range of systemic blood pressures.
- Autoregulation is generally effective over a wide range of blood pressures (typically MAP 50–150 mmHg; see Fig. 5.2), although this range may shift upwards in the context of chronic hypertension.
- In brain injury (traumatic or otherwise), autoregulation may be disrupted and close control of blood pressure becomes even more important.
- P_aCO_2 has a marked effect on cerebral blood flow (Fig. 5.3):
  - Hypercarbia causes cerebral vasodilation, increasing intracranial pressure.
  - Hypocarbia constricts the cerebral arteries, initially reducing intracranial pressure but potentially compromising the blood supply at extremely low CO_2 levels.

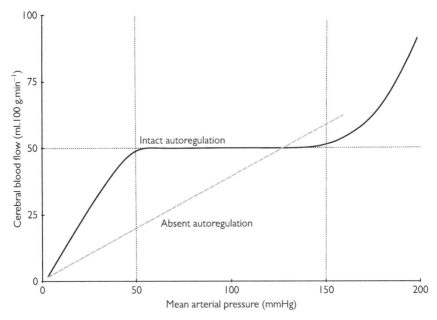

Fig. 5.2 Cerebral autoregulation of blood flow in relation to perfusion pressure.

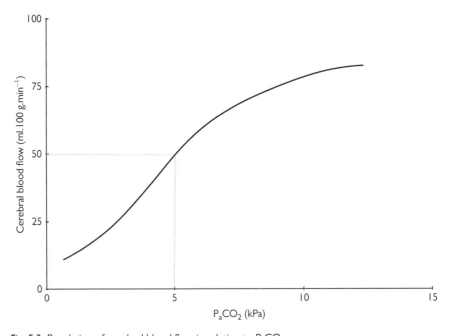

Fig. 5.3 Regulation of cerebral blood flow in relation to P_aCO_2.

- P_aO_2 has no significant effect on cerebral blood flow at normal levels but in hypoxia (P_aO_2 <8 kPa), cerebral blood flow increases exponentially causing a rise in intracerebral pressure (Fig. 5.4).

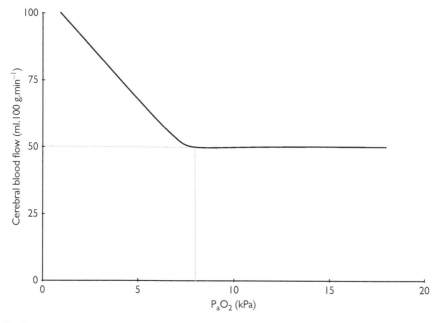

Fig. 5.4 Regulation of cerebral blood flow in relation to P_aO_2.

3.2.5 Consequences of raised intracranial pressure

- The normal range for ICP is between 0 and 10 mmHg, although this may transiently rise to 50 mmHg on coughing.
- Elevation of ICP impairs cerebral perfusion; the absolute value of ICP is not however as important as the difference between MAP and ICP in this respect.
- Extremes of ICP may not only compromise perfusion but can also lead to herniation of the brain:
  - Downward displacement of the diencephalon and midbrain leads to a drop in conscious level.
  - Further increase in ICP causes uncal herniation—herniation of the temporal lobe between brainstem and posterior fossa—resulting in pupillary dilation, ptosis, limited upward gaze (as the third cranial nerve is compressed), and extensor posturing.
  - Finally, tonsillar herniation occurs as the cerebellar tonsils are displaced through the foramen magnum; the consequence is haemodynamic instability (including the *Cushing's response* of hypertension and bradycardia), altered respiratory pattern, and ultimately brainstem death.

3.3 General management of traumatic brain injury

Initial management should be based upon advanced trauma life support principles with primary and secondary survey.

3.3.1 Airway management

- The airway should be secured in those patients:
  - Failing to obey commands
  - Who are combative
  - With failure of oxygenation or ventilation

- The choice of induction agent is controversial.
- A single transient episode of hypotension is associated with increased mortality in TBI patients; the use of hypotension precipitating anaesthetic agents, such as propofol or thiopental, is therefore undesirable, particularly in the multiply injured patient.
- Ketamine has the advantage of maintaining blood pressure but is traditionally contra-indicated in TBI due to a theoretical increase in ICP.
- The agent used therefore depends upon clinician preference and local policy.

3.3.2 Referral to neurosurgical services

- Box 5.1 outlines indications for referral to neurosurgical services.

Box 5.1 Indications for neurosurgical referral in traumatic brain injury

- Acute intracranial lesion on CT
- Persistent GCS <9 following resuscitation
- Confusion >4 hours
- Focal neurology
- Seizure without recovery
- Compound skull fracture
- Penetrating skull injury
- Cerebrospinal fluid leak

3.4 Prevention of secondary brain injury

3.4.1 Neuro-protective strategy

- The cornerstone of brain injury management in the ICU is avoidance of secondary injury.
- This so-called neuro-protective strategy is outlined in Table 5.8.

Table 5.8 Neuro-protective strategy

Monitoring and control of intracranial pressure	ICP monitoring
	Manipulation of parameters (described in Table 5.11
Maintain adequate oxygen delivery	Adequate MAP (sufficient to achieve CPP > 60 mmHg)
	P_aO_2 >13 kPa
	P_aCO_2 4–4.5 kPa
	Deep sedation/paralysis to avoid coughing and vomiting
Optimize cerebral venous drainage	30-degree head up
	Avoid tight endotracheal tube ties
	Avoid excessive PEEP
Minimize cerebral oedema	Na^+ 145–50 mmol.l^{-1}
Minimize $CMRO_2$	Avoid hyperthermia
	Prevent seizures

3.4.2 Intracranial pressure monitoring

- In the patient free from sedation, conscious level provides a means of monitoring ICP: a fall in GCS should prompt investigation for rising ICP:
  - Advantages: cheap, non-invasive, quick, and minimal expertise required.
  - Disadvantage: fall in GCS is a non-specific sign; cannot be reliably used in the context of sedation and therefore of little use in most TBI patients on ICU.
- CT brain allows intermittent estimation of ICP; CT findings suggestive of raised ICP include loss of CSF-filled spaces (decreased ventricular size and loss of sulci) and loss of grey-white differentiation:
  - Advantages: allows identification of focal lesions contributing to rising ICP with potential for intervention.
  - Disadvantages: non-continuous, requires transfer to CT, and requires expertise to interpret.
- ICP may be directly and continuously measured by placement of a catheter or transducer within the skull:
  - The most commonly encountered ICP monitor is the intraparenchymal transducer, often referred to as a 'bolt'.
    - Placed by means of a cranial bolt and sits within the parenchyma of the non-dominant hemisphere.
    - Relatively simple to insert, has a low risk of haemorrhage or infection, but once inserted cannot be re-calibrated and is therefore prone to drift.
  - An alternative is an extraventricular drain (EVD):
    - Usually surgically inserted into the ventricular system, this carries a greater risk of infection and haemorrhage.
    - Brings the advantages that it may be recalibrated, and also allows drainage of cerebrospinal fluid for either diagnostic purposes (e.g. culture) or therapeutics (management of hydrocephalus).
- The Brain Trauma Foundation recommends the use of invasive ICP monitoring in the following circumstances:
  - Moderate to severe head injury in those who cannot be neurologically assessed
  - Severe head injury (GCS <8) and abnormal CT brain
  - Or, severe head injury and normal CT brain, but with 2/3 of: age >40 years, systolic BP <90, and abnormal motor response in GCS
- ICP monitoring may also be utilized in the following non-traumatic problems:
  - Spontaneous intracranial haemorrhage complicated by coma
  - Anoxic brain injury (e.g. following cardiac arrest or drowning)
  - Hepatic encephalopathy and cerebral oedema associated with fulminant liver failure
  - Intracranial infections (e.g. meningitis or encephalitis)

3.4.3 The ICP waveform

- The ICP rises slightly with every heartbeat (Fig. 5.5; Table 5.9).
- The resultant pressure wave is divided into three components that provide information regarding brain compliance.
- As ICP rises, the amplitude of the ICP wave increases, but mean pressure remains the same. As the compliance of the brain decreases, P2>P1 and the wave broadens (Fig. 5.5).
- Monitoring of the ICP will reveal changes in the mean pressure over a period of time. _Lundberg_ first described these fluctuations in 1960: three distinct patterns (the Lundberg waves) are described in Table 5.10. Lundberg waves refer to the ICP over time rather than the morphology of individual ICP waveforms.

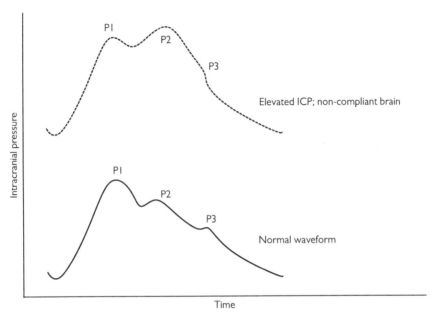

Fig. 5.5 Intracranial pressure waveform. Waveforms for both normal and non-compliant brains are demonstrated.

Table 5.9 Intracranial pressure waveform

P1	Percussion wave: arterial pressure transmitted from choroid plexus to ventricle
P2	Tidal wave: reflection of the pressure wave from the skull, affected by brain compliance
P3	Dicrotic wave—secondary to aortic valve closure

Table 5.10 Lundberg waves

Lundberg A waves	Slow vasogenic waves seen in patients with critical cerebral perfusion. Mean ICP of 50–100 mmHg reached, lasting for 5–10 min. Thought to be due to a reflex cerebral vasodilation in response to reduced MAP. The pressure plateaus when maximum vasodilation reached. May be terminated by increasing the MAP. These waves are always pathological and suggest decreased brain compliance.
Lundberg B waves	Occur in cycles of 30 seconds to 2 minutes. These transient increases of ICP to 20–30 mmHg above baseline are evidence of normal autoregulation. Observed in normal individuals; absence following head injury is poor prognostic sign.
Lundberg C waves	Occur in 4–8-minute cycles. Of no clinical importance.

3.4.4 Manipulation of intracranial pressure

- As a general rule targets are ICP <20 mmHg and CPP >60 mmHg.
- A rising ICP or falling CPP should prompt an urgent search for the cause.
- Blood pressure, respiratory parameters, and electrolytes should be normalized.

- Urgent CT may be required to identify surgical emergencies, such as hydrocephalus or expanding haematoma.
- Medical and surgical means of controlling ICP are described in Table 5.11.
- Steroids, which had been proposed as a means of reducing cerebral swelling and ICP, have been demonstrated to *increase* risk of mortality in TBI in the CRASH I study.

Table 5.11 Management of raised ICP

Surgical	Evacuation of mass lesion	Surgical evacuation of haematoma, if present.
	Drainage of CSF	CSF drainage by means of ventricular drain is most effective means of reducing elevated ICP secondary to hydrocephalus.
	Decompressive craniectomy	Used for the management of elevated ICP secondary to cerebral oedema. The DECRA trial demonstrated this technique to reduce ICP and ICU length of stay, but to produce worse neurological outcomes at 6 months. Its use is therefore controversial.
Medical	Hyperventilation (to P_aCO_2 <3.5 kPa)	Iatrogenic hyperventilation significantly reduces cerebral blood flow and thereby the volume of blood in the brain. Whilst this effectively reduces ICP (and may stall herniation) it can worsen cerebral perfusion. This is a temporary measure, pending definitive intervention.
	Osmotherapy— mannitol (0.5 g/kg over 15 min)	The osmotic diuretic mannitol increases plasma osmolality causing shift of water from the neurones into the plasma, thereby reducing cerebral oedema. Can theoretically enter the brain if blood–brain barrier damaged, worsening oedema. Causes an osmotic diuresis and potentially hypovolaemia. A temporary bridge to definitive management, use should be monitored via plasma osmolality levels (aim 310–320 mOsm/kg)
	Osmotherapy— hypertonic saline (aim Na^+ 145–155 mmol.l^{-1})	Infusion of NaCl 3% 2 ml/kg allows rapid increase in plasma Na^+ and therefore osmolality. This has a similar effect on the brain as mannitol. NaCl carries a lower risk of hypovolaemia and is less likely to cross the blood–brain barrier and cause worsening cerebral oedema; it can also be monitored more easily via the blood gas analyser. It does however require central venous access, can precipitate hyperchloraemic acidosis, and carries the theoretical risk of osmotic demyelination.
	Hypothermia	Has been demonstrated to reduce ICP but no clear demonstrable reduction in mortality. Associated with increased infection risk, coagulopathy, hypertension and bradyarrhythmias.
	Barbituate coma	Reduction in $CMRO_2$ by means of a thiopental infusion may reduce ICP. However, accumulation and subsequent prolonged half-life may make assessment of conscious level difficult.

3.4.5 Seizure prophylaxis in TBI

- Up to 25% of TBI patients will have early seizures (<7 days post-injury); up to 42% will have late seizures (beyond 7 days).
- Seizures theoretically increase ICP.

- Certain factors are known to be associated with a higher incidence of post-traumatic seizures:
  - Cortical contusion
  - Depressed skull fracture
  - Subdural haematoma
  - Extradural haematoma
  - Intracerebral haematoma
  - Penetrating head injury
  - GCS <10
- Anti-epileptic drugs reduce the incidence of seizures but have not been shown to improve long-term outcomes.

3.5 Other forms of neurological monitoring

3.5.1 Trans-cranial Doppler

- May be used to measure blood velocity through the Circle of Willis (usually the middle cerebral artery, as this carries 80% of blood flow).
- It may be used on a continuous or intermittent basis.
- It is operator-dependant and requires a degree of expertise to achieve meaningful results.
- Whilst it has a role in determining cerebral blood flow (CBF) in all brain pathologies, it is particularly useful in monitoring for vasospasm in subarachnoid haemorrhage.

3.5.2 Jugular venous bulb oximetry (SjVO$_2$)

- May be used intermittently or continuously to assess CBF.
- It works on the principle that a reduction in CBF will cause the brain to increase oxygen extraction. Therefore, assuming CMRO$_2$ remains constant, a fall in SjVO$_2$ below 60% reflects a reduction in CBF.
- It is a marker of global perfusion; SjVO$_2$ may be normal in the context of local hypoperfusion.
- It is not particularly specific for raised ICP, with up to half of measurements <50% false-positive results.
- The number of desaturations has, however, been shown to be a predictor of outcome.
- In practice, a fibre-optic oximeter, or a sampling catheter, is inserted into the internal jugular vein in a retrograde fashion and the tip advanced until in the jugular bulb (level with the mastoid air cells on lateral skull X-ray).

3.5.3 Near infra-red spectroscopy

- A continuous, non-invasive technique in which two oximeter probes are placed 4–7 cm apart on the scalp.
- Infra-red light is passed through a 10-ml volume of brain, allowing determination of regional oxygen saturation.
- Normal range is 60–80%. Measurements reflect local conditions only and it is difficult to differentiate between intracerebral and extra-cerebral tissues.

3.5.4 Brain tissue oxygenation

- Intracranial bolts may be adapted to incorporate multiple sensors in addition to the traditional ICP manometer; this may allow direct measurement of brain tissue oxygenation and metabolism.
- If a brain tissue oxygen sensor is inserted, oxygen from the surrounding 15 mm^3 of tissue diffuses to the oxygen-sensitive electrode, and the resultant current reflects oxygen tension. Normal range is 3.3–4 kPa.

3.5.5 Micro-dialysis catheter

- May be passed via the intracranial bolt into the parenchyma.
- Dialysate fluid continuously flows down the catheter. Low molecular weight substances in the parenchyma diffuse across the 20 kDa membrane and can be measured in the dialysate fluid.
- Of particular interest are the levels of lactate, pyruvate, and glucose: sensitive markers of brain hypoxia and ischaemia.
- A rise in the lactate/pyruvate ratio is associated with greater severity of injury and worse outcomes.
- Changes in the ratio appear to precede ICP rise and therefore potentially offer an earlier opportunity for intervention.

3.6 Predictors of outcome in traumatic brain injury

- Retrospective analysis of data from several TBI studies identified a number of factors associated with poor outcome:
  - Increasing age
  - Poor motor score on the GCS post resuscitation
  - Lack of pupil reactivity
  - CT head findings:
    - Worse outcomes with increasing Marshall CT grade (for which evidence of oedema, midline shift, and extra-axial blood all denote higher grade)
    - Worse outcome with presence of subarachnoid blood
  - Presence of hypoxia or hypotension
  - The existence of co-morbidities

3.7 Polyuria in brain injury

3.7.1 Differential diagnosis

- Alcohol
- Mannitol
- Cold diuresis
- Hyperglycaemia
- Diabetes inspidus
- Cerebral salt wasting

3.7.2 Investigation

- History and review of the notes may reveal recent ingestion of alcohol or administration of mannitol.
- Examination may reveal hypothermia or hyperglycaemia.
- Further investigation includes:
  - Plasma sodium
  - Urinary sodium
  - Plasma osmolality
  - Urinary osmolality

3.7.3 Diabetes insipidus

- Neurogenic diabetes insipidus may occur in the context of brain injury.
- Direct or indirect insult to the posterior pituitary impairs secretion of anti-diuretic hormone (ADH).

- As a consequence, free water is not reabsorbed in the collecting ducts of the kidney; a profound diuresis with inappropriate free water loss ensues.
- The patient is hypernatraemic with high plasma osmolality.
- Urinary osmolality is low.
- A urine output of several hundred ml.h^{-1} is common.
- Management:
  - Replacement of free water (dextrose 5%)
  - Intravenous DDAVP

3.7.4 Cerebral salt-wasting

- A neuroendocrine disorder associated with brain injury thought to relate to inappropriate release of naturetic peptide.
- Results in a salt-wasting diuresis.
- The patient is hyponatraemic with low plasma osmolality.
- Urine osmolality and sodium content is high.
- No specific treatment exists.
- Management involves fluid and sodium replacement.

FURTHER READING

Clifton GL, Miller ER, Choi SC, et al. Lack of effect of induction of hypothermia after acute brain injury. *New England Journal of Medicine* 2001; 344(8): 556–63.

Cooper DJ, Rosenfeld JV, Murray L, et al. Decompressive craniectomy in diffuse traumatic brain injury. *New England Journal of Medicine* 2011; 364(16): 1493–502.

CRASH I Investigators. Effect of intravenous corticosteroids on death within 14 days in 10 008 adults with clinically significant head injury (MRC CRASH trial): randomised placebo-controlled trial. *Lancet* 364(9442): 1321–8.

Edwards P, Arango M, Balica L, ettable 5.14 al. CRASH trial collaborators Final results of MRC CRASH, a randomized placebo-controlled trial of intravenous corticosteroid in adults with head injury–outcomes at 6 months. *Lancet* 2005; 365(9475): 1957–9.

Guidelines for the management of severe traumatic brain injury. *Journal of Neurotrauma* 2007; 24 (Suppl1).

Perel P, Arango M, Clayton T et al. Predicting outcome after traumatic brain injury: practical prognostic models based on large cohort of international patients. *British Medical Journal* 2008; 336(7641): 425–9.

---

4 Seizure disorders

4.1 General

4.1.1 Definition

- Status epilepticus (SE) is seizure activity for greater than 30 minutes, or recurrent seizures without return of consciousness between events; it can apply to any seizure type.

4.1.2 Incidence

- SE occurs in around 5% of epileptics at some point in their lives but has a higher incidence in children, those with learning disabilities, and in the presence of structural brain abnormalities.

4.1.3 Aetiology

- Presentation with *de novo* seizures should prompt the search for a cause (Table 5.12).

Table 5.12 Causes of seizure

Intracranial	Systemic
Infection (e.g. meningitis, encephalitis)	Drug toxicity (e.g. tricyclic antidepressants, aminophylline, calcineurin inhibitors)
Abscess	Alcohol withdrawal
Tumour (primary or metastasis)	Hypoglycaemia
Haemorrhage (intracerebral or extra-axial)	Hyponatraemia
	Hypoxia
Stroke	

4.2 Management

4.2.1 General principles

- The principles of management (Table 5.13) in SE are support of airway, breathing circulation, termination of seizures, and prevention of seizure recurrence, management of complications (Table 5.14), and treatment of underlying precipitants.
- Ensure a blood glucose is checked early as hypoglycaemia is an easily reversible cause of seizure.

Table 5.13 Management of status epilepticus

Initial	ABC approach
	Early glucose check
First line	Benzodiazepines
	• IV lorazepam (0.07 mg/kg up to max. 4 mg)
	▪ Rapid onset, long-acting and minimal risk of hypotension or respiratory depression
	• IV diazepam (10–20 mg)
	▪ Greater risk of hypotension and respiratory depression
Second line	Anti-epileptic medications
	• Phenytoin (18–20 mg/kg loading dose)
	▪ Administration <50 mg/min to avoid arrhythmias and hypotension, therefore not effective for 30 min
	▪ Fosphenytoin (15 mg/min) is an alternative that can be given at a 3x faster rate but is still associated with side-effects
	• Levetiracetam (500–3,000 mg daily)
	▪ The most commonly used anti-epileptic after phenytoin for management of SE. The absence of any significant side-effects or drug interactions makes this a popular drug in the critically ill.
Third line	General anaesthesia with endotracheal intubation
	• Thiopental (5–7 mg/kg)
	▪ A potent suppressor of seizure activity, this is the induction agent of choice for status epilepticus (SE)
	• Propofol (3–5 mg/kg)
	▪ Also supresses seizure activity. Case reports of propofol inducing seizure-like activity limit its popularity in SE

4.2.2 Complications

- Complications of prolonged seizures are listed in Table 5.14.

Table 5.14 Complications of status epilepticus

Cardiovascular	Tachycardia, hypertension, myocardial ischaemia
Respiratory	Aspiration pneumonitis, ARDS, pulmonary oedema
Metabolic	Rhabdomyolysis, hyperthermia
Neurological	Hypoxic brain injury
Drug-induced	Respiratory depression, arrhythmia, hypotension, gastroparesis

4.2.3 Monitoring and weaning of sedation

- Patients requiring intensive care admission for SE require electroencephalogram (EEG) monitoring (continuous or daily).
- The EEG is used primarily to identify ongoing seizure activity.
- If seizure activity persists, despite induction of general anaesthesia, sedative agents (thiopental, propofol, a benzodiazepine, or a combination of the three) are up-titrated until *burst suppression* is seen on the EEG.
- When the patient has been seizure-free for 24 hours and has been adequately loaded with an appropriate anti-epileptic agent, then anaesthetic agent is tapered.
- Failure to wake appropriately should prompt further EEG to rule out ongoing non-convulsive SE.
- It should be appreciated that thiopental and benzodiazepines, in the doses used in SE suppression, may take several days to fall below non-sedating levels in the plasma.

4.3 The electroencephalogram

4.3.1 General

- The electroencephalogram (EEG) is the summation of electrical activity in the brain, as measured by electrodes placed on the scalp.
- Most EEG activity represents activity of the pyramidal neurones of the cortex.

4.3.2 Role

- Roles in the intensive care include:
  - *Diagnosis*, with particular EEG patterns associated with a variety of conditions, including seizures (generalized, focal, myoclonic), encephalitis, encephalopathy, Creutzfeldt–Jakob disease, and subacute sclerosing panencephalitis.
  - *Monitoring*, for presence of ongoing seizure activity. Also of depth of sedation/awareness in non-neurological patients, particularly those requiring neuromuscular blocking agents. Monitoring may be conducted using bispectral index (BIS) technology—a modification of EEG technology designed for monitoring depth of anaesthesia in theatre; its use has not, however, been validated in the ICU.
  - *Prognostication*, as certain EEG patterns (burst suppression, generalized low voltage) are associated with poor neurological outcome in the context of anoxic brain injury.

4.3.3 Waveforms

- EEG waveforms are described in Table 5.15.

Table 5.15 The EEG waveform

Alpha waves (9–12 Hz)	Found primarily in occipital cortex, present when awake but eyes closed. May represent hypoxia if generalized and unchanged by stimulation.
Beta waves (13–20 Hz)	Fronto-temporal region, dominant when awake. Primary frequency in drug-induced coma.
Delta waves (0–4 Hz)	Occasionally seen in the awake adult. High-voltage delta waves represent metabolic encephalopathy.
Theta waves (4–8 Hz)	Dominant waveform in children; decrease with age.

5 Stroke and intracerebral haemorrhage

5.1 Stroke

5.1.1 Epidemiology

- Stroke is the third most common cause of death worldwide.
- 85% of strokes are ischaemic in aetiology and of those:
  - 35% the result of large artery thromboembolism
  - 24% cardiac in origin (atrial fibrillation, mural thrombus, infective endocarditis)
  - 18% small-vessel disease
  - Remainder due to vasculitis, arterial dissection, or of unknown aetiology

5.1.2 Presentation and immediate investigation

- Presentation of an ischaemic stroke is of a sudden onset focal neurological deficit, which, on examination, can be localized to a particular vascular territory.
- Focal neurology associated with altered conscious level, or severe headache, is suggestive of raised intracranial pressure and increases the likelihood of haemorrhage as a precipitant.
- Urgent neuroimaging is indicated to exclude bleed or space occupying lesion.
- If ischaemic stroke is the suspected diagnosis (ischaemia can rarely be confirmed on scan within the first few hours), reperfusion therapy should be considered.
- Blood glucose should be measured to exclude hypoglycaemia.

5.2 Approach to ischaemic stroke

5.2.1 General

- An ABC approach should be undertaken
- Early imaging
- Consideration of transfer to a specialist stroke unit, if appropriate facilities are not available locally

5.2.2 Reperfusion therapy

- Reperfusion therapy may be indicated in the treatment of ischaemic stroke.
- The American Society of Physicians recommends reperfusion with systemic tissue plasminogen activator (TPA), if the following conditions are met:
  - TPA can be delivered within 3 hours (grade 1A recommendation) or within 4.5 hours (grade 2C) of symptom onset
  - There is moderate to severe neuro-disability as a consequence of the stroke
  - There are no absolute contra-indications, i.e.:
    - Blood on CT
    - Severe hypertension

    ■ Surgery or trauma within 14 days

    ■ Known coagulopathy

- Direct intra-arterial thrombolysis may be performed up to 6 hours after the event, and is recommended as first line for acute basilar strokes.
- Aspirin should be started for all strokes within 48 hours; the initial dose should be administered as soon as haemorrhage is excluded on initial CT scan.
- The exception is in patients receiving TPA, in which case aspirin should be withheld until the 24 hours post-TPA scan demonstrates no bleed.
- Anticoagulation is not routinely recommended but should be considered in those with a cardiac cause of stroke from 2 weeks post-event onwards.

5.2.3 Surgical intervention

- *Decompressive craniectomy* may be considered in younger patients (<65 years) with large supra-tentorial infarcts with oedema.
- Removal of overlying skull leads to decrease in ICP, prevents herniation, and increases CPP.
- There is evidence that early (< 48 hours) decompression reduces mortality and improves functional outcome.

5.2.4 Intensive care admission

- Patients may be admitted to the ICU following stroke for a number of reasons (Table 5.16).

Table 5.16 Reasons for admission to ICU following stroke

	Reasons for ICU admission following stroke
Airway management	If altered consciousness is compromising airway patency
Neuro-monitoring	Post-thrombolysis
	Following stroke at high risk of neurological deterioration (brainstem, cerebellar, large haemorrhagic)
	Associated seizures
	Raised ICP
	Decreased GCS
Haemodynamic monitoring	Uncontrolled hypertension
	Arrhythmias
Other	Following surgical procedure
	Facilitate glycaemic control
	Management of complications (sepsis, pneumonia)

FURTHER READING

Jauch EC, Saver JL, Adams HP, et al. Guidelines for the early management of patients with acute ischemic stroke a guideline for healthcare professionals from the American Heart Association/American Stroke Association. *Stroke* 2013; 44(3): 870–947.

Tissue plasminogen activator for acute ischemic stroke. The National Institute of Neurological Disorders and Stroke rt-PA Stroke Study Group. *New England Journal of Medicine* 1995; 333(24): 1581–7.

Vahedi K, Hofmeijer J, Juettler E, et al. Early decompressive surgery in malignant infarction of the middle cerebral artery: a pooled analysis of three randomised controlled trials. *The Lancet Neurology* 2007; 6(3): 215–22.

5.3 Intracerebral haemorrhage

5.3.1 General

- Intracerebral haemorrhage accounts for only 10–30% of strokes but a disproportionate amount of death and disability.
- The majority of bleeds are related to hypertension and occur as a primary event (i.e. rupture of artery rather the bleeding from another pathology, such arterio-venous malformation or trauma).
- The pathology is tri-phasic:
  - The initial haemorrhage causes focal neurology in conjunction with evidence of raised ICP (vomiting, headache, decreased conscious state); dysautonomia, in the form of hypertension, tachycardia, fever, and hyperglycaemia, is common.
  - The haematoma expands, by often 30% of original size, for several hours; this phase is a major determinant of final outcome.
  - There follows peri-haematoma oedema from around 3 hours post-event and evolves over several days; this is believed secondary to the activation of the inflammatory response and clotting cascade, and disruption of the blood–brain barrier.
- CT brain is the initial investigation of choice but may be followed by angiography to identify vascular abnormalities underlying the bleed.

5.3.2 Management

- Intensive care management is aimed primarily at prevention of secondary neurological injury and therefore adheres to the principles of neuro-protection described for TBI.
- Specific considerations in spontaneous intracerebral haemorrhage include:
  - Reversal of anticoagulation:
    - Warfarin therapy is often a contributory factor in intracerebral haemorrhage.
    - Coagulopathy should be urgently reversed with vitamin K and clotting factor replacement, either in the form of fresh frozen plasma or prothrombin complex concentrate.
  - Haemostasis:
    - Recombinant factor VIIa has been investigated as a means of arresting bleeding in the non-anticoagulated patient.
    - Its use has been shown to reduce final haematoma size; however, the largest study in the field (FAST) failed to demonstrate any improvement in patient outcomes.
  - Clot evacuation:
    - Early surgical intervention for intracerebral haemorrhage is controversial.
    - The STITCH study demonstrated no benefit in evacuating supra-tentorial haematoma within the first 24 hours.
    - However, some subgroups showed a trend towards better outcomes (the young, large lobar haematomas, significant mass effect).

5.3.3 Outcomes

- At 6 months, 30–50% of patients are dead; less than 20% are independent.
- Predictors of poor outcome are large-volume bleed, old age, coma on presentation, need for ventilation, intraventricular extension, and posterior fossa haemorrhage.

FURTHER READING

Mayer SA, Brun NC, Begtrup K, et al. Efficacy and safety of recombinant activated factor VII for acute intracerebral hemorrhage. *New England Journal of Medicine* 2008; 358(20): 2127–37.

Mendelow AD, Gregson BA, Fernandes HM, et al. Early surgery versus initial conservative treatment in patients with spontaneous supratentorial intracerebral haematomas in the International Surgical Trial in Intracerebral Haemorrhage (STICH): a randomised trial. *Lancet* 2005; 365(9457): 387–97.

6 Subarachnoid haemorrhage

6.1 General

6.1.1 Aetiology

- Subarachnoid haemorrhage (SAH) occurs most commonly due to rupture of aneurysm (80%), with the vast majority (90–95%) lying in the anterior Circle of Willis.

6.1.2 Presentation

- Presentation is classically with sudden onset ('thunder-clap'), severe ('worst ever') headache, often associated with vomiting, meningism, focal neurology, and decreased conscious level.

6.1.3 Differential diagnosis

- The differential diagnosis includes migraine, tension headache, and stroke.
- Missed diagnosis is common and a high index of suspicion required.

6.2 Investigation

6.2.1 CT scan

- Urgent CT brain is the investigation of choice; fine cuts should be employed to minimize the risk of missed bleed.
- Characteristic findings are high-density material in the basal cisterns, and often throughout the cerebrospinal fluid.
- There may be associated cerebral oedema, hydrocephalus, or intraparenchymal blood.

6.2.2 Lumbar puncture

- CT scan is false-negative in a small number of SAH (2%); if SAH is suspected, negative CT should be followed, at least 6 hours post-symptom onset, by lumbar puncture with particular focus on opening pressure, red cell count, and the presence of xanthochromia (the degradation product of red cells in cerebrospinal fluid).

6.2.3 Vascular imaging

- On diagnosis of SAH, four vessel digital subtraction angiography or CT angiography is required to identify underlying aneurysm and determine the vascular anatomy in preparation for definitive management.

6.3 Scoring system

6.3.1 World Federation of Neurosurgeons system

- Severity of SAH is commonly clinically classified by the World Federation of Neurosurgeons grading (Table 5.17).

Table 5.17 World Federation of Neurosurgeons grading of subarachnoid haemorrhage

Grade	Description
1	GCS 15 with no motor deficit
2	GCS 13–14 with no motor deficit
3	GCS 13–14 with associated motor deficit
4	GCS 7–12 irrespective of motor function
5	GCS 3–6 irrespective of motor function

Adapted from *Journal of Neurology, Neurosurgery, and Psychiatry*, 51, Teasdale G et al., 'A universal subarachnoid hemorrhage scale: report of a committee of the World Federation of Neurosurgical Societies'. Copyright (1988) with permission from BMJ Publishing Group Ltd.

- Fisher system:
  - The Fisher system provides a radiological means of grading SAH (Table 5.18).

Table 5.18 Fisher scale of subarachnoid haemorrhage

Grade	Radiological appearance
I	No blood
II	Diffuse disposition of SAH without clots or layers of blood >1 mm
III	Localized clots and/or vertical layers of blood >1 mm thickness
IV	Diffuse or no subarachnoid blood but intracerebral or intraventricular clots

Adapted from *Neurosurgery*, 6, Fisher et al., 'Relation of cerebral vasospasm to subarachnoid hemorrhage visualized by computerized tomographic scanning', pp. 1-9. Copyright (1980) with permission from Wolters Kluwer Health, Inc.

6.4 Management

- The intensive care management of SAH is guided by the Neuro-Critical Care Consensus Guidelines (2011).
- Management should occur at a high-volume centre capable of urgent and definitive neurosurgical intervention.
- There are four main areas of management.

6.4.1 Effects of the haemorrhage

- The principles underpinning management of any neurological injury apply to SAH.
- Neuro-protective strategies should be employed.
- Blood pressure management may be problematic:
  - A MAP sufficient to maintain CPP is necessary; however, hypertension prior to securing the aneurysm increases the risk of rebleed.
  - It is recommended that systolic blood pressure should be maintained below 140 mmHg, whilst the aneurysm is unsecured.
  - Beta blockers are the agent of choice, as vasodilators may dilate cerebral vessels and increase ICP.

6.4.2 Early rebleeding

- The overall risk of rebleed is around 30%, the likelihood dependent upon the site of the aneurysm, presence of clot, degree of vasospasm, age, and sex.
- Mortality following rebleed is around 40%.
- Early repair of aneurysm significantly reduces the risk of rebleed.
- The aneurysm may be secured by either surgical clipping or endovascular coiling.
- The ISAT study reported better outcomes and lower resource use in coiling and this has become the modality of choice where technically feasible.
- Advantages and disadvantages of coiling and clipping are outlined in Table 5.19.
- The use of the anti-fibrinolytic agent tranexamic acid prior to coiling is believed to reduce the risk of rebleed; the duration should not exceed 72 hours.

Table 5.19 Advantages and disadvantages of endovascular coiling and surgical clipping

	Endovascular coiling	Surgical clipping
Advantages	Cheaper	More experience
	Less invasive	Ability to manage complications
	Better for posterior fossa lesions	Best for wide-necked aneurysm
	Less vasospasm	
	Option for intra-arterial nimodipine	
Disadvantages	Interventional radiology service required	Open procedure
	Some aneurysms not amenable to coiling	Requires general anaesthesia
	Requires anticoagulation	

6.4.3 Hydrocephalus

- Blockage of the ventricular system with blood can cause hydrocephalus and subsequently an increase in ICP.
- Hydrocephalus should be suspected in any SAH patient with a fall in GCS or change in pupillary response; CT will confirm the diagnosis.
- Hydrocephalus is managed by insertion of a drain:
  - Most commonly an extra-ventricular drain (EVD).
  - The EVD is typically inserted at 'Kocher's point', a landmark 2–3 cm from the midline and 1 cm anterior to the coronal suture, which allows access to the ventricle avoiding the motor cortex.
  - In the case of *communicating hydrocephalus*, in which drainage from the ventricular system into the spinal subarachnoid space continues, a lumbar ventricular drain may be preferred.

6.4.4 Vasospasm/delayed cerebral ischaemia (DCI)

- A common complication of SAH, DCI leads to ischaemic neurological injury.
- It commonly occurs between days 4 and 14, is angiographically evident in up to 70% of SAH, but only causes symptoms in around 30%.
- Prophylactic nimodipine (60 mg qid for 21 days) has been demonstrated to significantly reduce the incidence of DCI.
- Nimodipine may be administered enterally or intravenously; the former is associated with lower incidence of hypotension.
- A number of means of monitoring for DCI are available (Table 5.20).

Table 5.20 Monitoring for delayed cerebral ischaemia

Clinical	<ul><li>Drop in GCS, new focal neurology</li><li>Advantages: free, quick, easily repeatable</li><li>Disadvantages: subjective, assessment impaired by sedation, non-specific</li></ul>
Digital subtraction angiography	<ul><li>The gold standard</li><li>Allows simultaneous intervention if vasospasm detected</li><li>Requires specialist centre, transfer to radiology department, risk of arterial injury/haemorrhage, small risk of stroke</li></ul>
CT angiography	<ul><li>Allows examination of the brain parenchyma and delineation of cerebral vasculature</li><li>Avoids the need for arterial access</li><li>Unlikely to be as sensitive as DSA; does not allow for intervention</li></ul>
Transcranial Doppler	<ul><li>Quick, bedside test that measures arterial velocity</li><li>Velocity in the middle cerebral artery >200 cm.s^{-1} is suggestive of DCI. This may be confirmed by use of the Lindegaard index (middle cerebral artery velocity/external carotid velocity): an index >3 is strongly predictive of DCI.</li><li>Operator dependent</li></ul>
EEG	<ul><li>May demonstrate focal changes in keeping with vasospasm</li><li>Non-invasive bedside test</li><li>Requires expertise</li></ul>

- Risk factors for DCI include:
  - High Fisher grade
  - Smoker
  - Previous hypertension
  - Female
  - Coma on admission

6.4.5 Management of delayed cerebral ischaemia

- Strategies for the management of DCI are described in Table 5.21.

Table 5.21 Management of delayed cerebral ischaemia

Induced hypertension	Generally agreed that increasing blood pressure reduces the incidence and significance of vasospasm. Aneurysm must first be secured. Blood pressure can be titrated to clinical response (i.e. better neurology observed with higher MAP).
Hydration	Target euvolaemia. Supra-physiological hypervolaemia is probably not beneficial and may result in complications; hypovolaemia is probably harmful.
Intra-arterial nimodipine	Nimodipine may be administered intra-arterially during angiography.
Balloon angioplasty	Angiography offers the option of balloon dilatation of vessels in spasm.
Other proposed therapies	Other therapies proposed and undergoing investigation include magnesium sulphate, statins and intrathecal thrombolytic agents.

FURTHER READING

Connolly ES, Rabinstein AA, Carhuapoma JR, et al. Guidelines for the management of aneurysmal subarachnoid hemorrhage a guideline for healthcare professionals from the American heart association/American stroke association. *Stroke* 2012; 43(6): 1711–37.

Diringer MN, Bleck TP, Hemphill III JC, et al. Critical care management of patients following aneurysmal subarachnoid hemorrhage: recommendations from the Neurocritical Care Society's Multidisciplinary Consensus Conference. *Neurocritical Care* 2011; 15(2): 211–40.

Fisher C, Kistler J, Davis J. Relation of cerebral vasospasm to subarachnoid hemorrhage visualized by computerized tomographic scanning. *Neurosurgery* 1980; 6(1): 1–9.

Hillman J, Fridriksson S, Nilsson O, Yu Z, Säveland H, Jakobsson K-E. Immediate administration of tranexamic acid and reduced incidence of early rebleeding after aneurysmal subarachnoid hemorrhage: a prospective randomized study. *Journal of Neurosurgery* 2002; 97(4): 771–8.

Molyneux A, Group ISATC. International Subarachnoid Aneurysm Trial (ISAT) of neurosurgical clipping versus endovascular coiling in 2143 patients with ruptured intracranial aneurysms: a randomised trial. *Lancet* 2002; 360(9342): 1267–74.

Pickard J, Murray G, Illingworth R, et al. Effect of oral nimodipine on cerebral infarction and outcome after subarachnoid haemorrhage: British aneurysm nimodipine trial. *British Medical Journal* 1989; 298(6674): 636–42.

Teasdale G, Drake C, Hunt W, et al. A universal subarachnoid hemorrhage scale: report of a committee of the World Federation of Neurosurgical Societies. *Journal of Neurology, Neurosurgery, and Psychiatry* 1988; 51(11): 1457.

7 Neuromuscular disorders

7.1 Weakness on the intensive care

7.1.1 General

- Generalized weakness is common in intensive care, both as a cause for admission and as a sequalae of other illnesses.

7.1.2 Differential diagnosis

- The differential diagnosis is vast and pathology may lie anywhere from cerebrum to muscle (Table 5.22).

Table 5.22 Differential diagnosis of ICU weakness

Cerebral cortex	Vascular event
	Encephalopathy
Brainstem	Pontine infarction or haemorrhage
Spinal cord	Transverse myelitis
	Compression (tumour, abscess, or haemorrhage)
	Ischaemia
	Infection (CMV, mycoplasma, legionella, herpes)
	Motor neurone disease
	Poliomyelitis

Peripheral nerves	Guillian–Barre syndrome
	Critical illness polyneuropathy
	Eaton–Lambert syndrome
	Uraemia
	Mononeuropathies
Neuromuscular junction	Myasthaenia gravis
	Botulism
	Residual neuromuscular blocking agent
Muscle fibre	Steroid myopathy
	Electrolyte derangement ($\downarrow PO_4$ or K^+; $\uparrow Mg^{2+}$)
	Critical illness myopathy
	Disuse atrophy
	Polymyositis

7.2 Myasthaenia gravis

7.2.1 General

- Myasthaenia gravis (MG) is an autoimmune disorder characterized by autoantibodies against the nicotinic acetylcholine receptor at the neuromuscular junction.
- The resultant weakness is classically distributed in the facial and bulbar muscles but can also affect respiratory function.
- The hallmark of MG is fatiguability: repeated effort in any muscle group leads to rapidly progressive weakness, and symptoms typically worsen towards the end of the day.
- Thymic hyperplasia is common; thymoma occurs in around 10%; thymectomy often leads to long-term remission.
- MG is associated with several other autoimmune disorders, including rheumatoid arthritis, systemic lupus erythematosus, and pernicious anaemia.

7.2.2 Investigation

- Investigation is by means of a Tensilon test in which the acetylcholine-esterase inhibitor edrophonium (Tensilon) is administered.
- Improvement in symptoms in response to the resultant increase in acetylcholine at the neuromuscular junction is sensitive but not particularly specific for MG.
- Tensilon tests must be medically supervised with access to resuscitation equipment, given the potential for severe cholinergic side-effects, particularly profound bradycardia.
- Electromyography (EMG) provides a more accurate investigation.
- Repetitive nerve stimulation demonstrates reduction in muscle action potential.
- Serum antibodies against acetylcholine receptors can be measured.

7.2.3 Management

- MG is usually well controlled with a combination of:
  - Acetylcholine potentiation (via the long-acting acetylcholine-esterase inhibitor pyridiostigmine)
  - Immunosuppression (steroids and azathioprine)

7.2.4 Myasthenic crisis

- This is a rapid and life-threatening deterioration in disease state.
- Common precipitants include:
  - Intercurrent illness
  - Pregnancy
  - Drug issues (gentamicin, morphine, suxamethonium, and pethidine have all been implicated)
  - Surgery
- Myasthenic crises are commonly referred to intensive care for either respiratory failure, or an airway at risk due to bulbar palsy.
- The specific therapies for myasthenic crisis are:
  - High-dose steroids (50–100 mg prednisolone/24 hours or equivalent)
  - Plus either *plasma exchange* (5x 3 l exchange over 2 weeks) or *intravenous immunoglobulin* (5-day course)

7.3 Guillian–Barre syndrome

7.3.1 General

- Gullian–Barre syndrome (GBS) is an autoimmune disease believed to be the result of antibodies produced against pathogens (Box 5.2) cross-reacting with neuronal myelin sheaths.
- The result is demyelination of peripheral nerves.

Box 5.2 Pathogens associated with Gullian–Barre syndrome

Campylobacter (40%)

Mycoplasma (5%)

Cytomegalovirus (15%)

Epstein–Barr virus

HIV

7.3.2 Clinical features

- GBS manifests as a symmetrical, ascending neuropathy progressing over just a few days.
- Motor symptoms predominate but sensory impairment does occur.
- Prodromal illness (typically diarrhoea) is common and neurological symptoms are often heralded by back pain and vague paraesthesia.
- Examination reveals a symmetrical polyneuropathy; absence of reflexes is universal.
- Autonomic involvement is common: arrhythmia, postural hypotension, sweating, and urinary retention are all features of GBS.
- The diagnosis is largely clinical; supporting investigations, however, include characteristic EMG and cerebrospinal fluid obtained from lumbar puncture with an isolated rise in protein.

7.3.3 Management

- Intensive care involvement relates to respiratory impairment (30% of GBS patients require ventilator support) and autonomic instability.
- Ventilation:
  - The key determinant of the need for ventilator support is the forced vital capacity (FVC).

- This should be performed on admission and 4-hourly thereafter.
- An FVC of 20 ml/kg or less necessitates transfer to a critical care area; FVC of 15 ml/kg or less warrants endotracheal intubation and mechanical ventilation.
- Induction of anaesthesia may be complicated by the autonomic dysfunction (large blood pressure swings and bradycardia may be encountered).
- Suxamethonium should be avoided lest it precipitate life-threatening hyperkalaemia in the presence of muscle denervation.
- Specific management:
  - *Plasma exchange* (3–5 treatments over 5–8 days; 40 ml/kg exchange per session); this may not be well tolerated in the presence of autonomic instability and comes with the risks of central vascular access and connection to an extracorporeal circuit.
  - The alternative is *intravenous immunoglobulin*: as effective as plasma exchange, it avoids the risks of vascular access but is more expensive and increases the risk of venous thrombus.
- Steroids have *no role* in the treatment of GBS and indeed appear to increase mortality.

7.4 Critical illness myoneuropathy

7.4.1 General

- Weakness in the critically ill patient may be the result of a pre-existing neuromuscular disorder, a previously undiagnosed neuromuscular disorder, or as a complication of their critical illness.
- Critical illness myoneuropathy (CIMN) is a diagnosis of exclusion, when all other causes of peripheral weakness (Table 5.22) have been discounted.
- It is an under-recognized phenomenon, which is believed to affect between 25% and 80% of critically ill patients; of those patients with a critical care stay longer than 28 days, 90% will exhibit EMG evidence of neuromuscular abnormality 5 years later.
- The mechanism is poorly understood; a combination of microcirculatory damage, direct neurotoxicity, and cytokine-mediated injury has been proposed.
- Several risk factors have been proposed (Box 5.3).

Box 5.3 Risk factors for critical illness myoneuropathy

Sepsis
Corticosteroids
Neuromuscular blocking agents
Hyperglycaemia
Electrolyte derangement ($\downarrow K^+, PO_4^-, Mg^{2+}$)
Immobility

7.4.2 Clinical features and diagnosis

- Diagnosis is difficult.
- CIMN should be suspected in any intensive care patient with unexplained weakness; difficulty in ventilatory wean being often the first indicator of weakness.
- Presentation is variable:
  - Motor deficit is usually symmetrical but ranges from mild weakness to quadriplegia.
  - The face is usually spared.
  - Reflexes are typically reduced or absent.
  - Around 50% of patients exhibit sensory loss.

- Investigation should begin by excluding alternative diagnoses:
  - Imaging of brain and spinal cord is necessary to exclude a central cause for the symptoms.
  - EMG is useful: it either allows identification of alternative diagnoses or will yield the typical pattern of CIMN (reduced action potential with normal conduction velocity).
  - Muscle biopsy is not routinely performed but should be undertaken if needed, for cases of diagnostic uncertainty; typically demonstrates a reduced actin/myosin ratio in CIMN.

7.4.3 Prevention and treatment

- No specific treatment exists for CIMN; prevention is preferable (Box 5.4).
- Most will require prolonged respiratory wean but complete functional recovery can be expected in around 70% of patients.
- Some will, however, remain disabled, with impairment ranging from mild sensory impairment to complete functional dependence.

Box 5.4 Prevention of critical illness myoneuropathy

Aggressive treatment of sepsis

Tight glucose control

Avoidance of steroids

Avoidance of neuromuscular blockers

Minimize sedative use

Regular physiotherapy

Optimize nutrition

8 Delirium

8.1 General

8.1.1 Features

- Delirium is common in the intensive care population affecting in excess of 80% of patients. It is a syndrome characterized by:
  - Disturbance in consciousness with reduced ability to focus attention.
  - Change in cognition or a perceptual disturbance not accounted for by pre-existing cognitive impairment.
  - Onset over a short period of time (hours to days) and a fluctuating course.
  - Evidence from history, examination, and investigation of a physical precipitant.

8.1.2 Associated factors

- Delirium is associated with:
  - Increased length of stay
  - Increased cost; increased mortality
  - Increased need for nursing home placement
  - Long-term cognitive dysfunction

8.2 Delirium assessment

8.2.1 Subtypes

- There are three subtypes of delirium:
    - Hyperactive delirium, which manifests as agitation, restlessness, and attempts to remove tubes and lines.
    - Hypoactive delirium, characterized by withdrawal, flat affect, apathy, lethargy, and reduced responsiveness.
    - Mixed delirium in which patients fluctuate between the two.
- Mixed and hypoactive are most common in the intensive care.

8.2.2 Screening

- Recognition of delirium is often difficult unless active screening is undertaken.
- The most commonly employed tool for identification of delirium is the confusion assessment monitor in ICU (CAM-ICU) (Box 5.5):
    - A four-point scale
    - Suitable for non-verbal patients, so long as RAAS is greater than or equal to −3

Box 5.5 CAM-ICU.

CAM-ICU
1. Acute change or fluctuating course of mental status: • Is there a change from mental status baseline? OR   • Has the patient's mental state fluctuated in the last 24 hours?
2. Inattention: • *Squeeze my hand when I say the letter 'A'.*   • Read the following sequence of letters: S A V E A H A A R T   • Errors: no squeeze on letter 'A'; squeeze on letters other than A
3. Altered level of consciousness: • Current RASS   • RASS other than zero is considered positive
4. Disorganized thinking: • Will a stone float on water?   • Are there fish in the sea?   • Does one pound weigh more than two?   • Can you use a hammer to pound a nail?
1 error is considered as positive

Adapted from *Critical Care Medicine*, 29, Ely et al., 'Evaluation of delirium in critically ill patients: validation of the Confusion Assessment Method for the Intensive Care Unit (CAM-ICU)', pp.1370–1379. Copyright (2001) with permission from Wolters Kluwer Health, Inc.

- Patients positive in both steps 1 and 2, and either 3 or 4, are considered to be CAM-ICU positive and therefore delirious.

8.3 Risk factors and prevention

8.3.1 Risk factors

- Recognized risk factors are outlined in Table 5.23.

Table 5.23 Risk factors for delirium

Pre-existing factors	Intensive care factors
Increasing age	High APACHE score
Pre-existing cognitive impairment	Mechanical ventilation
Alcohol, drug, or nicotine dependence	Metabolic acidosis
Hypertension	Coma
Emergency surgery or trauma	Steroids
	Sepsis
	Benzodiazepines

8.3.2 Prevention

- Prevention of delirium is based upon avoidance of precipitating factors when possible.
- Avoidance of benzodiazepines, with preferential use of propofol and α2 agonists (e.g. clonidine) if sedation is required.
- Attention should be paid to:
  - Good sleep hygiene
  - Maintenance of a normal sleep–wake cycle
  - Removal of unnatural stimuli, where possible (e.g. early de-escalation of monitoring)
  - Involvement of family
  - Early mobilization
  - Frequent orientation

8.4 Treatment

8.4.1 Contributing causes

- Consideration should be given to potentially reversible, contributing causes:
  - Hypoxia
  - Hypoglycaemia
  - Uraemia
  - Sepsis
  - CNS infection
  - Urinary retention
  - Alcohol or substance withdrawal

8.4.2 Pharmacological management

- The mainstay of management is the anti-psychotic agents (either typical, e.g. haloperidol, or atypical, e.g. quetiapine).
- There is no convincing evidence that anti-psychotic agents have a role in the *prevention* of delirium.
- There is weak evidence that they may reduce the duration of delirium and ICU stay.

- Anti-psychotics offer a degree of control in hyperactive patients at risk of harm.
- Dexmedetomidine may offer an alternative treatment but there is limited evidence supporting its role in the management of established delirium.

FURTHER READING

Devlin JW, Roberts RJ, Fong JJ, et al. Efficacy and safety of quetiapine in critically ill patients with delirium: a prospective, multicenter, randomized, double-blind, placebo-controlled pilot study. *Critical Care Medicine* 2010; 38(2): 419–27.

Ely EW, Margolin R, Francis J, et al. Evaluation of delirium in critically ill patients: validation of the Confusion Assessment Method for the Intensive Care Unit (CAM-ICU). *Critical Care Medicine* 2001; 29(7): 1370–9.

National Institute for Clinical Excellence. Delirium: diagnosis, prevention and management. *NICE Clinical Guideline* 2010; 103.

Page VJ, Ely EW, Gates S, et al. Effect of intravenous haloperidol on the duration of delirium and coma in critically ill patients (Hope-ICU): a randomised, double-blind, placebo-controlled trial. *Lancet Respiratory Medicine* 2013; 1(7): 515–23.

Pandharipande P, Shintani A, Peterson J, et al. Lorazepam is an independent risk factor for transitioning to delirium in intensive care unit patients. *Anesthesiology* 2006; 104(1): 21–6.

Reade MC, Finfer S. Sedation and delirium in the intensive care unit. *New England Journal of Medicine* 2014; 370(5): 444–54.

Zaal IJ, Devlin JW, Peelen LM, Slooter AJ. A systematic review of risk factors for delirium in the ICU. *Critical Care Medicine* 2015; 43(1): 40–7.

---

9 Central nervous system infections

9.1 General

- CNS infections are uncommon but are associated with high mortality, morbidity, and long-term disability.
- Presentation is often vague and therefore a high index of suspicion is required.

9.1.1 Types of central nervous system infections

- Meningitis
- Encephalitis
- Pyogenic infections
    - Brain abscesses
    - Empyema

9.2 Cerebral spinal fluid analysis

9.2.1 Lumbar puncture

- A key investigation in patients presenting with unexplained neurological symptoms or sepsis.
- Contra-indications:
    - Infection in overlying skin
    - Thrombocytopaenia (in the absence of other risk factors for bleeding, a platelet count of $>50 \times 10^9$ is generally accepted as safe for lumbar puncture)

- Coagulopathy and anticoagulation:
  - An INR >1.5 should be corrected prior to procedure.
  - Intravenous unfractionated heparin should be off for between 2 and 4 hours prior to lumbar puncture and should not be restarted for 1 hour post-procedure.
  - 12 hours between *prophylactic* low molecular weight heparin dose and procedure; 24 hours between *therapeutic* low molecular weight heparin and procedure; should be withheld for 24 hours post-procedure.
- Raised intracranial pressure or presence of space occupying lesion:
  - A lumbar puncture should not be performed if there is suspicion of raised intracranial pressure or space occupying lesion.
  - A CT or MRI scan should be undertaken to look for evidence of raised intracranial pressure prior to lumbar puncture if:
    - Altered level of consciousness
    - Focal neurology
    - History of CNS lesions
    - Immunosuppression
    - Clinical evidence of raised intracranial pressure
- Ideally, lumbar puncture and CSF sampling should occur prior to administration of antimicrobials (as this slightly decreases the yield of CSF culture); delay to lumbar puncture should not, however, delay antimicrobials (as early administration is associated with improved outcomes); blood culture taken at time of intravenous cannulation provides an alternative means of microbiological diagnosis.

9.2.2 CSF analysis

- Samples should be sent for:
  - Microscopy:
    - Cell count
    - Gram stain
  - Culture and sensitivity
  - Biochemistry
    - Protein
    - Glucose (send simultaneous plasma glucose)
  - Possible antigen studies:
    - *Pneumococcus*
    - *Meninococcus*
    - Group B *Streptococcus*
    - *Haemophilus influenzae*
  - In patients at risk, send for tuberculosis analysis
  - In the immunocompromised, India ink stain for *Cryptococcus*
- Bacterial meningitis (<-> denotes normal range)
  - WCC: neutrophils↑; lymphocytes <->
  - Glucose (CSF:blood ratio) <0.4
  - Protein >1 g.l^{-1}
- Viral meningitis
  - WCC: neutrophils<->; lymphocytes↑
  - Glucose (CSF:blood ratio) >0.6 (normal)
  - Protein 0.4–1.0 g.l^{-1}

- Tuberculosis or fungal meningitis
  - WCC: Neutrophils<->; Lymphocytes↑↑
  - Glucose (CSF:blood ratio) <0.3
  - Protein 1–5 g.l⁻¹
- Subarachnoid haemorrhage
  - Presence of red blood cells; number of cells don't decrease on consecutive bottles (as would be the case if blood arose from the lumbar puncture itself).
  - Spinning of CSF will reveal xanthochromia in subarachnoid haemorrhage.

9.2.3 Red cells and impact upon interpretation of WCC

- Red blood cells in the CSF sample indicate the presence of blood; whilst this may occur secondary to a subarachnoid haemorrhage, the most common explanation is a 'traumatic tap'.
- If blood has entered the CSF, then it stands to reason that this contains both red cells and white cells; the challenge in analysis is determining what proportion of the WCC arises from blood in the CSF, and what proportion relates to meningeal inflammation.
- The contribution of blood to the CSF WCC can be determined from the ratio of WCC to red cell count (RCC) in the patient's full blood count:

$$\text{Predicted CSF WCC} = \text{CSF RCC} \times \frac{\text{FBC WCC}}{\text{FBC RCC}}$$

- By subtracting the predicted CSF WCC from the actual CSF WCC, the contribution of meningeal inflammation may be determined.
- As a general rule of thumb—based upon a typical WCC:RCC ratio in the FBC—expect 1 additional white cell per mm³ for every 1,000 red cells per mm³.

9.3 Meningitis

9.3.1 General

- May be subdivided by:
  - Circumstance
    - Spontaneous
    - Post-traumatic
    - Post-neurosurgical
  - Organism
    - Bacterial
    - Viral
    - Fungal
    - Tuberculosis
    - Aseptic (e.g. autoimmune or malignancy)

9.3.2 Risk factors

- Age—the young are at greater risk.
- Environment—those living in close proximity to others (e.g. student halls, military barracks) are at increased risk of meningococcus.
- Travellers to sub-Saharan Africa during the dry season and Mecca for pilgrimage are at increased risk of meningococcus.

- Breach in the skull (e.g. neurosurgery or open skull fracture) increases the risk of *Staphylococcal* meningitis.
- Otitis media, pneumonia, or impaired defence against encapsulated organisms (e.g. asplenia) increase the risk of *Pneumococcal* meningitis.

9.3.3 Causative organisms by age

- The incidence of particular causative organisms varies with age.
- Neonatal:
  - *E. coli*
  - *Listeria monocyogenes*
  - Group B *Streptococcus*
- Children:
  - *Niserria meningitides (meningococcus)*
  - *Streptococcus pneumoniae (pneumococcus)*
  - *Haemophilus influenza*
- Adults:
  - *Neisserria meningitides*
  - *Streptococcus pneumoniae*
- Elderly:
  - *Streptococcus pneumoniae*
  - *Niserria meningitides*
  - *Listeria monocytogenes*
- Viral meningitis
  - Include:
    - *Echovirus*
    - *Enterovirus*
    - Mumps
    - *Herpes simplex* virus
    - *Cytomegalovirus*
    - *Epstein Barr* virus
    - *Varicella zoster* virus

9.3.4 Investigation

- CT brain
  - Identification of alternative diagnoses
  - Identification of raised intracranial pressure
  - Meningeal enhancement suggestive of meningitis
- Lumbar puncture
  - Biochemistry
  - Microscopy, cell count, and Gram stain
  - Culture and sensitivity
  - Viral PCR
  - +/− additional tests (see Section 9.2)

9.3.5 Management

- Organ support as required for altered level of consciousness and associated sepsis response.

- Antibiotics
  - Appropriate intravenous antibiotics should be given early (within first 30 min).
  - High-dose ceftriaxone is appropriate as a single agent in previously well, young adults.
  - If at risk of *Listeria* (e.g. elderly), amoxicillin should be added.
- Steroids
  - Administration of dexamethasone 0.15 mg.kg^{-1} prior to antibiotics is associated with a significant reduction in the incidence of hearing loss and neurological sequelae in bacterial meningitis of all aetiology; a mortality reduction with steroids has been reported in pneumococcal meningitis.
- Public health
  - Personal protection for healthcare professionals.
  - Liaison with public health is essential (meningococcus is a 'notifiable disease' in the UK).
  - Antibiotic prophylaxis should be offered to close contacts:
    - Those in prolonged close contact with the index case for the 7 days preceding admission (e.g. living and sleeping in the same household or institution, e.g. barracks/dormitories, and partners).
    - Those with transient close contact, if they have been exposed to respiratory secretions around time of admission to hospital.
  - Prophylaxis should *not* be routinely offered:
    - Colleagues or classmates
    - Friends
    - Kissing on cheek or mouth
    - Food or drink sharing
    - Travelling in the same vehicle
  - Antibiotic prophylactic options include:
    - Single-dose 500 mg ciprofloxacin (which does not interact with other drugs such as the contraceptive pill) or
    - Rifampicin 600 mg bd for 2 days (which may interact with the contraceptive pill)
    - Single dose of azithromycin 500 mg is recommended for pregnant women.
  - The patient and close contacts should be offered appropriate vaccination.

9.4 Encephalitis

9.4.1 *General*

- Inflammatory process affecting the brain parenchyma
- Most commonly viral in aetiology
  - *Herpes simplex* virus (most common)
  - Influenza
  - *Epstein–Barr* virus
  - HIV
  - *Enterovirus*
  - Measles
- Rarely bacterial
  - *Tuberculosis*
  - *Listeria*
  - *Syphilis*

- Occasionally autoimmune
    - Anti-NMDA receptor encephalitis (associated with teratomas)
    - Acute disseminated encephalomyelitis (typically secondary to infections, both viral (e.g. influenza, measles) and bacterial (e.g. *Salmonella, Pertussis*)

9.4.2 Features and investigation

- Presentation is often vague with a combination of neurological symptoms, particularly affecting higher functions.
- Investigation includes:
    - Full infective work up
    - Lumbar puncture
    - CT or MRI brain (HSV encephalitis demonstrates characteristic changes in the temporal lobes, although a negative scan does not exclude the diagnosis)

9.4.3 Treatment

- Supportive care
- Specific to cause
    - Acyclovir for suspected or confirmed HSV encephalitis (early administration is associated with better outcomes).
    - Immunomodulation (e.g. steroids, intravenous immunoglobulin, or plasma exchange) may be required for autoimmune processes.

FURTHER READING

Beckham JD, Tyler KL. Neuro-intensive care of patients with acute CNS infections. *Neurotherapeutics* 2012; 9(1): 124–38.

Brouwer MC, McIntyre P, Prasad K, van de Beek D. Corticosteroids for acute bacterial meningitis. *Cochrane Database of Systematic Reviews* 2013; 6: Cd004405.

Layton KF, Kallmes DF, Horlocker TT. Recommendations for anticoagulated patients undergoing image-guided spinal procedures. *American Journal of Neuroradiology* 2006; 27(3): 468–70.

Ramsay M. Guidance for public health management of meningococcal disease in the UK. *Health Protection Agency* 2012.

Simon DW, Da Silva YS, Zuccoli G, Clark RS. Acute encephalitis. *Critical Care Clinics* 2013; 29(2): 259–77.

Van Veen JJ, Nokes TJ, Makris M. The risk of spinal haematoma following neuraxial anaesthesia or lumbar puncture in thrombocytopenic individuals. *British Journal of Haematology* 2010; 148(1): 15–25.

Infection

CONTENTS

1 Principles of infection

Infection is a common cause for ICU admission and a common complication of critical illness.

1.1 Risk factors for infection in the critically ill

1.1.1 Patient factors

- Loss of natural barriers:
  - Tracheal intubation
  - Vascular access
  - Open wounds
- Reduction in immune function:
  - Drug-induced immunosuppression
  - Disease-induced immunosuppression
  - Nutritional state

1.1.2 Environmental factors (on the ICU)

- Relative overcrowding:
  - Multiple complex patients in one area
- Multiple staff contacts:
  - Complex patients requiring input from many professionals

1.1.3 Organisms

- Resistant organisms more common in the ICU environment:
  - High antibiotic use
  - Infection itself more common

1.2 Biomarkers of infection

- Most intensive care patients are inflammatory at some point in their admission.
- Not all inflammation is secondary to sepsis.

- It is desirable to differentiate between infective and non-infective causes of an inflammatory response, primarily for the purposes of antibiotic stewardship.
- 'Traditional' markers, such as white cell count and c-reactive protein (CRP), have no capacity to differentiate between infective and non-infective inflammation.
- The 'ideal' biomarker of infection would:
  - Differentiate between infective and non-infective causes
  - Rise and fall in line with clinical picture, with minimal time-lag
  - Allow quantification of the severity of infection

1.2.1 Procalcitonin

- Procalcitonin (PCT) is the precursor to calcitonin, synthesized in the thyroid C cells.
- In presence of bacterial infection, PCT is synthesized in neurohumeral tissues throughout the body.
- PCT is relatively specific to bacterial infection, although short-lived, small rises are seen in the context of major trauma and surgery.
- PCT rises as early as 4 hours post-bacteraemia, compared to 36 hours with CRP.
- The area under the Receiver Operator Curve for a PCT >2ng.ml^{-1} in diagnosis of bacterial infection has been reported as 0.82.
- Interpretation of the PCT result, and decisions regarding antibiotics, must however be made in the context of the clinical picture.

1.2.2 Broad-range bacterial PCR (16s)

- This test utilizes polymerase chain-reaction techniques to identify the ribosomal RNA of bacteria.
- The need to grow bacteria in the laboratory is therefore negated; this is particularly useful for those organisms resistant to *in vitro* growth.
- The test can be applied to any sample (blood, sputum, pleural fluid, etc.).

1.2.3 β-D Glucan

- β-D glucan is a component in most fungal cells walls.
- Detection of β-D glucan in plasma is highly suggestive of invasive fungal infection.

1.2.4 Galactomannan

- Galactomannan is a component of the cell wall of *Aspergillus* sp.
- Detection of galactomannan in plasma is highly suggestive of invasive *Aspergillus*.

1.3 Failure to respond to treatment

- Apparent failure of infection to respond to treatment may be due to numerous factors.

1.3.1 Patient-related

- Co-morbidity:
  - Directly impeding recovery from infection (e.g. bronchial neoplasm in non-resolving pneumonia)
  - Indirectly impeding recovery from infection (e.g. neuromuscular weakness in non-resolving pneumonia)
- Immunosuppression:
  - Pathological (e.g. HIV)
  - Pharmacological (e.g. immunosuppressant medication; bone marrow suppression)
- Ongoing contamination of sterile site (e.g. micro-aspiration; enteral leak)

1.3.2 Antibiotic-related

- Wrong antibiotic:
  - Bacteria not sensitive
  - Inadequate tissue penetration to the site of infection
- Inadequate dose or frequency leading to sub-therapeutic plasma levels.
- Antibiotic inactivation by bacteria (e.g. beta lactamase).

1.3.3 Disease-related

- Non-bacterial infection.
- Non-infective inflammatory process.
- Unrecognized secondary infection.
- Lack of source control.
- Development of collection (e.g. empyema in pneumonia, abscess in pancreatitis).

1.4 Infection control

- Prevention and management of resistant organisms.

1.4.1 Organizational

- Antibiotic policy:
  - Narrow spectrum
  - Limited formulary for non-specialist staff
  - Infectious disease/microbiology involvement
- Surveillance and eradication.
- Audit and quality assurance.

1.4.2 Local

- Avoidance of inappropriate antibiotics.
- Rigorous hand washing.
- Contact precautions.
- Cohorting of infected patients.

FURTHER READING

Dupuy A-M, Philippart F, Péan Y, et al. Role of biomarkers in the management of antibiotic therapy: an expert panel review: I–currently available biomarkers for clinical use in acute infections. *Annals of Intensive Care* 2013; 3(1): 22.

Kibe S, Adams K, Barlow G. Diagnostic and prognostic biomarkers of sepsis in critical care. *Journal of Antimicrobial Chemotherapy* 2011; 66(Suppl 2): ii33–40.

---

2 Antibiotics

2.1 Principles of antibiotics in intensive care

- Antimicrobials are a class of agents used to kill or suppress microorganisms.
- Antibiotic is a specific term for a substance produced by a microorganism, which has the capacity to kill or inhibit the growth another microorganism.

2.1.1 Roles of antibiotics

- Treatment of infection:
    - Empirical
    - Targeted
- Prophylaxis:
    - Selective digestive decontamination
- Non-antimicrobial role:
    - E.g. erythromycin as a prokinetic

2.1.2 Principles of use

- Right agent—ideally guided by direct microbiological evidence; empirical therapy should be guided by local infection and resistance patterns.
- Right time—early, within 1 hour of severe sepsis recognition.
- Right duration—empirical antibiotics should be switched as early as possible.

2.1.3 Pharmacology of antibiotics in critical illness

- Pharmacokinetics studied primarily in healthy volunteers.
- Critical illness impacts upon:
    - Absorption:
        - Gut oedema
        - Impaired gut function
        - Impaired splanchnic blood flow
    - Distribution:
        - Oedema and extra-corporeal circuits increase volume of distribution
    - Protein binding (which Impacts upon half-life and free drug availability):
        - Reduced protein availability
        - Acid–base derangement
        - Variable drug binding to extra corporeal circuits
    - Clearance:
        - Hepatic impairment reduces metabolism
        - Biliary obstruction impairs hepatic excretion
        - Renal impairment reduces renal excretion

2.1.4 Antibiotic dosing regimens

- The desired plasma levels vary between antibiotic classes but tend to fall into one of three patterns:
    - *Maximum concentration dependent (Cmax:MIC):*
        - E.g. aminoglycosides, metronidazole
        - Efficacy dependent upon the peak plasma concentration
        - Bolus dosing regimen
    - *Time above 'minimum inhibitory concentration (MIC)' dependent (T>MIC):*
        - E.g. penicillins, carbapenems, linezolid, clindamycin
        - Efficacy dependent upon the proportion of time with plasma concentrations greater than MIC
        - Frequent dosing or continuous infusion utilized
    - *Time and concentration dependent:*
        - E.g. quinolones
        - Area under the curve above the MIC line is the most important marker of efficacy (AUC:MIC)

2.1.5 Antibiotic resistance

- May be inherent or acquired:
    - Inherent—a natural resistance (e.g. the outer membrane surrounding Gram-negative bacteria is impenetrable to many antibiotics).
    - Acquired—the modification of existing genetic material to provide resistance.
- Mechanisms include:
    - Inactivation of antibiotic by bacterial enzyme, either degradation of the antibiotic or modification of activity (e.g. beta-lactamase).
    - Decreased target site penetration (e.g. impaired bacterial penetration or active efflux from the cell).
    - Altered target site (e.g. alteration of the protein binding site in MRSA confers resistance to penicillins).
- Resistance mechanisms are frequently encoded in bacterial plasmids and therefore potentially transmissible between bacteria (horizontal gene transfer).

2.2 Beta lactams

2.2.1 General

- Most commonly used group of antibiotics.
- Defined by the presence of a 'beta-lactam ring' within molecular structure.

2.2.2 Pharmacokinetics

- Absorption
    - Variable
    - Many beta lactams are available only in the parenteral form.
- Distribution
    - Variable protein binding:
        - Ampicillin 20%
        - Flucloxacillin 90%
    - Generally good tissue penetration but requires inflammation to penetrate central nervous system or bone.
- Metabolism
    - Excreted mostly unchanged.
- Excretion
    - Relatively short half-life (generally 1 hour or less with normal renal function).
    - Primarily renal excretion.
    - Probenecid blocks active tubular excretion and therefore increases plasma levels of most beta lactams.
    - Dose adjustment may be required in renal impairment, particularly benzylpenicillin and piperacillin.
    - Clearance via RRT is variable; dependent upon degree of protein binding (e.g. ampicillin undergoes greater clearance with RRT than flucloxacillin).
    - Plasma concentration of beta-lactams should be 4–5 times MIC and plasma levels should be maintained as long as possible between doses.
    - For this reason, in ICU beta lactams are often delivered as infusion rather than bolus dose.

2.2.3 Pharmacodynamics

- Bactericidal—beta-lactam ring binds to and inhibits bacterial transpeptidases thereby inhibiting cell wall synthesis:

- Gram-positive bacteria
  - Beta lactams weaken the thick glycopeptide wall, killing bacteria.
  - Synergistic effect with aminoglycosides (beta lactams will allow better aminoglycoside penetration).
  - They lack post-antibiotic effect.
- Gram-negative bacteria
  - Beta lactams weaken the thin glycopeptide wall and liposacharide envelope.
  - Cell death dependent upon osmotic influx of water.

2.2.4 Adverse effects

- Hypersensitivity—allergy in approximately 10% of cases; anaphylaxis in approximately 0.01% of cases.
- Encephalopathy—benzylpenicillin, particularly when CNS levels high (i.e. large doses in meningitis, renal dysfunction, and probenecid use).
- Reduction in seizure threshold—particularly benzylpenicillin and the carbapenems.
- Rash—particularly ampicillin; 10% of patients, rises to 95% in infectious mononucleosis.
- Gastrointestinal—diarrhoea; 0.3–0.7% incidence of pseudomembranous colitis.

2.2.5 Penicillins

- Further subdivided into:
  - Narrow-spectrum penicillins—e.g. benzypenicillin
  - Narrow-spectrum penicillins with beta-lactamase resistance—e.g. flucloxacillin
  - Extended spectrum penicillins—e.g. ampicillin
  - Anti-pseudomonas penicillins—e.g. piperacillin
- Benzylpenicillin:
  - Narrow spectrum.
  - Inactivated by gastric acid, therefore must be administered parenterally.
  - Typically effective against a wide range of Gram-positive bacterial, Gram-negative cocci, and some Gram-negative bacilli.
  - Typically ineffective against *Staphylococcus, Haemophilus influenza*, and *Pseudomonas spp.*
- Flucloxacillin:
  - A synthetic penicillin with moderate resistance to beta lactamase.
  - Well absorbed via oral route.
  - More effective than benzylpenicillin against *Staphylococcus*; less effective against other Gram-positive cocci.
  - Highly protein bound; limited clearance on RRT.
  - Can cause cholestatic jaundice.
- Ampicillin/amoxicillin:
  - Same range of effectiveness as benzylpenicillin, with greater Gram-negative bacilli cover (*Haemophilus influenza spp., Salmonella, Escherichia coli, Enterococcus faecalis*—although increasing resistance to the latter).
  - Amoxicillin provides superior bioavailability (therefore may be administered orally); also bactericidal to Gram-negative bacteria at lower concentrations.
  - The addition of clavulanic acid to amoxicillin irreversibly inhibits a wide range of beta lactamases and reduces the MIC.
- Piperacillin:
  - Broader spectrum but less potent than benzylpenicillin.

- Particularly effective against *Pseudomonas spp.*, *Serratia*, and *Citrobacter*.
- Beta-lactamase sensitive, therefore combined with beta-lactamase inhibitor tazobactam (which, unlike clauvanic acid, has no intrinsic anti-microbial activity).

2.2.6 Cephalosporins

- Cephalosporins are a broad and widely used group of beta-lactam antibiotics.
- Cephalosporins combine a beta-lactam ring with a hydrothiazide ring.
- Less susceptible to beta lactamase.
- Wide distribution, particularly effective at crossing inflamed membranes (e.g. ceftriaxone and inflamed meninges).
- Classified into successive generations; with each successive generation, Gram-positive cover is maintained, Gram-negative cover improves; some later generations demonstrate activity against *Pseudomonas spp.*
    - First-generation cephalosporins:
        - E.g. cefradine
        - Effective against beta-lactamase producing *Staphylococci, Streptococci*, and anaerobic Gram-positive cocci.
    - Second-generation cephalosporins:
        - E.g. cefuroxime
        - More resistant to beta lactamase; increased Gram-negative activity (*H. influenza, Neisseria gonorrhoeae, Klebsiella pneumoniae*, and *Enterobacter spp.*).
        - Widespread resistance to *E. faecalis, Acinobacter, Serratia*, and *Pseudomonas spp.*
        - Useful agents for abdominal cover but additional anaerobic cover required.
    - Third-generation cephalosporins:
        - E.g. ceftriaxone, cefotaxime.
        - Improved Gram-negative cover but slightly less effective against Gram-positive bacteria.
        - Typically effective against *Acinetobacter* and *Serratia*.
        - Ceftazidime is effective against *Pseudomonas*, although limited *Staphylococcus* cover.
        - The long half-life of ceftriaxone allows once daily dosing.
    - Fourth-generation cephalosporins:
        - Cefepime
        - Similar Gram-negative cover to ceftazidime (including anti-pseudomonal cover) but better Gram-positive cover.
    - Fifth-generation cephalosporins:
        - Ceftaroline
        - Similar Gram-positive and negative cover to cefotaxime but with activity against methicillin-resistant *Staphylococcus aureus*.

2.2.7 Carbapenems

- The broadest spectrum of any antimicrobial with Gram-positive, Gram-negative aerobic and anaerobic cover.
- Best administered as prolonged infusions (3 hours).
- Imipenem:
    - Very broad spectrum (although only moderate cover for *Citrobacter, Enterobacter spp.* and *Serratia*).
    - Partially metabolized by renal dehydropeptidase; cilastatin given concurrently to block this metabolic pathway.

- Excreted unchanged in urine; accumulates in renal failure; dose alteration required with renal replacement therapy.
- Hepatotoxicity—self-limiting rise in transaminase levels and cholestatic jaundice occur in 5–10% of patients; may be latency of onset of several days; acute liver failure has been reported.
- Meropenem:
  - Similar profile to imipenem but does not require concurrent cilastatin administration.
  - Some increase in Gram-negative cover but reduction in Gram-positive cover.

2.3 Macrolides

2.3.1 General

- Similar range of activity to penicillins:
  - Most Gram-positive bacteria
  - *N. meningitides*
  - *H. influenza*
  - Some anaerobes
  - Also have specific cover against *Mycoplasma pneumoniae* and *Legionella*

2.3.2 Pharmacokinetics

- Absorption
  - Good oral bioavailability.
- Distribution
  - Good lung but limited CSF penetration.
  - Variable protein binding.
- Metabolism
  - Metabolized primarily by the liver.
- Excretion
  - Significant amount excreted unchanged, therefore dose reduction required in kidney injury.

2.3.3 Pharmacodynamics

- Primarily bacteriostatic.
- Bind to the 50s ribosomal subunit preventing replication.

2.3.4 Adverse effects

- Gastrointestinal effects common (nausea, diarrhoea, hepatic dysfunction); prokinetic effect, which may be used for therapeutic purposes.
- Cardiovascular—prolong QT interval.
- Drug interaction—augment the effect of theophylline, warfarin, and digoxin.

2.3.5 Specific agents

- Erythromycin:
  - Parent compound.
  - Marked gastrointestinal effects: commonly used as a prokinetic agent (including prior to gastroscopy for suspected haemorrhage to improve visualization).
- Clarithromycin:
  - Fewer gastrointestinal effects.
  - Superior activity against *Streptococcus, Listeria*, and *Legionella* than erythromycin.

- Azithromycin:
  - Improved bioavailability.
  - Longer half-life allows once daily dosing.
  - Better Gram-negative cover.

2.4 Aminoglycosides

2.4.1 General

- A large group of antibiotics, of which only gentamicin, amikacin, neomycin, and tobramycin are in routine clinical use.
- Wide Gram-negative cover.
- Some Gram-positive cover (e.g. *Staphylococci*, some *Streptococci*).
- No anaerobic activity.
- Synergistic activity with beta lactams and vancomycin.

2.4.2 Pharmacokinetics

- Absorption
  - No absorption from gastrointestinal tract, therefore parenteral only.
- Distribution
  - Large polar molecules.
  - Low protein binding (20–30%).
  - Distribution is limited; poor intracellular, CSF, and sputum penetration.
- Metabolism
  - Not metabolized.
  - Aminoglycoside molecules are large and polar; active transport is required to access bacterial cells. Transport mechanisms may be inhibited by:
    - Divalent cations (Mg^{2+}, Ca^{2+})
    - Acidosis
    - Hypoxia
- Excretion
  - Excreted unchanged in urine.

2.4.3 Pharmacodynamics

- Bactericidal.
- Bind to the ribosomal 30s subunit, blocking protein synthesis.
- They have significant post-antibiotic effect.
- Administered as single doses with extended interval dosing.

2.4.4 Adverse effects

- Narrow therapeutic range.
- Ototoxicity may occur if significant aminoglycoside accumulation in the perilymph; risk is related to peak plasma concentrations and increased by renal dysfunction and concurrent use of furosemide.
- Nephrotoxicity: acute tubular necrosis occurs in up to 37% of intensive care patients given gentamicin.
- Muscular weakness—aminoglycosides reduce the pre-junctional release and post-junctional sensitivity of acetylcholine at the neuromuscular junctions; effect of non-depolarizing muscle relaxants is extenuated; aminoglycosides should be avoided in myasthenia gravis.

2.5 Quinolones

2.5.1 General

- See individual agents for cover (Section 2.5.5).

2.5.2 Pharmacokinetics

- Absorption
  - Good absorption, reduced by concurrent administration of magnesium, calcium, and iron.
- Distribution
  - Wide distribution with excellent penetration of the CSF.
  - Limited protein binding.
- Metabolism
  - Limited metabolism.
- Excretion
  - Largely excreted unchanged.

2.5.3 Pharmacodynamics

- Bactericidal.
- Inhibits subunit of DNA-gyrase.
- They some significant post-antibiotic effect.

2.5.4 Adverse effects

- Reduction of seizure threshold.
- Nausea, vomiting, and abdominal pain.
- Haemolysis in the presence of glucose-6-phosphatase deficiency.
- Interaction, e.g. increases plasma theophylline levels.

2.5.5 Specific agents

- Ciprofloxacin:
  - Most commonly used quinolone.
  - Broad Gram-negative cover, including *Pseudomonas*; some Gram-positive cover (*Streptococcus, Enterococcus*).
  - Available in oral and intravenous preparations.
  - Agent of choice for anthrax (with clindamycin) and pneumonic plague.
- Norfloxacin:
  - Oral only.
  - Prophylaxis against spontaneous bacterial peritonitis in patients with cirrhosis.
- Levofloxacin:
  - Intravenous agent.
  - Similar cover to ciprofloxacin with improved pneumococcal cover.
  - Effective against legionella.

2.6 Metronidazole

2.6.1 General

- Potent inhibitor of obligate anaerobes and protozoa.
  - Active against *Clostridium spp.*, *Bacteroides spp.*, *Treponema pallidum*, and *Campylobacter*

2.6.2 Pharmacokinetics

- Absorption
  - Well absorbed with almost 100% oral bioavailability.
- Distribution
  - Minimal protein binding.
  - Wide distribution including CSF, prostate, pleural fluid, cerebral abscess.
- Metabolism
  - Metabolized to active compounds by liver.
- Excretion
  - Excreted in urine.
  - Half-life of active drug unchanged in renal insufficiency.

2.6.3 Pharmacodynamics

- Unclear; thought to be related to the nitro-group.
- Bacterial strand breakage leads to cell death.

2.6.4 Adverse effects

- Nausea.
- Rarely rash, pancreatitis, peripheral nephropathy.

2.7 Glycopeptides

2.7.1 General

- Naturally occurring compounds, active against virtually all Gram-positive bacteria.
- Large molecular size prevents penetration of the lipid layer of Gram-negative bacteria.

2.7.2 Pharmacokinetics

- Absorption
  - Not absorbed, therefore parenteral route is the only route in treatment of systemic infections (teicoplanin licensed for intra-muscular use).
  - Enteral route for gastrointestinal infections.
- Distribution
  - Variable protein binding.
  - Bone and CSF penetration of vancomycin is very poor; better with teicoplanin.
- Metabolism
  - No metabolism.
- Excretion
  - Excreted largely unchanged in urine.
  - Variable half-life.
  - Narrow therapeutic range.
  - Monitoring of plasma levels required.
- Peak plasma level is governed by the dose; trough level is governed by the interval.

2.7.3 Pharmacodynamics

- Bactericidal: glycopeptide synthase inhibitor.
- Glycopeptide cannot therefore be formed in the bacterial walls.

2.7.4 Adverse effects

- Renal—toxicity is rare but more common with concurrent gentamicin administration.
- Ototoxicity—reported but very rare if excess peaks are avoided.
- Phlebitis—dilute preparations should be used for peripheral administration.
- 'Red man syndrome'—precipitated by histamine release, manifests as hypotension tachycardia and diffuse erythematous rash; avoided by limiting rate of administration.
- Haematological—neutropaenia and thrombocytopaenia have been reported.

2.7.5 Specific agents

- Vancomycin:
  - Commonly used empirical agent in the treatment of hospital-acquired infection, owing to activity against methicillin-resistant *Staphylococcus aureus* (MRSA).
  - Administered as bolus or preferably as a continuous infusion (the latter is preferable in the critical care environment).
  - Oral (or rectal) administration for treatment of *C. difficile*.
- Teicoplanin:
  - Similar profile to vancomycin.
  - Longer duration of action and greater potency.
  - Twice daily loading for 48 hours, then once daily administration (increased to alternate day administration in renal dysfunction).
  - Resistance is more common than vancomycin (25% resistance to *Staphylococcus* epidermis).
  - May be given via intra-muscular route.
  - Better bone and CSF penetration.
  - Fewer side-effects than vancomycin.

2.8 Lincosamides

2.8.1 General

- Clindamycin is a semi-synthetic agent, highly active against Gram-positive bacteria, particularly anaerobes.
- Also has activity against *falciparum malaria* and *Pneumocystis jirovici*.
- Demonstrates suppression of the toxin production in toxin-elucidating strains of *Staphylococcus* and *Streptococcus*.

2.8.2 Pharmacokinetics

- Absorption
  - Good oral bioavailability.
- Distribution
  - Generally good penetration, particularly bone and joint.
  - Poor CSF penetration.
- Metabolism
  - Hepatic, to both active and inactive metabolites.
- Excretion
  - Primarily in urine, some biliary excretion.
  - Half-life increased in renal dysfunction, limited removal with renal replacement therapy.

2.8.3 Pharmacodynamics

- Primarily bacteriostatic; bactericidal against some strains of *Staphylococcus* and *Streptococcus*.

- Acts upon the 50s ribosomal subunit, thus disrupting protein synthesis.
- May therefore compete with macrolide antibiotics and chloramphenicol for binding site.

2.8.4 Adverse effects

- Gastrointestinal effects common. Up to 30% incidence of diarrhoea; increased risk of *C. difficile* infection.
- Also associated with fever, rash, eosinophilia, and thrombocytopaenia.

2.9 Oxazolidinones

2.9.1 General

- Linezolid is a novel antibiotic agent.

2.9.2 Pharmacokinetics

- Absorption
  - 100% oral bioavailability.
- Distribution
  - Limited protein binding, therefore good penetration into all compartments.
- Metabolism
  - Hepatic metabolism to inactive metabolites.
- Excretion
  - Urinary excretion of inactive metabolites.
  - Doesn't require dose adjustment in renal or hepatic failure.
  - Plasma levels reduced by high-flux renal replacement therapy.

2.9.3 Pharmacodynamics

- Bacterial protein synthesis inhibitor via the 50s ribosomal subunit but no cross-reactivity with other protein synthesis inhibitors.
- Supresses bacterial toxin production.

2.9.4 Adverse effects

- Diarrhoea and nausea most common (4%).
- Thrombocytopaenia, peripheral neuropathy, and lactic acidosis reported.

3 Antivirals

3.1 Guanosine analogues

3.1.1 General

- Acyclovir and gancyclovir are commonly used guanosine analogues.
- Active against *Herpes Simplex* (HSV), *Varicella Zoster* (VSV) and *Epstein–Barr* (EBV) viruses. Gancyclovir also has activity against *Cytomegalovirus* (CMV).

3.1.2 Pharmacokinetics

- Absorption
  - Unpredictable absorption and limited oral bioavailability (around 25%).
- Distribution
  - Low protein binding (15%) and therefore wide distribution including CSF.

- Metabolism
  - Partial hepatic metabolism.
- Excretion
  - Active tubular renal excretion (blocked by probenecid).
  - Risk of accumulation (and associated neuro-toxicity) in renal failure.

3.1.3 Pharmacodynamics

- Acyclovir:
  - Converted by thymidine kinase to acyclovir monophosphate and then acyclovir triphosphate in infected cells.
  - Thymidine kinase is not present in CMV-infected cells, hence the lack of efficacy against this virus.
  - Acyclovir triphosphate is then incorporated into viral DNA as a surrogate for deoxyguanosine triphosphate; this results in viral DNA chain termination.
- Gancyclovir:
  - Phosphorylation is catalysed by a viral kinase encoded within the CMV virus; therefore effective against CMV.

3.1.4 Adverse effects

- Extravasation may lead to thrombophlebitis and ulceration.
- Renal impairment, secondary to crystallization of acyclovir in the renal tubules; associated with dehydration and rapid administration of drug.
- Neurological effects, including tremors, confusion seizures, and coma; associated with rapid administration and accumulation of drug.
- Bone-marrow suppression is associated with gancyclovir.

3.1.5 Specific agents

- Acyclovir
- Gancyclovir
- Valgancyclovir—the orally administered prodrug of gancyclovir

3.2 Neuraminidase inhibitors

3.2.1 General

- Includes oseltamivir, zanamivir, and peramivir.
- Indicated in the prevention and treatment of influenza.

3.2.2 Pharmacokinetics

- Absorption
  - Good oral bioavailability of oseltamivir, even in critical illness.
  - Zanamivir is available as an intravenous preparation, if the enteric route is not available or treatment failure in critically ill patients.
  - An inhaled powder preparation of zanamivir is available; however, this is not amenable to nebulization and is not therefore suitable for use in ventilated patients; an aqueous solution may be nebulized via the ventilator but this is unlicensed.
- Distribution
  - Widely distributed.
- Metabolism
  - First pass metabolism converts the majority of oseltamivir to its active metabolite.
- Excretions
  - Renally cleared, therefore dose adjustment is necessary in renal failure.

3.2.3 Pharmacodynamics

- Neuraminidase inhibitors are sialic acid analogues, which competitively inhibit the enzyme neuraminidase on the surface of host cells; in so doing, the release of new virions from infected cells is prevented; the spread of infection within the host is thus reduced.

3.2.4 Adverse effects

- Nausea and vomiting are the most commonly reported side-effect with oseltamivir.
- Neuropsychiatric disturbance has been reported in children, but is rare.

4 Antifungals

4.1 Azoles

4.1.1 General

- Subdivided into:
  - Triazoles
    - Fluconazole; itraconazole; voriconazole.
  - Imidazoles
    - Ketoconazole; micoconazole.
- Generally active against:
  - *Candida*
  - *Coccidiodes*
  - *Cryptococcus*
  - *Histoplasma*
  - Some active against *Aspergillus* (itraconazole, micoconazole, voriconazole).

4.1.2 Pharmacokinetics

- Absorption
  - Typically good.
  - Fluconazole has 100% oral bioavailability.
- Distribution
  - Fluconazole has minimal protein binding and therefore good CNS penetration.
  - Other drugs within the class are highly protein bound and therefore have poor CSF penetration.
- Metabolism
  - Hepatic metabolism to inactive compounds.
- Excretion
  - Biliary excretion.
  - Dose adjustment in renal failure unnecessary.

4.1.3 Pharmacodynamics

- Blockage of 14 α demethylation disrupts synthesis of ergosterol: a key component of the fungal membrane.
- Direct ergosterol damage may occur at higher drug levels.

4.1.4 Adverse effects

- Drug interactions (e.g. enhances the effect of warfarin).
- Gastrointestinal irritation.
- Inhibition of steroid synthesis.

4.2 Polyenes (amphotericin B)

4.2.1 General

- Amphotericin B is the only polyene in clinical use.
- Isolated from *Streptomyces nodosus* in 1959.
- It is a broad-spectrum antifungal, including activity against:
  - *Aspergillus*
  - *Candida*
  - *Cryptococcus*
- Resistance is rarely a problem.

4.2.2 Pharmacokinetics

- Absorption
  - Systemic treatment is by intravenous administration only.
  - Local installation is described (e.g. intraperitoneal, intrathecal, intravitreal).
- Distribution
  - Highly protein bound and therefore limited penetration into CSF and urine.
- Metabolism
  - Metabolized in the liver with no active metabolites.
- Excretion
  - No adjustment required in renal or hepatic impairment.

4.2.3 Pharmacodynamics

- Binds to the ergosterol component of fungal cell walls and creates pores.
- Increasing doses leads to larger pore formation and more rapid fungal death.

4.2.4 Adverse effects

- Amphotericin infusion associated with a number of symptoms, including nausea and vomiting; muscle pain; chills and rigors; and thrombophlebitis.
- More significant side-effects include blood dyscrasias, seizures, hypokalaemia, hypomagnesaemia, and hyperchloraemic acidosis.
- Of particular concern is the associated renal failure. This occurs in up to 80% of recipients. Increased likelihood with high initial doses, in the presence of other nephrotoxins, and in hypovolaemia.

4.2.5 Liposomal preparations

- Allows administration of higher doses with reduced incidence of renal dysfunction.
- No difference in efficacy.
- Significantly more expensive.

4.3 Echinocandins

4.3.1 General

- Three semi-synthetic echinocandins are available:
  - Caspofungin, micafungin, and anidulofungin.
- They have broad antifungal activity, with less resistance in *Candida* species than the azoles.

4.3.2 Pharmacokinetics

- Variable kinetics, and therefore difference in dosing schedules between different members of the class.

- Absorption
  - Poor oral absorption, therefore intravenous administration only.
- Distribution
  - Highly protein bound and large molecular weight, therefore limited distribution to CSF, urine, or the eye.
- Metabolism
  - Echinocandins are not metabolized by the cytochrome p450 system and there is therefore less risk of drug interaction than is found in other systemic antifungals.
  - Caspofungin and anidulofungin degrade spontaneously; micafungin is metabolized hepatically via catechol O-methytransferase and hydroxylation.
- Excretion
  - Dose adjustment in renal failure is not necessary.

4.3.3 Pharmacodynamics

- Inhibit the 1,3/3-D-glucan synthase enzyme, thereby inhibiting cell wall synthesis.

4.3.4 Adverse effects

- Generally better tolerated, with fewer side-effects than other systemic antifungals.
- Reported problems include elevated liver enzymes, delayed hypersensitivity reactions, and gastrointestinal side-effects.

5 Sepsis

5.1 Definitions

- The definition of sepsis has undergone a number of revisions over the last few decades.
- These definitions have been driven by various committees, formed by the European Society of Intensive Care Medicine, the Society for Critical Care Medicine, the American Thoracic Society, and the American Society of Chest Physicians.
- Several key definitions have emerged.

5.1.1 Systemic inflammatory response syndrome (SIRS)

- The definition of SIRS was expanded significantly in the most recent consensus statement of 2013.
- Recent observational data have questioned the sensitivity and validity of the SIRS criteria in detecting and evaluating sepsis.*
- The diagnosis of SIRS requires the presence of 'some' of the following:
  - General variables:
    - Fever (>38°C)
    - Hypothermia (core temperature <36°C)
    - Heart rate (90 bpm or more than two standard deviations (SD) above the normal value for age)
    - Tachypnoea (respiratory rate >20 breaths per minute)
    - Altered mental status
    - Significant oedema or positive fluid balance (20 ml.kg^{-1} over 24 hours)
    - Hyperglycaemia (plasma glucose >7.7 mmol.l^{-1}) in the absence of diabetes
  - Inflammatory variables:
    - Leukocytosis (WCC>12 x 10^3/l)

---

* The 2016 revised definition of sepsis recommended that SIRS be replaced by a modification of the SOFA score; see Singer et al (Further reading) for full explanation.

- Leukopenia (WCC <4 x 10^3/l)
- Normal WCC with greater than 10 % immature forms
- Plasma C-reactive protein more than two SD above the normal value
- Plasma procalcitonin more than two SD above the normal value

- Haemodynamic variables:
  - Arterial hypotension (SBP <90 mmHg, MAP <70 mmHg, or an SBP decrease >40 mmHg)
- Organ dysfunction variables:
  - Arterial hypoxaemia (P_aO_2/F_iO_2 ratio <300 mmHg or <40 kPa)
  - Acute oliguria (urine output <0.5 ml.kg.hour^{-1} for at least 2 hours despite adequate fluid resuscitation)
  - Creatinine increase (>44.2 µmol.l^{-1})
  - Coagulation abnormalities (INR >1.5 or a PTT >60 s)
  - Ileus (absent bowel sounds)
  - Thrombocytopenia (platelet count <100 x 10.l^{-9})
  - Hyperbilirubinaemia (plasma total bilirubin >70 µmol.l^{-1})
- Tissue perfusion variables:
  - Hyperlactataemia (>1 mmol.l^{-1})
  - Decreased capillary refill or mottling

5.1.2 Infection
- Presence of organisms in a normally sterile tissue.

5.1.3 Bacteraemia
- Presence of viable live bacteria in blood.

5.1.4 Sepsis
Sepsis is defined as life-threatening organ dysfunction caused by a dysregulated host response to infection.

Organ dysfunction is traditionally defined by SIRS; in 2016 the SOFA score was suggested as an alternative definition.

5.1.5 Severe sepsis
- Infection associated with one of the following:
  - Sepsis-induced hypotension (defined as systolic blood pressure <90 mmHg; MAP <70 mmHg; or drop in systolic blood pressure by >40 mmHg)
  - Lactate above upper limits of laboratory normal
  - Urine output <0.5 ml.kg.hour^{-1} for more than two hours despite adequate fluid resuscitation
  - Acute lung injury with P_aO_2/F_iO_2 ratio <250 mmHg (or 33.3 kPa) in the absence of pneumonia as infection source
  - Acute lung injury with P_aO_2/F_iO_2 ratio <200 mmHg (or 26.6 kPa) in the presence of pneumonia as infection source
  - Creatinine >176.8 µmol.l^{-1}
  - Bilirubin >34.2 µmol.l^{-1}
  - Platelet count <100 x 10.l^{-9}
  - Coagulopathy (INR >1.5)

5.1.6 Septic shock
- Persistent sepsis-induced hypotension (MAP <65mmHg; necessitating vasopressor therapy) or persistent lactate (>2 mmol.l^{-1}) despite volume resuscitation.

5.1.7 Multi-organ dysfunction syndrome

- Progressive organ dysfunction to the point that life cannot be sustained without organ support.

5.2 Pathophysiology of septic shock

- Systemic sepsis represents an imbalance in pro- and anti-inflammatory processes. It has been described as a malignant intravascular inflammation.
- The normal immune response to infection involves:
  - Recognition of foreign material by the innate immune system (including mast cells, dendritic cells, and natural killer cells).
  - The release of pro-inflammatory mediators (tumour necrosis factor alpha, TNFα; interleukin 1, IL-1), chemotactic agents (intercellular adhesion molecule 1, ICAM-1; vascular cell adhesion molecule 1, VCAM-1), and nitric oxide.
- Sepsis occurs when this inflammatory response expands beyond the localized site of infection.
- High concentrations of TNFα and IL-1 in the circulation lead to widespread inflammation, activation of the complement system, a pro-coagulant state, endothelial dysfunction, microvascular compromise, and ultimately end organ dysfunction.

5.3 Management of severe sepsis and septic shock

- In recent years, the Surviving Sepsis Campaign has heavily influenced management of severe sepsis and septic shock.
- The first iteration of the Surviving Sepsis Guidelines emerged in 2004 and has been updated in 2008 and 2013.
- These represent the consensus opinion of a group of authors drawn from a range of European and North American organizations, based upon recent evidence.

5.3.1 Surviving sepsis guidelines*

- Key elements of the surviving sepsis guidelines, include:
- Resuscitation:
  - 'Protocolized and quantitative'
  - Goal-directed:
    - CVP 8–12 mmHg
    - MAP >65 mmHg
    - Urine output >0.5 ml.kg^{-1} per hour
    - Superior vena cava oxygen saturation (ScvO$_2$) >70%
    - Normal lactate
- Screening:
  - Screening for sepsis, and early identification, allows earlier intervention with improved outcomes.
- Diagnosis:
  - At least two sets of blood cultures from separate sites.
  - Culture of other fluids and tissues, where appropriate.
  - Cultures prior to antibiotics, providing this will not delay antibiotics by more than 45 minutes.
  - Imaging to identify site of infection with potential for source control.
- Antibiotics:
  - Effective intravenous antibiotics should be administered within 1 hour of recognition of severe sepsis or septic shock.

* Adapted from *Critical Care Medicine*, 41, Dellinger R et al., 'Surviving Sepsis Campaign: International Guidelines for Management of Severe Sepsis and Septic Shock: 2012'. Copyright (2013) with permission from Wolters Kluwer Health, Inc.

- There is compelling evidence that the greater the duration between recognition of septic shock and administration of appropriate antibiotics, the higher the mortality.
- Frequent reassessment of antimicrobial needs with a view to de-escalation.

- Source control:
  - Actively seek the need for source control, and if identified, aim for intervention within 12 hours.
- Prevent additional infection:
  - The use of selective oral decontamination and selective digestive decontamination are suggested.
  - Oral chlorhexadine gluconate is recommended for oropharyngeal decontamination.
  - These are in addition to careful infection control practice.
- Fluid therapy:
  - First-line recommended fluid therapy is crystalloid.
  - Fluid therapy in severe sepsis and septic shock has been the subject of a number of recent large trials (see discussion of specific therapies in Section 5.4.4).
- Vasopressors:
  - All patients on vasopressors should have an arterial catheter placed.
  - Should be used to achieve a mean arterial pressure of 65 mmHg.
  - Noradrenaline is the first choice vasopressor.
  - Adrenaline is recommended as a second vasopressor agent.
  - Vasopressin (at low dose, 0.03 units.min^{-1}) may be of use in raising blood pressure and reducing catecholamine dose.
  - Dopamine is reserved as a vasopressor for selected cases (such as relative bradycardia), but should not be used for perceived renal protective properties.
- Inotropes:
  - Dobutamine is recommended in addition to vasopressors if:
    - There is evidence of myocardial dysfunction.
    - Hypoperfusion persists despite adequate filling and adequate MAP.
    - Inotropy should not be used to elevate cardiac output to supranormal levels.
- Corticosteroids:
  - In patients whom fluid replacement and vasopressors alone are insufficient to achieve blood pressure targets, intravenous administration of 200 mg hydrocortisone per day is suggested (see specific therapies in Section 5.4.5).

FURTHER READING

Dellinger RP, Levy MM, Rhodes A, et al. Surviving Sepsis Campaign: international guidelines for management of severe sepsis and septic shock, 2012. *Intensive Care Medicine* 2013; 39(2): 165–228.

Kumar A, Roberts D, Wood KE, et al. Duration of hypotension before initiation of effective antimicrobial therapy is the critical determinant of survival in human septic shock. *Critical Care Medicine* 2006; 34(6): 1589–96.

Pinsky MR, Matuschak GM. Multiple systems organ failure: failure of host defense homeostasis. *Critical Care Clinics* 1989; 5(2): 199–220.

Singer M, Deutschman CS, Seymour CW, et al. The third international consensus definitions for sepsis and septic shock (Sepsis-3). *JAMA : the journal of the American Medical Association* 2016; 315(8): 801–10.

5.4 Discussion of specific therapies

5.4.1 Goal-directed therapy

- The use of goal-directed sepsis resuscitation is based largely upon the single-centre Rivers study, which demonstrated a significant reduction in mortality (30.5% vs 46.5%) with the introduction of protocolized, quantitative, goal directed therapy.
- Three multi-centre studies in the UK, USA, and Australasia (PROMISE, PROCESS, and ARISE) have failed to reproduce these results.
- Limitations of the original Rivers paper include:
  - Non-blinded
  - Unclear which of the many interventions were effective
  - Single centre in an urban US hospital
  - Surprisingly high mortality in the control arm
- Explanations for failure to reproduce results in subsequent multi-centre studies include:
  - The lessons learned from the Rivers study are already so widely disseminated that no discernable difference exists between the control and intervention arms. This is illustrated by the early administration of antibiotics in both arms.
  - The low mortality in the control arm may have caused the studies to be underpowered.

5.4.2 Target blood pressure

- The Surviving Sepsis campaign suggests targeting a MAP of 65 mmHg.
- The SEPSISPAM study was a multi-centre trial, which randomized patients with septic shock refractory to fluid resuscitation to a target MAP of 65–70 mmHg or 85–90 mmHg.
- No mortality benefit was demonstrated in the higher blood pressure group.
- The study was underpowered to detect mortality due to a higher than predicted survival.
- There was greater use of vasopressors and a higher incidence of atrial fibrillation in the high blood pressure group.
- In sub-group analysis of patients with chronic hypertension, the higher blood pressure group had a lower incidence of AKI and less frequently required renal replacement therapy.

5.4.3 Pharmacological haemodynamic support

- Evidence relating to vasopressors and inotropes in sepsis is discussed in Chapter 2, Section 3.1.

FURTHER READING

Asfar P, Meziani F, Hamel J-F, et al. High versus low blood-pressure target in patients with septic shock (SEPSISPAM). *New England Journal of Medicine* 2014; 370(17): 1583–93.

Mouncey PR, Osborn TM, Power GS, et al. Trial of early, goal-directed resuscitation for septic shock. *New England Journal of Medicine* 2015; 372(14): 1301–11.

Peake SL, Delaney A, Bailey M, et al. Goal-directed resuscitation for patients with early septic shock. *New England Journal of Medicine* 2014; 371(16): 1496.

Rivers E, Nguyen B, Havstad S, et al. Early goal-directed therapy in the treatment of severe sepsis and septic shock. *New England Journal of Medicine* 2001; 345(19): 1368–77.

Yealy DM, Kellum JA, Huang DT, et al. A randomized trial of protocol-based care for early septic shock. *New England Journal of Medicine* 2014; 370(18): 1683–93.

5.4.4 Fluid therapy

- Several randomized trials comparing different resuscitation fluids have been conducted in recent years. These are outlined in Table 6.1.

Table 6.1 Trials examining resuscitation fluids

Title	Authors	Comparisons	Conclusions
A comparison of albumin and saline for fluid resuscitation in the intensive care unit (SAFE study)	Finfer et al.	0.9% NaCl vs 4% human albumin solution in 6997 intensive care patients requiring volume resuscitation.	No difference in 28-day mortality, length of ICU or hospital stay, time of mechanical ventilation, or time on renal replacement therapy. Subgroup analysis suggested worse outcome with albumin in traumatic brain injury. Non-significant trend towards better outcome in patients with severe sepsis.
Intensive insulin therapy and pentastarch resuscitation in severe sepsis (VISEP study)	Brunkhorst et al.	Two by two study comparing intensive vs normal insulin therapy and hydroxyethyl starch vs Ringer's lactate for fluid resuscitation in severe sepsis.	Starch associated with a higher rate of AKI and need for renal replacement therapy. Trial stopped early due to the high rate of hypoglycaemia in the intensive insulin group.
Hydroxyethyl starch or saline for fluid resuscitation in intensive care (CHEST study)	Myburgh et al.	Hydroxyethyl starch vs 0.9% NaCl in patients admitted to an intensive care unit and requiring volume resuscitation.	No difference in 90-day mortality but increase in need for renal replacement therapy in the starch group.
Assessment of hemodynamic efficacy and safety of 6% hydroxyethylstarch 130/0.4 vs 0.9% NaCl fluid replacement in patients with severe sepsis: the CRYSTMAS study.	Guedet et al.	Hydroxyethyl starch vs 0.9% NaCl in 196 patients with severe patients; primary endpoint of haemodynamic stability.	Haemodynamic stability achieved more quickly and with less fluid in the hydroxyethyl starch group. No difference in mortality or incidence of acute kidney injury.
Hydroxyethyl starch 130/0.42 versus Ringer's acetate in severe sepsis (6S study)	Perner et al.	Hydroxyethyl starch vs Ringer's acetate in 804 patients with severe sepsis.	Increased 90-day mortality in the starch group; also an increased risk of renal failure.

Effects of fluid resuscitation with colloids vs crystalloids on mortality in critically ill patients presenting with hypovolemic shock: the CRISTAL randomized trial.	Annane et al.	Colloids (of any kind) vs crystalloids (of any kind) in 2,857 critically ill, hypovolaemic patients. Most had concurrent sepsis.	No difference in 28-day mortality. Decrease in 90-day mortality in the colloid group: suggested by the study authors to be used as hypothesis generating point rather than evidence for change of practice.
Mortality after fluid bolus in African children with severe infection (FEAST study)	Maitland et al.	3,141 Sub-Saharan African children (60 days to 12 years) with febrile illness and evidence of shock were randomized to saline bolus, albumin bolus, or no bolus fluid therapy.	Significant decrease in 48-hour mortality amongst the no-bolus group. The use of bolus fluid therapy in this specific patient group is therefore brought into question.
Albumin replacement in patients with severe sepsis or septic shock (ALBIOS study)	Caironi et al.	1,818 patients with severe sepsis randomized to albumin replacement (to achieve plasma albumin levels >30 g/dl) or no albumin.	No difference in 28- or 90-day mortality in the predefined analysis. Post hoc subgroup analysis suggested a reduction in 90-day mortality in patients with septic shock at enrolment.

FURTHER READING

Annane D, Siami S, Jaber S, et al. Effects of fluid resuscitation with colloids vs crystalloids on mortality in critically ill patients presenting with hypovolemic shock: The cristal randomized trial. *Journal of the American Medical Association* 2013; 310(17): 1809–17.

Brunkhorst FM, Engel C, Bloos F, et al. Intensive insulin therapy and pentastarch resuscitation in severe sepsis. *New England Journal of Medicine* 2008; 358(2): 125–39.

Caironi P, Tognoni G, Masson S, et al. Albumin replacement in patients with severe sepsis or septic shock. *New England Journal of Medicine* 2014; 370(15): 1412–21

Finfer S, Bellomo R, Boyce N, French J, Myburgh J, Norton R. A comparison of albumin and saline for fluid resuscitation in the intensive care unit. *New England Journal of Medicine* 2004; 350(22): 2247–56.

Guidet B, Martinet O, Boulain T, et al. Assessment of hemodynamic efficacy and safety of 6% hydroxyethylstarch 130/0.4 vs. 0.9% NaCl fluid replacement in patients with severe sepsis: the CRYSTMAS study. *Critical Care* 2012; 16(3): R94.

Maitland K, Kiguli S, Opoka RO, et al. Mortality after fluid bolus in African children with severe infection. *New England Journal of Medicine* 2011; 364(26): 2483–95.

Myburgh JA, Finfer S, Bellomo R, et al. Hydroxyethyl starch or saline for fluid resuscitation in intensive care. *New England Journal of Medicine* 2012; 367(20): 1901–11.

Perner A, Haase N, Guttormsen AB, et al. Hydroxyethyl starch 130/0.42 versus Ringer's acetate in severe sepsis. *New England Journal of Medicine* 2012; 367(2): 124–34.

5.4.5 Corticosteroids

- The belief that severe sepsis occurs as a result of excess inflammation, and may be associated with adrenal axis dysfunction, has raised the possibility that steroids may improve outcomes.
- Two key trials examined this theory:
  - The 'Annane' study:
    - This multi-centre French study examined the effect of 7 days of hydrocortisone and fludrocortisone on patients with septic shock within 8 hours of onset of hypotension, in comparison to placebo.
    - Prior to commencement of study drug, a Synthacthen test was undertaken; those patients who failed to respond by increasing plasma cortisol levels were labelled as having 'relative adrenal insufficiency' (RAI).
    - In those patients with RAI, the administration of hydrocortisone and fludrocortisone resulted in a reduction in 28-day mortality and faster resolution of shock.
    - In patients *without* RAI, no difference in mortality or duration of shock was observed.
  - CORTICUS
    - An international multi-centre trial that randomized patients with septic shock to receive hydrocortisone or placebo within 72 hours of the onset of hypotension.
    - A synthacthen test was performed prior to commencement to identify those with RAI.

- There was no difference in mortality between the groups, regardless of whether patients had RAI.
  - Resolution of shock was quicker in the steroid group but the incidence of secondary infection was also increased.
- The difference in conclusions between CORTICUS and the Annane study may be due to:
  - The Annane population had higher severity of illness score.
  - CORTICUS stopped early due to slow recruitment and, as a consequence, was underpowered.
- Systematic review of the use of a prolonged (~7 days) course of low dose (~200 mg of hydrocortisone per 24 hours) steroid in septic shock suggests reduced mortality.

FURTHER READING

Annane D, Sébille V, Charpentier C, et al. Effect of treatment with low doses of hydrocortisone and fludrocortisone on mortality in patients with septic shock. *Journal of the American Medical Association* 2002; 288(7): 862–71.

Annane D, Bellissant E, Bollaert P-E, et al. Corticosteroids in the treatment of severe sepsis and septic shock in adults: a systematic review. *Journal of the American Medical Association* 2009; 301(22): 2362–75.

Sprung CL, Annane D, Keh D, et al. Hydrocortisone therapy for patients with septic shock. *New England Journal of Medicine* 2008; 358(2): 111.

5.4.6 Activated protein C

- An inappropriate pro-coagulant response is believed to contribute to the severe sepsis syndrome.
- Protein C—a key inhibitor in the pro-coagulant process—has been found to be deficient in severe sepsis.
- Infusion of recombinant activated protein C (APC) was therefore proposed as a means of inhibiting the deleterious pro-coagulant process.
- Two randomized control trials examined the use of APC in severe sepsis:
  - PROWESS
    - A large, multi-centre study comparing APC to placebo in patients with SIRS and organ failure.
    - 28-day mortality was reduced in the APC group (24.7% vs 30.8%); APC was particularly beneficial in those with greater illness severity scores.
    - Bleeding was increased in the APC group.
  - Subsequent observational studies (namely ADDRESS and ENHANCE) produced equivocal results and therefore a second large-scale randomized control trial was conducted:
  - PROWESS-SHOCK
    - A large multicentre trial comparing APC to placebo in patients with SIRS and shock.
    - No mortality benefit with APC but increased risk of bleeding.
  - APC was withdrawn from the market on the basis of PROWESS-SHOCK.

FURTHER READING

Abraham E, Laterre P-F, Garg R, et al. Drotrecogin alfa (activated) for adults with severe sepsis and a low risk of death. *New England Journal of Medicine* 2005; 353(13): 1332–41.

Bernard GR, Vincent J-L, Laterre P-F, et al. Efficacy and safety of recombinant human activated protein C for severe sepsis. *New England Journal of Medicine* 2001; 344(10): 699–709.

Bernard GR, Margolis BD, Shanies HM, et al. Extended evaluation of recombinant human activated protein C United States Trial (ENHANCE US): a single-arm, phase 3B, multicenter study of drotrecogin alfa (activated) in severe sepsis. *CHEST Journal* 2004; 125(6): 2206–16.

Martí-Carvajal A, Solà I, Gluud C, Lathyris D, Cardona A. Human recombinant activated protein C for severe sepsis and septic shock in adult and paediatric patients. *Cochrane Database of Systematic Reviews* 2012; Dec 12; 12: CD004388. doi: 10.1002/14651858.CD004388. pub6.

Ranieri VM, Thompson BT, Barie PS, et al. Drotrecogin alfa (activated) in adults with septic shock. *New England Journal of Medicine* 2012; 366(22): 2055–64.

5.4.7 Other therapies

- Beta blockade
  - Tachycardia is associated with worse outcomes in septic shock.
  - It has been suggested that rather than simply being a marker of greater physiological derangement, tachycardia may itself contribute to the pathological process.
  - One open label pilot randomized control study has compared the use of esmolol infusions to control heart rate between 80 and 94 bpm with standard therapy.
  - Whilst heart rate and cardiac output were reduced in the esmolol group, markers of tissue perfusion were maintained.
  - The mortality in the esmolol group was significantly lower, although the limitations of this single-centre study make this finding suitable for hypothesis generation only.
- Heparin
  - The antithrombotic properties of heparin have been proposed as beneficial.
  - Retrospective data suggested the use of heparin in sepsis to have a mortality benefit; this was not however borne out in a randomized control trial.
- Statins
  - The anti-inflammatory properties of statins have been postulated as beneficial in sepsis.
  - Two meta-analyses, however, conclude there to be no mortality benefit in the introduction of *de novo* statins in sepsis; continuation of statins should be considered on a case-by-case basis, as they may be associated with an increased risk or renal and hepatic dysfunction.
- Extracorporeal clearance of cytokines and toxins
  - High-dose haemofiltration in sepsis is discussed in Chapter 3, Section 2.3.2.1; the IVOIRE study demonstrated no survival benefit in the use of high-dose compared to standard-dose haemofiltration.
  - The use of absorbent extracorporeal membranes should increase removal of cytokines but evidence relating to outcomes is conflicting.
  - Plasma exchange has been proposed as a means of cytokine removal but high level evidence of efficacy is lacking.

- Intravenous immunoglobulin
  - Immunoglobulins are glycoproteins produced by plasma cells; these are components of the adaptive immune system that display a wide range of receptors specific to pathogens to which the individual has previously been exposed.
  - Intravenous immunoglobulin (IVIg) preparations are derived from the plasma of over 1,000 blood donors; the large number of donors—and the diverse pathogens to which the cohort have been exposed—provides a broad range of antibodies within the preparation.
  - Numerous biological rationale for the administration of IVIg in sepsis:
    - Recognition and clearance of bacterial pathogens
    - Recognition and clearance of bacterially produced toxins
    - Scavenging of host inflammatory mediators:
      - 'Upstream' (e.g. transcription factor)
      - 'Downstream' (e.g. cytokines)
    - Direct anti-inflammatory effects
    - Attenuation of lymphocyte apoptosis
  - Clinical trials of IVIg in sepsis are heterogeneous.
  - Meta-analysis of high-quality trials at low risk of bias fails to demonstrate mortality benefit with the use of IVIg.
  - IVIg is associated with a higher risk of thromboembolic disease, renal dysfunction, and anaphylaxis.

FURTHER READING

Deshpande A, Pasupuleti V, Rothberg MB. Statin therapy and mortality from sepsis a meta-analysis of randomized trials. *The American Journal of Medicine* 2014; 128 (4): 410–417.e1.

Jaimes F, De La Rosa G, Morales C, et al. Unfractioned heparin for treatment of sepsis: a randomized clinical trial (The HETRASE Study). *Critical Care Medicine* 2009; 37(4): 1185–96.

Joannes-Boyau O, Honoré PM, Perez P, et al. High-volume versus standard-volume haemofiltration for septic shock patients with acute kidney injury (IVOIRE study): a multicentre randomized controlled trial. *Intensive Care Medicine* 2013; 39(9): 1535–46.

Morelli A, Ertmer C, Westphal M, et al. Effect of heart rate control with esmolol on hemodynamic and clinical outcomes in patients with septic shock: a randomized clinical trial. *Journal of the American Medical Association* 2013; 310(16): 1683–91.

Shankar-Hari M, Spencer J, Sewell WA, Rowan KM, Singer M. Bench-to-bedside review: Immunoglobulin therapy for sepsis-biological plausibility from a critical care perspective. *Critical Care* 2012; 16(2): 206.

Thomas G, Hraiech S, Loundou A, et al. Statin therapy in critically-ill patients with severe sepsis: a review and meta-analysis of randomized clinical trials. *Minerva Anestesiologica* 2015; 81(8): 921–930.

---

6 Specific infections

6.1 Influenza

6.1.1 General

- Influenza is an acute respiratory illness caused by the influenza A, B, or C virus.
- Influenza strains are subdivided based upon differences in two glycoprotein surface markers: the HA and NA.

- Influenza A is more transmissible than B and C, and is therefore responsible for epidemics and pandemics.
- Transmission is by large droplets; prolonged or close contact with an infected individual is generally required.
- The average incubation period is 2 days.
- Viral shedding can be detected in respiratory samples for 1 to 2 days prior to onset of symptoms.

6.1.2 Features and complications

- Clinical features include:
  - Respiratory:
    - Coryzal symptoms
    - Breathlessness
    - Cough
  - Constitutional:
    - Fever
    - Myalgia
    - Headache
- Complications are more common in:
  - The elderly
  - Pregnancy
  - Obesity
  - Immunocompromised
  - Those with chronic disease
- Complications include:
  - Secondary bacterial respiratory infection (classically *Staphylococcus aureus*)
  - Direct viral pneumonitis
  - Rhabdomyolysis

6.1.3 Management

- The intensive care management of influenza infection is primarily supportive.
- Neuramidase inhibitors are used for treatment of the underlying infection.
- Public Health England recommends the use of neuramidase inhibitors in the following patients:
  - Any patient with confirmed or suspected influenza (A or B) infection in whom:
    - Admission to critical care is required or
    - There is evidence of lower respiratory tract infection or
    - There is evidence of central nervous system infection or
    - Significant exacerbation of underlying disease
- First-line treatment of influenza A on ICU is enteral oseltamivir at the standard dose (75 mg bd); a higher dose regimen may be appropriate for influenza B but discussion with local virologists is recommended.
- Patients should be isolated and barrier-nursed; staff should wear appropriate personal protective equipment.

6.2 Malaria

6.2.1 General

- Malaria is one of the most common causes of fever in the returned traveller, affecting predominantly young and middle-aged adults.

- Whilst anti-malarial pharmacological prophylaxis is effective, compliance is often poor.
- Almost all severe, imported malarial disease is due to *Plasmodium falciparum*:
  - Around 10% of the cases in UK are severe
  - Mortality from *P. falciparum* is around 1%
  - Other malarial pathogens are *P. ovale*, *P. vivax*, and *P. malariae*; these rarely cause severe disease

6.2.2 Diagnosis and severity

- Malaria is diagnosed by means of blood film (thick films have high sensitivity; thin films are more specific and allow quantification for parasitaemia).
- Markers of severe infection described by the World Health Organization are:
  - Cerebral malaria, as characterized by impaired consciousness or coma, convulsions, or both
  - Acute respiratory distress syndrome.
  - Circulatory collapse.
  - Jaundice in the setting of other organ dysfunction.
  - Haemoglobinuria.
  - Abnormal spontaneous bleeding.
  - Laboratory features of severe falciparum infection:
    - Hypoglycaemia (<2.2 mmol.l^{-1})
    - Severe anaemia (Hb <50 g.l^{-1}; packed cell volume $<15\%$)
    - Metabolic acidosis (plasma bicarbonate <15 mmol.l^{-1} or pH <7.35)
    - Hyperparasitaemia (2% in low-intensity transmission areas or 5% in areas of high stable malaria transmission intensity)
    - Hyperlactataemia (lactate 5 mmol.l^{-1})
    - Acute kidney injury (serum creatinine 265 μmol.l^{-1})

6.2.3 Intensive care management

- The most common reasons for critical care admission are:
  - Cerebral malaria
  - Acute kidney injury
  - Acute respiratory distress syndrome
- Intravenous quinine has been the mainstay of treatment for many years:
  - Side-effects include:
    - Tinnitus, blurred vision
    - Causes hypoglycaemia, therefore plasma glucose must be regularly monitored
    - Prolongs the QT interval therefore regular ECGs are required
  - Relative resistance is increasing, particularly in South-East Asia.
- Artesunate has been demonstrated to be more effective but its availability is often limited to specialist centres.
- Supportive management includes:
  - Management in a specialist centre.
  - A restrictive fluid strategy is typically employed in severe malaria (to minimize the risk of lung injury and cerebral oedema); care should, however, be taken not to 'under-resuscitate', and goal-directed fluid therapy may provide a pragmatic means of achieving sufficient volume replacement.

- Respiratory failure may be the consequence of an ARDS secondary to endothelial dys-function; superadded bacterial infection is also reported; standard ARDS ventilator man-agement should be employed.
- Cerebral involvement of malaria (GCS <9 with other causes excluded): mechanisms are unclear but cerebral oedema is a contributing factor; no specific treatment has been shown to be effective; supportive therapy is indicated.
- Acute kidney injury is managed with standard renal support.

- Prognosis in developed health systems is generally good (mortality for *P. falciparum* <1%) but is significantly worse resource poor health systems.
- Markers of worse prognosis in the ICU population include:
  - Older age.
  - Neurological involvement.
  - High parasite count.

6.3 HIV

6.3.1 General

- 100,000 people in the UK are believed to be living with HIV infection (around 1.5 per 1,000 population), one in five of whom are currently undiagnosed.
- There were 490 deaths of patients with HIV in the UK in 2012.
- Patients diagnosed early can expect normal life-expectancy.

6.3.2 Natural history of HIV

- Viral transmission
- Seroconversion
- Chronic infection:
  - Asymptomatic, latent period.
  - AIDS:
    - CD4 count <200 cells per µl or
    - AIDS defining illness (see Box 6.1)
  - Advanced HIV/AIDS:
    - CD4 count <50 cells per µl

Box 6.1 AIDS defining illnesses

- HIV wasting syndrome
- *Pneumocystis jirovecii pneumonia*
- Recurrent severe bacterial pneumonia
- Chronic *herpes simplex* infection (orolabial, genital, or anorectal of more than 1 month's duration or visceral at any site)
- Oesophageal candidiasis (or candidiasis of trachea, bronchi or lungs)
- Extrapulmonary tuberculosis
- Kaposi's sarcoma
- *Cytomegalovirus* infection (retinitis or infection of other organs)
- Central nervous system toxoplasmosis
- HIV encephalopathy
- Extrapulmonary cryptococcosis, including meningitis

Box 6.1 *continued*

- Disseminated non-tuberculous mycobacterial infection
- Progressive multifocal leukoencephalopathy
- Chronic cryptosporidiosis (with diarrhoea)
- Chronic isosporiasis
- Disseminated mycosis (coccidiomycosis or histoplasmosis)
- Recurrent non-typhoidal *Salmonella* bacteraemia
- Lymphoma (cerebral or B-cell non-Hodgkin) or other solid HIV-associated tumours
- Invasive cervical carcinoma
- Atypical disseminated leishmaniasis
- Symptomatic HIV-associated nephropathy or symptomatic HIV-associated cardiomyopathy

Adapted from *WHO* 2007. World Health Organisation Definitions. HIV/AIDS Programme. http://www.who.int/entity/hiv/pub/guidelines/WHO%20HIV%20Staging.pdf

6.3.3 Highly active antiretroviral treatment (HAART)

- HAART described the standard treatment for HIV infection.
- A combination of at least three drugs is used to supress HIV replication.
- Classes of antiretroviral agents:
  - Entry inhibitors (e.g. enfuvirtide)
  - Nucleoside and nucleotide reverse transcriptase inhibitors (e.g. zidovudine, abacavir, tenofovir, emtricitabine)
  - Non-nucleoside reverse transcriptase inhibitors (e.g. efavirenz, etravirine).
  - Integrase inhibitors (raltegravir, elvitegravir)
  - Protease inhibitors (lopinavir, indinavir)
- Combination therapy increases efficacy and reduces the likelihood of resistance.
- Examples include:
  - Truvada (tenofovir and emtricitabine)
  - Atripla (efavirenz, tenofovir, and emtricitabine)
- The timing of initiation of initiation of antiretroviral therapy is debated.
- Those with CD4 count <200 cells per μl are generally considered to benefit, as the risk of opportunistic infection will be reduced by therapy.
- Treating those with higher CD4 counts has a public health advantage and reduces the rate of progression of HIV-related cardiovascular and neurological disease.
- Disadvantages to early treatment are cost, side-effects of therapy, and the lack of trial data demonstrating benefit.

6.3.4 Immune reconstitution inflammatory syndrome (IRIS)

- IRIS is an inflammatory process, associated with worsening of existing infectious processes, which occurs on initiation of antiretroviral therapy.
- This phenomenon is most commonly associated with *Tuberculosis, Cryptococcus, Pneumocystis,* or *Cytomegalovirus* infection.
- A rise in CD4 count occurring with antiretroviral treatment leads to a sudden increase in the natural inflammatory response leading to systemic inflammatory symptoms, and associated local tissue involvement at the site of existing infection.

- Risk factors for IRIS include:
  - Low CD4 count at initiation of treatment
  - Significant response to antiretroviral treatment
  - Presence of opportunistic infection
- IRIS is of particular concern for those patients admitted to the intensive care unit with an opportunistic infection, a new diagnosis of HIV infection, and a low CD4 count.
- The risk of IRIS must be taken into account when contemplating the timing of HAART initiation.
- It is recommended that HAART may be commenced within 2 weeks of antimicrobial therapy for the opportunistic infection.
- Steroids may have some role in supressing the immune response and have been proposed as a means of both preventing and treating IRIS; use is however controversial and specific to underlying infection and should be guided by an HIV specialist.

6.3.5 HIV and AIDS on the intensive care unit—epidemiology

- The disease processes necessitating ICU admission in the HIV population has changed over the course of the last 30 years:
  - Admissions early in the existence of HIV were primarily related to end-stage, AIDS-defining illnesses, such as *Pneumocystis jiroveci* pneumonia.
  - With advances in HAART and significant improvement in HIV disease control, around half of ICU admissions in HIV positive patients are unrelated to the HIV infection.
  - Bacterial infections are responsible for more pneumonia in HIV patients than *Pneumocystis jirovecii*.
  - Opportunistic infections now tend to be seen primarily in patients with previously undiagnosed HIV infection.
- Survival of HIV-infected patients now approaches that of non-HIV-infected patients.
- Epidemiological studies that examine ICU survival in this population are, however, limited by the multiple confounding factors that may accompany HIV infection.

6.3.6 Specific considerations regarding the HIV-positive patient in the ICU

- Antiretroviral therapy:
  - Timing of initiation (and associated risk of IRIS)
  - Drug interactions (of which there are many)
  - Difficulty with enteral access and absorption (most antiretroviral agents are only available for the enteral route)
- The management of opportunistic infection:
  - Pneumocystis jiroveci pneumonia (PJP):
    - *Pneumocystis* is classified as a fungus and remains one of the most commonly encountered opportunistic infections on the ICU.
    - Patients with a CD4 count of <200 cells per µl are at risk.
    - Classically presents as progressive dyspnoea and cough.
    - Associated with a classical chest X-ray appearance of diffuse bilateral infiltrates.
    - Beta D glucan levels are typically elevated.
    - Diagnosis is based upon immunofluorescence staining +/− polymerase chain reaction.
    - First-line therapy is with co-trimoxazole; alternative agents include primaquine.
    - Steroids (usually in the form of prednisolone) should be given to all patients on the ICU with PJP infection.

- Cryptococcal meningitis:
    - *Cryptococcus neoformans* can produce an invasive fungal infection of the meninges.
    - Presentation is with headache and general decline.
    - Definitive diagnosis is with culture of *Cryptococcus* in CSF; interim analysis of CSF typically reveals low white cells, low glucose, and moderately elevated protein; a positive India ink stain is suggestive of *Cryptococcus*.
    - There are no specific associated neuroradiological findings.
    - First-line treatment is amphotericin B in combination with flucytosine for the initial phase; fluconazole provides a cheaper, less problematic alternative for the long-term consolidation phase.
- *Toxoplasmosis* encephalitis:
    - *Toxoplasmosis* may occur in up to 30% of patients with a CD4 count <100 cells per µl.
    - Presentation is with neurological symptoms, primarily confusion, headache, and fever.
    - Patients will be *Toxoplasmosis gondii* IgG antibody positive in serum; neuroimaging classically demonstrates multiple ring enhancing lesions.
    - Initial treatment is with pyrimethamine, sulfadiazine, and calcium folinate.
    - Concurrent dexamethasone is indicated in those with evidence of intracranial pressure effect.

6.4 Botulism

6.4.1 General

- Botulism is the clinical manifestation of *Clostridium botulinum* infection.
- Classically a consequence of ingesting contaminated foods, the incidence is increasing due to wound infections, particularly in the context of intravenous drug abuse.

6.4.2 Clostridium botulinum

- A spore-forming Gram-positive anaerobic rod.
- Heat resistant.
- Found in soil, vegetables, fish, putrid food.
- Toxin-producing:
    - 8 toxins identified (toxins A, B, and E associated with human disease)
    - Denatured at >80°C
    - Very potent (1 g of toxin could potentially kill millions of humans)
- Absorbed via the mucous membranes and spread in blood.

6.4.3 Pathophysiology and clinical features

- Botulinum toxin binds to a specific receptor at the acetylcholine transmission site leading to an irreversible blockade of acetylcholine release; this leads to impaired transmission at:
    - Neuromuscular junctions:
        - Progressive descending paralysis with **no** sensory involvement
        - Respiratory compromise
        - Cranial nerve involvement, often early due to the relatively high frequency of depolarization:
            - Diplopia
            - Dysarthria
            - Dysphonia

- Autonomic ganglia and parasympathetic terminals:
    - Nausea, vomiting
    - Abdominal distension and ileus
    - Dry mouth
    - Urinary retention
    - Absent pupillary reflexes
    - Hypotension, with normal heart rate
- Differential diagnosis includes:
    - Miller–Fisher syndrome: a descending paralysis but limbs tend to be affected before respiratory muscles.
    - Myasthenia gravis: no autonomic features.
    - Eaton–Lambert syndrome: no opthalmoplegia and weakness improves with exercise.

6.4.4 Investigation
- Classically: mouse lethality bioassay—injection of sample into laboratory mouse peritoneum, observation for signs of botulism, observation of response to anti-toxin.
- Specific assays now available.
- Nerve conduction studies demonstrate reduced amplitude of muscle action potentials.
- Markers of respiratory function (such as Forced Vital Capacity) should be tracked to determine need for respiratory support.

6.4.5 Management
- Management is primarily supportive.
- No specific antibiotic for botulinum. Appropriate cover should be provided for concurrent infection; aminoglycosides should be avoided due to their association with neuromuscular junction blockade.
- Trivalent equine anti-toxin may be effective, if given early; carries a risk of anaphylaxis.

6.5 Tetanus
6.5.1 General
- A rare disease, which is the consequence of infection with *Clostridium tetani*.

6.5.2 Clostridium tetani
- Gram-positive, anaerobic, spore-forming bacteria, commonly found in soil and human faeces.
- Incubation period of between 7 and 10 days.

6.5.3 Pathophysiology and clinical features
- Tetanus toxin inhibits neurotransmitter release from presynaptic GABA inhibitory interneurons; this leads to uninhibited motor and sympathetic nerve activity.
- Followed by clinical features, which progress over 2–3 weeks:
    - Locked jaw (the presenting feature in the majority of patients)
    - Tonic contractions of the skeletal muscles, spasmodic episodes:
        - Rigid abdomen
        - Intermittent apnoea/airway obstruction as respiratory system impaired by spasms
        - Dysphagia

- Autonomic instability:
  - Tachycardia
  - Labile blood pressure
  - Sweating
  - Irritability
- Differential diagnosis includes:
  - Dystonic syndromes (e.g. neuroleptic malignant syndrome)
  - Strychnine poisoning

6.5.4 Investigation and management

- No specific diagnostic test exists.
- Antibiotics:
  - Metronidazole is widely recommended but has no proven benefit.
  - Consideration should be given to the possibility of concurrent infection with another organism and appropriate antimicrobial cover commenced.
- Debridement of affected wound.
- Antitoxin:
  - Human tetanus immune toxin should be administered by the subcutaneous or intramuscular route; some should be infiltrated around the wound.
  - Antitoxin will only affect unbound toxin and not that already bound to nerves.
- Tetanus toxoid:
  - To confer active immunity (does not reliably emerge following tetanus infection).
  - Course of three injections, distant from the antitoxin injection site.
- Supportive measures:
  - Spasms:
    - Benzodiazepines
    - Anaesthesia
    - In severe cases, muscle relaxants
  - Autonomic dysfunction:
    - Magnesium sulphate
    - Beta blockade

6.6 Necrotizing fasciitis

6.6.1 General

- Necrotizing fasciitis (NF) is an uncommon, life-threatening, fulminant infection of soft tissues.
- Incidence in developed nations is less than 5 cases per 100,000 per year.
- Mortality is quoted as around 25%.

6.6.2 Classification

- NF is typically classified on the basis of microbiological grounds:
  - Type I (polymicrobial):
    - Accounts for the majority (70%) of cases.
    - Slower progression, therefore more opportunity for diagnosis and intervention, and better outcomes.
    - An average of four organisms are isolated in infected tissue.
    - Typically a combination of Gram-positive (often *Streptococcus*), Gram-negative (e.g. *Enterobacter, E. coli, Klebsiella, Proteus*), and anaerobic organisms (e.g. *Clostridium* spp., *Bacteroides* spp.).

- Type II (group A streptococcal infection +/− *Staphylococcus*)
  - Typically affects the extremities
  - Associated with a toxic shock syndrome (see Toxin-producing bacteria in Section 6.7).
- Type III (related to infection with *Vibrio* spp.) and Type IV (related to *Candida*) are very uncommon but associated with a high mortality.

6.6.3 Risk factors

- Risk factors are related to:
  - Relatively immunocompromised (diabetes, steroid use, underlying malignancy, malnutrition).
  - Chronic disease (renal failure, peripheral vascular disease).
  - Disruption of skin integrity (intravenous drug use, trauma, surgery, childbirth).

6.6.4 Diagnosis

- It is important to differentiate NF from cellulitis:
  - Cellulitis begins at the junction between dermis and epidermis; NF begins between sub-cutaneous fat and deep dermis.
  - As a result of the differing depths of infection, erythema and oedema are earlier signs in cellulitis than NF. A purple-blue appearance to skin may be seen in the early stages of NF.
  - NF is more painful; apparently disproportionate pain is one of the cardinal symptoms of NF.
- Diagnosis of NF is clinical, but may be retrospectively confirmed by histology from surgical samples.
- Imaging may demonstrate evidence of gas in the tissues, particularly in Type I NF. This is a specific, but insensitive sign.

6.6.5 Treatment

- Supportive therapy, as for any severe sepsis.
- Early and adequate surgical debridement, with care to remove all necrotic tissue; amputation may be required in NF of the limb; multiple debridement over a period of days is often required.
- Antibiotic therapy must take into account tissue penetration, the potential for multiple organisms, and the possibility of a toxin-producing *Streptococcus*:
  - Tazobactam and piperacillin or a carbopenem provide broad cover against Gram-positive, Gram-negative, and anaerobic organisms.
  - Clindamycin provides additional cover against group A *Streptococcus* with the additional benefit of an anti-toxin effect.
- Additional therapy of uncertain efficacy includes:
  - Intravenous immunoglobulin, as a means of managing toxin production (see Section 5.4.7).
  - Hyperbaric oxygen therapy as a means of enhancing the bactericidal effect of neutrophils. This is reported beneficial in *Clostridium* spp. infections but is of uncertain efficacy with other organisms. Hyperbaric therapy is available in a limited number of centres and carries significant logistical difficulties.

6.7 Toxin-producing bacteria

- Many bacteria produce toxins: enzyme-like proteins with biological activity.
- Some toxins are specific in their action (e.g. tetanus toxin, botulinum toxin).

- Some toxins are broad in their action and cause widespread inflammation (e.g. staphylococcal and streptococcal toxins).
- Endotoxins (or lipopolysaccharides) are inherent components of bacterial structure found primarily in Gram-negative organisms; multiplication or destruction of the bacteria causes release of endotoxin and contributes to the symptoms of Gram-negative infection. Endotoxins promote a profound inflammatory response by direct interaction with the immune system.
- Exotoxins are proteins secreted by bacteria and may act by one of a number of mechanisms including:
  - Super-antigens: endotoxin directly activates the immune system leading to a massive release of cytokines; may occur with *Staphylococcus aureus* associated toxic shock syndrome and group A *Streptococcus* infection.
  - Pore formation: insertion of the endotoxin into the host cell membrane leads to pore formation and cell lysis; may occur with *Streptococcus pneumoniae* and *Clostridium perfringens*.
  - Intracellular: the endotoxin enters the cell and alters cellular bio-activity, e.g. the cholera toxin activates adenylate cyclase increasing cyclic GMP and resulting in excretion of water, sodium, potassium, and bicarbonate ions into the intestinal lumen.
- Linezolid and clindamycin have toxin-suppressing properties.

FURTHER READING

Akgün KM, Huang L, Morris A, Justice AC, Pisani M, Crothers K. Critical illness in HIV-infected patients in the era of combination antiretroviral therapy. *Proceedings of the American Thoracic Society* 2011; 8(3): 301–7.

Davoudian P, Flint NJ. Necrotizing fasciitis. *Continuing Education in Anaesthesia, Critical Care & Pain* 2012: doi: 10.1093/bjaceaccp/mks033.

Johnstone C, Hall A, Hart IJ. Common viral illnesses in intensive care: presentation, diagnosis, and management. *Continuing Education in Anaesthesia, Critical Care & Pain* 2014; 14(5): 213–9.

Marks M, Gupta-Wright A, Doherty J, Singer M, Walker D. Managing malaria in the intensive care unit. *British journal of anaesthesia* 2014; 113(6): 910–21.

Public Health England. *PHE Guidance on use of Antiviral Agents for the Treatment and Prophylaxis of Influenza (2014–15)*, 2014. https://www.gov.uk/government/uploads/system/uploads/attachment_data/file/400392/PHE_guidance_antivirals_influenza_2014-15_5_1.pdf

World Health Organization Guidelines Approved by the Guidelines Review Committee. *Guidelines for the Treatment of Malaria*. Geneva: World Health Organization Copyright (c) World Health Organization, 2010.

World Health Organization Definitions. HIV/AIDS Programme. 2007. http://www.who.int/entity/hiv/pub/guidelines/WHO%20HIV%20Staging.pdf

7 Nosocomial infections

7.1 Clostridium difficile

- *Clostridium difficile* is discussed in Chapter 4, Section 6.2.1.

7.2 Multidrug-resistant organisms*

7.2.1 General

- Multidrug-resistant organisms (MDRO) are microorganisms (primarily bacteria) that are resistant to antimicrobial agents to which they would be expected to be responsive.
- MDROs may be associated with:
    - Contamination: microbial attachment without proliferation.
    - Colonization: microbial attachment and proliferation within the host but no inflammatory response.
    - Infection: an inflammatory response to the presence of microorganisms.
- Whilst the clinical manifestations of MDRO infection are comparable to the sensitive strain of the pathogen, treatment options may be severely limited.
- MDRO infections are associated with increased risk of mortality, length of hospital stay, and cost to the healthcare system.
- The epidemiology of MDRO varies depending upon geographical location (with some countries experiencing far higher rates of MDRO infection) and location within the hospital (ICUs have higher rates than other wards; tertiary ICUs have higher rates still; long-term care facilities experience high rates of MDRO colonization, although not infection).

7.2.2 Minimizing transmission

- Transmission of MDRO is influenced by several factors:
    - Availability of vulnerable patients: patients vulnerable to both colonization and infection are those with severe underlying disease—particularly disease that impairs the immune response—and those with indwelling medical devices.
    - Selective pressure: widespread use of broad-spectrum antibiotics risks 'selecting out' resistant strains of bacteria.
    - Colonization pressure: the larger the number of colonized patients within an institution, and the longer a non-colonized patient is exposed to those who are colonized, the greater the risk of transmission.
    - Existence of, and adherence to, infection-control measures: transmission by hands of health professionals is probably the primary route of transmission in healthcare facilities; poor adherence to hand hygiene and other rudimentary infection-control practices increases the risk of transmission.
- The Centre for Disease Control recommends several measures for minimizing transmission of MDRO (Siegal et al. 2006):
    - Administrative support
        - Effective control of MDROs requires an organization-wide response with infection control a part of organizational ethos. Sufficient resources for an effective response must be made available.
    - Education
        - A robust education programme that encourages behaviour change by improving understanding of MDROs. Examples include promotion of hand hygiene and antimicrobial prescribing.
    - Judicious use of antimicrobial agents
        - Approaches include use of narrow-spectrum antibiotics when feasible and reserving broad-spectrum antibiotics for severe infections in which the pathogen is

* Adapted from *American Journal of Infection Control*, 35, Siegal et al, 'Management of multidrug-resistant organisms in health care settings', pp.S165-S193. Copyright (2007) with permission from Elsevier.

unknown; avoiding the treatment of contaminants; limiting duration of course; optimizing pharmacokinetics of antibiotics (i.e. ensuring appropriate plasma levels).

- MDRO surveillance:
  - Surveillance allows detection of emerging MDRO pathogens, provides epidemiological data, and allows the effectiveness of interventions to be tested. Active surveillance for asymptomatic colonization (e.g. by routine throat and rectal swabs on ICU admission) allows detection of colonized patients, institution of contact precautions, and, for some pathogens, the institution of suppression therapy.
- Infection–control measures include:
  - *Standard precautions* for all patients: scrupulous hand hygiene, aprons and gloves for patient contact.
  - *Contact precautions* for patients identified as being colonized or infected by a potentially pathogenic organism: a side room is optimal, gown and gloves for patient contact are necessary.
  - *Cohorting*: if a single room is not available, cohorting of patients colonized or infected with the same MDRO may be an acceptable alternative.
- Environmental measures:
  - Medical equipment and surfaces are potential reservoirs of infection. A robust cleaning policy, appropriately trained housekeeping staff, and intermittent environmental cultures may reduce the risk of contamination.
- Decolonization:
  - Methicillin resistant *Staphylococcus aureus* is the only MDRO for which decolonization has been consistently proven to be successful. Various combinations of antimicrobial soaps (e.g. chlorhexidine), topical antibiotics (e.g. nasal mupirocin) and systemic antibiotics (e.g. enteral rifampicin) are used.

7.2.3 Methicillin-resistant Staphylococcus aureus (MRSA)

- The most commonly identified MDRO in hospitals.
- Increasingly found in the community setting.
- A genetic alteration within MRSA leads to a change in the penicillin-binding protein; beta-lactam antibiotics cannot effectively bind the bacterium.
- Glycopeptides and oxazolidinones are effective alternative antibiotics.

7.2.4 Vancomycin-resistant Enterococcus (VRE)

- An increasingly common and problematic healthcare-associated infection.
- Risk factors for VRE include:
  - Previous antibiotic exposure, particularly vancomycin and cephalosporins
  - Prolonged hospitalization, in particular ICU admission
  - Co-morbidities, particularly transplant, end-stage renal disease, cancer
  - Long-term intravenous access; enteral tube
  - Prevalence of VRE colonized patients in the hospital/ICU
  - Low staff-to-patient ratios
- Resistance occurs due to modification of the glycopeptide-binding sites on enterococci.
- Genes encoding resistance may spread from VRE to MRSA.
- Multiple subtypes of resistance, which vary in sensitivity to alternative antibiotics (e.g. Van A is vancomycin and teicoplanin-resistant; Van B is teicoplanin-sensitive).
- The oxazolidinone linezolid is an effective alternative for all subtypes.

7.2.5 Multidrug-resistant Gram-negative bacilli

- Defined as Gram-negative bacilli resistant to more than two antimicrobial agents.
- Typically resistant to penicillins, cephalosporins, fluroquinolones, and aminoglycosides; some strains are also resistant to carbapenems.
- *Pseudomonas aeruginosa* is the most common example in North America.
- *Acinetobacter baumannii* is resistant to most antimicrobials, carbapenems are usually effective but resistant strains are emerging; under such circumstances, tigecycline may offer the only effective option.
- Carbapenem-resistant enterobacteriaceae (CRE)(enterobacteriaceae include *Klebsiella* sp. and *Escherichia coli*) produce carbapenemase enzymes, deactivating the antibiotic; alternative agents include tigecycline, amikacin, and colistin. These are also known as extended-spectrum beta-lactamase (ESBL)-producing enterobacteriaceae.
- *Stenotrophomonas maltophila*: co-trimoxazole is the only reliably effective antibiotic.

FURTHER READING

Luyt C-E, Bréchot N, Trouillet J-L, Chastre J. Antibiotic stewardship in the intensive care unit. *Critical Care* 2014; 18(5): 480.

Siegel JD, Rhinehart E, Jackson M, Chiarello L, Committee HICPA. Management of multidrug-resistant organisms in health care settings, 2006. *American Journal of Infection Control* 2007; 35(10): S165–93.

7.3 Catheter-related bloodstream infections

7.3.1 General

- Vascular access is ubiquitous to intensive care patients.
- Vascular access, in particular central venous catheters (CVC), carries an inherent risk of bloodstream infection.
- Catheter-related bloodstream infection is associated with risk of harm to the patient and significant financial burden to healthcare systems.
- Four routes are recognized for catheter infection:
  - Migration of skin organisms along the skin tract formed by the catheter; most common route in short-term catheters.
  - Contact contamination of the catheter or injection hub by hands or equipment and subsequent intra-luminal migration of pathogen.
  - Haematogenous spread to catheter from a distant site of infection.
  - Contaminated infusate.

7.3.2 Definitions and diagnosis

- The definitions surrounding catheter-related infections are not straightforward.
- Vascular catheters may be defined by:
  - Type of vessel: peripheral or central; arterial or venous.
  - Lifespan: temporary, short-term; permanent, long-term.
  - Site of insertion: jugular, subclavian, femoral, peripheral.
  - Pathway from skin to vessel: tunnelled, non-tunnelled.
  - Length: long, short.
  - Additional features: number of lumens; antibiotic, antiseptic or heparin impregnated.

- Laboratory confirmed bloodstream infection (LCBSI):
  - Either:
    - The presence of one or more recognized *pathogens* in blood cultures, or
    - If the isolated bacterium is a common skin commensal, it must be isolated from two or more blood cultures separate in time, and be associated with fever (>38°C), chills or hypotension.
- Catheter-related infections:
  - Central line *associated* bloodstream infection (CLABSI) is a pragmatic definition applicable to clinical practice and screening programmes, it is defined as:
    - Bloodstream infection
    - The presence of a CVC within the 48 hours preceding blood culture, and
    - Absence of another apparent source of the bacteraemia
  - Catheter-related bloodstream infection (CRBSI) is a more complex definition, which requires a higher standard of evidence and the ability of the laboratory to perform quantitative analysis of blood culture, it is defined as:
    - Bloodstream infection
    - The presence of a CVC within the 48 hours preceding blood culture, and
    - Either:
      - A positive quantitative CVC blood culture (>10 colony forming units per ml) whereby the same organism is isolated from blood drawn from the CVC (or on the CVC tip) and in peripheral blood, or
      - Simultaneous quantitative blood cultures with a >5:1 ratio of colony forming units between CVC and peripheral cultures
  - CRBSI is typically reserved for research studies.

7.3.3 Risk factors

- Patient
  - Immunocompromised
  - Severity of illness
  - Loss of skin integrity (e.g. burns)
- Duration of insertion
  - The incidence of infection increases with time; the duration associated with significant increase in infection rates varies with the type of line, with peripheral lines, and pulmonary artery catheters becoming prone to infection at an earlier stage than central lines.
- Line
  - Insertion site
    - Femoral lines carry the highest risk of infection; subclavian lines the lowest.
  - Material
    - Catheters impregnated with antimicrobials (chlorhexidine/silver sulfadiazine) or antibiotics (minocycline/rifampicin) are associated with a reduction in catheter-related bacteraemia.
    - The Centre for Disease Control recommends the use of impregnated catheters if the rate of line infection exceeds that of comparable units, despite a comprehensive programme for CLABSI reduction.
    - Heparin-bonded lines reduce the risk of catheter-related thrombosis, which may, in turn, reduce the risk of infection.

7.3.4 Bundles of care

- In 2006 Provonst et al. reported the use of a CVC insertion and care 'bundle', which combined five evidence-based interventions aimed at reducing the incidence of CLABSI; a reduction in CLABSI from 7.7 to 1.4 per 1,000 CVC days was reported.
- The original bundle consisted of:
  - Hand washing.
  - Full barrier precautions during insertion.
  - Cleaning skin with chlorhexidine.
  - Avoidance of the femoral vein as a site of insertion.
  - Removing catheters when no longer necessary.
- In addition to these technical elements, a number of non-technical interventions were implemented:
  - The bundle was introduced as part of a general education programme relating to a culture of safety.
  - Checklists were encouraged.
  - CVC carts were implemented.
  - Staff were empowered to challenge unsafe behaviour and terminate line insertion if recommended steps were not implemented.
- Subsequent British examination of implementation of a similar CVC bundle by Bion et al. demonstrated a steady decrease in CVC infection rate to a level similar to the post-intervention rate reported by Provonst.
- Analysis of the British data suggested that the reduction in infection rates could not be attributed solely to the introduction of the designated CVC bundle.
- This may demonstrate the difficulty in experimental work relating to complex phenomenon (such as bundles and behaviour) being tested in a dynamic clinical environment.

7.3.5 Other high-grade recommendations relating to CVC

- Use subclavian over jugular over femoral lines.
- Avoid subclavian lines in patients likely to require long-term dialysis as there is a risk of subclavian stenosis—this may have implications for future long term dialysis access.
- Chlorhexidine in conjunction with alcohol is associated with a lower risk of BSI than iodine-based solutions.
- The use of chlorhexidine-impregnated sponges appears to reduce the risk of line infection and BSI.
- Dressings should be semi-permeable to prevent build-up of moisture.
- Use ultrasound to insert CVC:
  - Reduce mechanical complications.
  - Reduce number of punctures.
  - Appears to reduce the rate of CLABSI.
- Replace catheters inserted in an emergency (and in which aseptic technique cannot be guaranteed) as soon as practical.
- Use catheter with the minimum number of required ports.
- Consider antibiotic (e.g. rifampicin and minocycline) or antimicrobial (e.g. chlorhexidine and silver sulphadalazine) impregnated lines if CLABSI rates remain high despite best practice, if lines are expected to remain *in situ* for greater than 7 days, or the patient is at particular risk of infection (e.g. immunocompromised).
- Do NOT routinely replace CVCs to prevent infection.

- Do NOT remove or replace CVCs on the basis of fever alone; clinical judgement should be used.
- Administration sets should be changed regularly: between 72 hours and 7 days for crystalloid solutions; every 24 hours for lipid-containing solutions (propofol, TPN).

FURTHER READING

Australia and New Zealand Intensive Care Society. Central Line Insertion and Maintenance Guideline, 2012. http://www.anzics.com.au/Downloads/ANZICS.

Bion J, Richardson A, Hibbert P, et al. 'Matching Michigan': a 2-year stepped interventional programme to minimise central venous catheter-bloodstream infections in intensive care units in England. *BMJ Quality & Safety* 2012; doi: 10.1136/bmjqs-2012-001325.

Frasca D, Dahyot-Fizelier C, Mimoz O. Prevention of central venous catheter-related infection in the intensive care unit. *Critical care* 2010; 14(2): 212.

O'Grady N, Alexander M, Burns L, Dellinger E, Garland J, Heard S. Guidelines for the Prevention of Intravascular Catheter-Related Infections. Centers for Disease Control and Prevention 2011. http://www.cdc.gov/hicpac/pdf/guidelines/bsi-guidelines-2011.pdf.

Pronovost P, Needham D, Berenholtz S, et al. An intervention to decrease catheter-related bloodstream infections in the ICU. *New England Journal of Medicine* 2006; 355(26): 2725–32.

Veenstra DL, Saint S, Saha S, Lumley T, Sullivan SD. Efficacy of antiseptic-impregnated central venous catheters in preventing catheter-related bloodstream infection: a meta-analysis. *Journal of the American Medical Association* 1999; 281(3): 261–7.

7.4 Ventilator-associated pneumonia[*]

7.4.1 General

- Ventilator-associated pneumonia (VAP) is a nosocomial infection occurring over 48–72 hours post-tracheal intubation.
- It is common, with a reported incidence of up to 27% of all mechanically ventilated patients.
- The risk of VAP is highest in the early stage of mechanical ventilation.
- The associated mortality may be as high as 50%.

7.4.2 Definition

- There is no universally agreed definition for VAP.
- The Centre for Disease Control define pneumonia as:
  - Radiological signs (two or more serial chest X-rays with at least one of the following):
    - New or progressive and persistent infiltrate
    - Consolidation
    - Cavitation
  - Clinical signs (at least one of the following):
    - Fever (temperature >38°C with no other recognized cause)
    - Leucocytosis or leucopenia
    - For adults 70 years or older, altered mental status with no other recognizable cause

---

[*] Data from Infection Control, 29, 2008, Coffin et al., 'Strategies to prevent ventilator-associated pneumonia in acute care hospitals', pp. S31–S40.

- And at least two of the following:
  - New onset of purulent sputum, or change in character of sputum, or increased respiratory secretions, or increased suctioning requirements.
  - New-onset or worsening cough, or dyspnoea or tachypnoea.
  - Crackles or bronchial breath sounds.
  - Worsening gas exchange.
- Microbiological criteria (optional) (at least one of the following):
  - Positive growth in blood culture not related to another source of infection.
  - Positive growth in culture of pleural fluid.
  - Positive quantitative culture from bronchoalveolar lavage ($\geq 10^4$ colony forming units.ml^{-1}) or protected specimen brushing ($\geq 10^3$ colony forming units.ml^{-1}).
  - 5% or more of cells with intracellular bacteria on direct microscopic examination of Gram-stained bronchoalveolar lavage fluid.
  - Histopathological evidence of pneumonia.
- Development of the above criteria in a patient with a tracheal tube in situ for greater than 48 hours would constitute VAP.

7.4.2.1 Mechanism and risk factors

- The presence of a tracheal tube increases the risk of nosocomial pneumonia by up to 21-fold; potential mechanisms include:
  - Microaspiration around the cuff (or during intubation).
  - Bacterial biofilm developing within the tracheal tube.
  - Impaired ciliary activity and clearance of mucous.
  - Positive pressure ventilation driving bacteria into the respiratory tree.
- Additional risk factors include:
  - High severity of illness
  - Immunosuppression
  - Chronic lung disease
  - ARDS
  - Reintubations
  - Increased gastric pH (including the use of gastric acid supressing medications)
  - Supine position
  - Enteral nutrition
  - Intra-cuff pressure <20 mmHg

7.4.3 Microbiology

- The pathogen varies dependent upon the duration of hospital admission and ventilation.
- Early VAP (within 72 hours of admission):
  - Common community pathogens:
    - *Streptococcus pneumoniae*
    - *Haemophillus influenzae*
    - *Staphylococcus aureus*
    - *Klebiella pneumoniae*
    - *Escherichia coli*
- Later VAP (over 72 hours):
  - Higher incidence of Gram-negative bacteria; higher incidence of antibiotic resistance.

- Common pathogens include:
    - *Pseudomonas aeruginosa*
    - *Methicillin-resistant Staphylococcus aureus*
    - *Acinetobacter*
    - *Stenotrophomonas maltophilia*

7.4.4 Prevention

- Strict hand-washing policy.
- Oral care with chlorhexidine.
- Head of bed angle >30 degrees.
- Subglottic suction.
- Maintaining cuff pressure >20 mmHg.
- Consideration of silver/antibiotic coated tubes.
- Extubation at earliest opportunity, with strategies to facilitate early extubation (e.g. daily sedation interruption).
- Avoid re-intubation.
- Selective oral and digestive decontamination.

7.4.5 Decontamination of the digestive tract

- Decontamination of the digestive tract may constitute one of several strategies:
- Selective digestive decontamination (SDD):
    - A strategy aimed at reducing the incidence of VAP.
    - It seeks to prevent both endogenous and exogenous infection but eradication of both 'normal' and abnormal potentially pathogenic organisms.
    - Classically consists of four components:
        - Enteral antimicrobials: poorly absorbed agents applied as a gel to the oropharynx and bolused down a nasogastric tube; typically tobramycin, polymixin E and amphotericin B.
        - Parenteral antibiotic: a short (4-day) course of an anti-pseudomonal (typically cephalosporin) is administered to eradicate potentially pathogenic admission bacteria.
        - Strict hygiene practice.
        - Regular surveillance cultures from rectum and throat, to monitor the effectiveness of the SDD and to detect the emergence of resistant organisms.
- Selective oral decontamination (SOD)
    - Administration of poorly absorbed antimicrobials as paste to the mouth but no nasogastric or parenteral component.
- Topical oropharyngeal antiseptic agents
    - Refers to the use of chlorhexidine gel or solution to the oropharynx.
- Many randomized control trials, systematic reviews, and meta-analyses have been published relating to decontamination of the digestive tract; the majority of this work has been conducted in continental Europe.
- Both SOD and SDD have been demonstrated to reduce the incidence of respiratory tract infection (number needed to treat of 4), bacteraemia, and mortality (number needed to treat of 18); the results relating to antiseptic decontamination of the oropharynx are equivocal.

- Despite the mortality benefit associated with SDD and SOD, uptake outwith continental Europe has been limited; a number of reasons have been proposed:
    - There is concern regarding the development of antimicrobial resistance; this is not supported by the trials, which have demonstrated reduction in rate of colonization by highly resistant organisms.
    - The external validity of the research has been questioned: the majority of studies have been performed in regions with low levels of antibiotic resistance; the efficacy of SOD and SDD in areas of higher antibiotic resistance is unclear.
    - SOD and SDD are relatively resource intense procedures, particularly for nursing staff undertaking drug preparation and administration, and laboratory staff conducting surveillance cultures.

FURTHER READING

Coffin SE, Klompas M, Classen D, et al. Strategies to prevent ventilator-associated pneumonia in acute care hospitals. *Infection Control* 2008; 29(S1): S31–40.

Drakulovic MB, Torres A, Bauer TT, Nicolas JM, Nogué S, Ferrer M. Supine body position as a risk factor for nosocomial pneumonia in mechanically ventilated patients: a randomised trial. *Lancet* 1999; 354(9193): 1851–8.

Kalanuria AA, Zai W, Mirski M. Ventilator-associated pneumonia in the ICU. *Critical Care* 2014; 18(2): 208.

Liberati A, D'Amico R, Pifferi S, Torri V, Brazzi L, Parmelli E. Antibiotic prophylaxis to reduce respiratory tract infections and mortality in adults receiving intensive care. *Cochrane Database of Systematic Reviews* 2009; (4): Cd000022.

National Institute for Health and Clinical Excellence. *Technical Patient Safety Solutions for Ventilator-Associated Pneumonia in Adults*. www.nice.org.uk/nicemedia/pdf/PSG002Guidance.pdf

Price R, MacLennan G, Glen J. Selective digestive or oropharyngeal decontamination and topical oropharyngeal chlorhexidine for prevention of death in general intensive care: systematic review and network meta-analysis. *British Medical Journal* 2014; 348: g2197.

Weinstein RA, Bonten MJ, Kollef MH, Hall JB. Risk factors for ventilator-associated pneumonia: from epidemiology to patient management. *Clinical Infectious Diseases* 2004; 38(8): 1141–9.

CHAPTER 7

Haematology

CONTENTS

1 Anaemia and transfusion medicine

1.1 Anaemia

1.1.1 General

- Anaemia is common in the critically ill and will affect most patients during their ICU stay.
- It is defined by the World Health Organization as haemoglobin (Hb) of:
    - ≤120 g.l⁻¹ in women
    - ≤130 g.l⁻¹ in men
    - Severe anaemia is defined as Hb ≤80 g.l⁻¹

1.1.2 Aetiology and investigation

- Common causes of anaemia in ICU include:
    - Blood loss, including haemorrhage (although haemorrhage accounts for only 20% of transfusions in ICU)
    - Blood sampling
    - Impaired erythropoiesis as a result of critical illness (e.g. sepsis)
    - Haemodilution
    - Extracorporeal therapies
- Other causes include:
    - B12/folate deficiency
    - Iron deficiency
    - Myelodysplastic syndromes
    - Anaemia of chronic disease
    - Coeliac disease/malabsorption
    - Haemolysis
    - Drugs

- In many cases, investigation will not be required as the cause will be obvious (e.g. haemorrhage, recent major surgery).
- Some investigative measures include:
  - Thorough and systematic history and examination, including drug history (e.g. NSAIDs and occult gastrointestinal bleeding).
  - Mean Corpuscular Volume (MCV):
    - Macrocytosis encountered in B12/folate deficiency, chronic alcohol excess, haemolysis, myelodysplasia, hypothyroidism, and liver disease.
    - Microcytic picture commonly encountered in chronic iron deficiency.
  - Blood film, B12/folate, ferritin and iron studies—can be difficult to interpret in ICU as serum ferritin increases in acute illness, while serum iron can decrease.
  - Raised lactate dehydrogenase (LDH) and reticulocyte count can be suggestive of haemolysis.

1.2 Red cell transfusion in the absence of major haemorrhage

1.2.1 Red cell transfusion in the general ICU population

- Up to half of all ICU patients will require a red cell transfusion during their ICU stay.
- Red cell transfusion in critically ill patients is not a benign intervention and is associated with increased risk of death, infection, and prolonged length of critical care stay.
- The British Committee for Standards in Haematology (BCSH) currently recommend the following practices with regard to blood and blood transfusion:*
  - Transfusion threshold of 70 g.l^{-1} in the general ICU population
  - Consideration of the use of blood-conservation devices for blood sampling
  - Routine use of erythropoietin (EPO) and iron therapy is not currently recommended
- The transfusion threshold described above, and much of current ICU transfusion practice, is traditionally based on the results of the multi-centre RCT Transfusion Requirements in Critical Care (TRICC) study.
- This study compared a liberal vs restrictive blood transfusion protocol:
  - Transfusion threshold of 100 g.l^{-1} vs 70 g.l^{-1}
  - There were significantly fewer transfusions in the restrictive group
  - There was also a trend towards decreased mortality in the restrictive group.
  - The study was underpowered. It was conducted prior to the routine leukodepletion of blood products and therefore the findings may not be applicable to current practice.
- Current evidence/guideline-based best practice in red cell transfusion in specific situations is outlined in Table 7.1; in cases where there is an absence of recent high-quality evidence the reader should defer to the BCSH red cell transfusion guideline.

Table 7.1 Red cell transfusion targets in special circumstances

Circumstance	Recommendation	Evidence/guideline
Septic shock	Aim Hb >70 g.l^{-1}	TRISS Study, Holst et al. NEJM, 2014—no difference in outcomes between liberal (90 g.l^{-1}) and restrictive (70 g.l^{-1}) transfusion thresholds Higher thresholds used in 'Rivers' style EGDT not associated with improved outcomes—ARISE/PROCESS/PROMISE Studies all NEJM 2014-2015
Post-elective cardiac surgery	Aim Hb >90 g.l^{-1}	'Liberal or restrictive transfusion after cardiac surgery', Murphy et al. NEJM, 2015—slightly increased mortality in restrictive group
Upper GI bleeding	Aim Hb >70 g.l^{-1}	'Transfusion strategies for acute upper GI bleeding', Villanueva et al. NEJM, 2013: Improved survival overall for all cause GI bleeding using restrictive (70 g.l^{-1}) strategy when compared to liberal strategy (90 g.l^{-1}). Within cirrhotic group effect seen in Child-Pugh A and B, but not C.
Traumatic brain injury (TBI)	Target range 70–90 g.l^{-1}	BCSH Guideline, Grade 2D evidence
TBI with evidence of cerebral ischaemia	Aim Hb >90 g.l^{-1}	BCSH Guideline, Grade 2D evidence
Subarachnoid haemorrhage	Target range 80–100 g.l^{-1}	BCSH Guideline, Grade 2D evidence
Ischaemic stroke	Aim Hb >90 g.l^{-1}	BCSH Guideline, Grade 2D evidence
Critical illness in context of stable chronic ischaemic heart disease	Aim Hb >70 g.l^{-1}	BCSH Guideline, Grade 2B evidence
Acute coronary syndromes	Aim Hb >80–90 g.l^{-1}	BCSH Guideline, Grade 2C evidence
Liberation from mechanical ventilation/weaning	Do not use transfusion to aid weaning if Hb >70 g.l^{-1}	BCSH Guideline, Grade 2D evidence

1.3 Adverse effects of red cell transfusion

1.3.1 Age of red cells and transfusion

- It had been postulated that transfusion of older red cells may have potentially deleterious effects.
- The 2015 multi-centre RCT 'Age of transfused blood in critically ill adults', however, showed no difference in 90-day mortality with transfusion of fresh red cells (i.e. stored for <8 days) when compared to standard issue red cells.
- Similar results were seen in a study looking at this issue in patients undergoing cardiac surgery.

1.3.2 Transfusion associated cardiac overload (TACO)

- Clinical features:
    - Acute respiratory distress
    - Tachycardia
    - Hypertension
    - Pulmonary oedema
    - Positive fluid balance post-transfusion
- Risk factors:
    - Hypoalbuminaemia
    - Renal impairment
    - Pre-transfusion fluid overload
- Frequency:
    - 1 in every 357 red cell units transfused
- Treatment:
    - Supportive measures
    - Diuretics

1.3.3 Transfusion-related acute lung injury (TRALI)

- Clinical features:
    - Acute pulmonary oedema within 6 hours of transfusion associated with P_aO_2/F_iO_2 <300 mmHg (40 kPa)
    - Bilateral pulmonary infiltrates, in absence of suspected left atrial hypertension
- Risk factors:
    - Products donated by multiparous women
    - Non-leukodepleted blood
- Frequency:
    - 1 in every 1,271 transfusions (more frequent after FFP, less frequent with cryoprecipitate)
- Treatment:
    - Supportive critical care measures and reporting of incident to relevant body with subsequent investigation

1.3.4 Other risks

- Infection:
    - Bacterial (from contamination of product)
    - Viral (e.g. HIV, hepatitis B and C)
    - Prion disease (e.g. Creutzfeld–Jacob disease)

- Haemolytic reaction:
    - ABO incompatibility (wrong blood to wrong patient)
    - Minor incompatibility
- Allergy:
    - Up to anaphylaxis
- Hypothermia
- Immune sensitization

1.4 Haemolysis

1.4.1 Definition and categorization

- Haemolysis is the premature destruction of red blood cells.
- Haemolysis is a common occurrence in the critically ill.
- It may be divided into:
    - Acquired
        - Immune mediated
        - Non-immune mediated
    - Congenital

1.4.2 Aetiology

Common aetiology in the intensive care includes:
- Mechanical destruction:
    - Renal replacement circuit
    - ECMO circuit
    - Intra-aortic balloon pump
    - Ventricular assist device
- Sepsis:
    - May be immune mediated with any infection
        - Some specific infections associated with haemolysis are *Clostridium perfringens*, Bartonellosis and Malaria.
- Drug-induced:
    - May be immune mediated or a direct effect of the drug
- Microangiopathic haemolysis (MAHA) e.g.:
    - Disseminated intravascular coagulation
    - Thrombotic thrombocytopaenic purpura
    - Haemolytic uraemic syndrome
- Red cell enzyme deficiency (congenital) e.g.:
    - Glucose-6-phosphate dehydrogenase deficiency
    - Pyruvate kinase deficiency
- Haemaglobinopathies (congenital) e.g.:
    - Sickle disease
    - Thalassaemia

1.4.3 Investigation

- Confirmation of haemolysis
    - Blood film for spherocytes and reticulocytes (reticulocyte count >1.5%); may reveal abnormal forms specific to a particular form of haemolytic anaemia
    - Unconjugated (indirect) bilirubin is increased in the presence of haemolysis

- LDH is elevated
- Haptoglobin is decreased
- Investigation of aetiology
  - Direct antigen (Coombs') test is positive in autoimmune acquired anaemia
  - Haemoglobin electrophoresis, if haemoglobinopathy is suspected
  - Coagulation profile for evidence of DIC
  - Renal function, if concurrent AKI, consider haemolytic uraemic syndrome
  - Plasma free Hb, which is elevated if mechanical destruction of red cells

1.4.4 Management

- Supportive care
- Involvement of a haematologist

FURTHER READING

Hebert PC, Wells G, Blajchman MA et al. A multicenter, randomized, controlled clinical trial of transfusion requirements in critical care. *New England Journal of Medicine* 1999; 240: 409–417.

Holst LB, Haase N, Wettersley J et al. Lower versus higher hemoglobin threshold for transfusion in septic shock. *New England Journal of Medicine* 2014; 371: 1381–91.

Joint UK blood transfusion and tissue transplantation service professional advisory committee. *Handbook of Transfusion Medicine*, 2013. http://www.transfusionguidelines.org.uk/transfusion-handbook

Lacroix J, Hebert PC, Fergusson DA et al. Age of transfused blood in critically ill adults. *New England Journal of Medicine* 2015; 372: 1410–18.

Steiner ME, Ness PM, Assman SF et al. Effects of red-cell storage duration on patients undergoing cardiac surgery. *New England Journal of Medicine* 2015; 372: 1419–29.

Murphy GJ, Pike K, Rogers CA et al. Liberal or restrictive transfusion after cardiac surgery. *New England Journal of Medicine* 2015. 372(11):997–1008.

Retter A, Wyncoll D, Pearse R et al. Guidelines on the management of anaemia and red cell transfusion in adult critically ill patients. *British Journal of Haematology* 2013; 160(4): 454–64.

Villanueva C, Colomo A, Bosch A at al. Transfusion strategies for acute upper gastrointestinal bleeding. *New England Journal of Medicine* 2013; 368: 11–21.

2 Major haemorrhage and massive transfusion

2.1 Definitions

2.1.1 Definitions of major haemorrhage

- Loss of >1 blood volume within 24 hours
- Loss of half of total blood volume within 3 hours
- Bleeding rate of >150 ml/min
- Bleeding with physiological derangement illustrated by systolic BP <90 mmHg or heart rate >110 beats per minute.

2.1.2 Definitions of massive transfusion

- Transfusion of >10 units of blood within 24 hours, or
- Transfusion of one blood volume within 24 hours.
- Most research and evidence within this sphere is within the context of trauma, particularly trauma on the battlefield.
- The observations that severely injured patients present with established coagulopathy (acute coagulopathy of trauma) and that large volume crystalloid infusion in the context of massive haemorrhage may be deleterious, have led to a move towards a concept of 'damage-control resuscitation'; this is described further in Chapter 8, Section 1.3.

2.2 Acute coagulopathy of trauma

- Coagulopathy in trauma has traditionally been attributed to the combination of acidosis, hypothermia, dilutional effects of crystalloid and packed red cell transfusion, and consumptive processes such as DIC.
- More recent work suggests acute coagulopathy of trauma is the consequence of tissue hypoperfusion mediated via the protein c pathway and hyper-fibrinolysis.
- It is associated with poor outcomes and requires early recognition and aggressive therapy.

2.3 Healthcare response to major haemorrhage

- A high index of suspicion is required to instigate early management of major haemorrhage and to avoid further deterioration.

2.3.1 Organization

- Use of major haemorrhage protocols with multidisciplinary response and protocol led administration/delivery of transfusion packs is associated with improved outcomes.
- Early, definitive control of surgical bleeding is essential.

2.3.2 Blood product ratios

- Early and aggressive volume expansion with blood products (including plasma and platelets) is key.
- The recent PROPPR (Holcomb et al, *JAMA*, 2015) study compared ratios of transfusion of plasma:platelets:packed red cells. The ratios studied where 1:1:1 and 1:1:2 (where 1 UK 'pool' of platelets contains 6 units of platelets). The study showed no overall difference in mortality at 24 hours or 30 days; however, more patients in the 1:1:1 group achieved haemostasis within 24 hours and fewer died due to exsanguination within 24 hours.

2.3.3 Hypothermia and acidosis

- Correction/avoidance of hypothermia and acidosis is important and a blood-warming device should be used.

2.3.4 Calcium

- Monitoring of ionized calcium and subsequent administration of calcium may be required—this is due to the inclusion of citrate in transfused blood as an anticoagulant.
- Excess citrate can lead to metabolic alkalosis and free hypocalcaemia. Massive brisk transfusion is required to induce this; however, patients with liver disease or ischaemic liver injury are at particular risk.

2.3.5 Antifibrinolysis

- Tranexamic acid inhibits plasminogen and thereby inhibits fibrinolysis.
- Tranexamic acid has been demonstrated to significantly reduce mortality from bleeding when given early in trauma-associated haemorrhage (CRASH-II).
- It also has a role in reducing transfusion requirements in cardiac and orthopaedic surgery.

2.3.6 Recombinant factor VII

- Factor VII combines with platelets and tissue factor to generate a 'thrombin burst' resulting in fibrin clot formation.
- High-quality evidence regarding the efficacy of recombinant factor VII in the setting of major haemorrhage is lacking, although case reports relating to refractory haemorrhage are encouraging.
- It is expensive and associated with a significant increase in the incidence of arterial (in particular coronary) thrombus.
- It is, however, used in some settings on a 'case by case' basis on the advice of haematologists with an interest in bleeding/coagulopathy.

FURTHER READING

Bawazeer M, Ahmed N, Izadi H et al. Compliance with a massive transfusion protocol (MTP) impacts patient outcome. *Injury* 2015; 46(1): 21–8.

Holcomb JB, Jenkins D, Rhee P et al. Damage control resuscitation: directly addressing the early coagulopathy of trauma. *Journal of Trauma* 2007; 62(2): 307–10.

HolcombJB, Tilley BC, Baraniuk S et al. Transfusion of plasma, platelets, and red blood cells in a 1:1:1 vs a 1:1:2 ratio and mortality in patients with severe trauma. The PROPPR randomized clinical trial. *Journal of American Medical Association* 2015; 313(5): 471–82.

Shakur H, Roberts I, Bautista R et al. Effects of tranexamic acid on death, vascular occlusive events, and blood transfusion in trauma patients with significant haemorrhage (CRASH-2): a randomised, placebo-controlled trial. *Lancet* 2010; 376(9734): 23–32.

---

3 Thrombocytopaenia

Thrombocytopenia is common in the ICU and affects approximately 50% of all ICU patients. It is associated with increased mortality and is a marker of illness severity.

3.1 Definitions and diagnostic criteria

3.1.1 Definition

- Platelet count <150 × 10^9/l
- Considered severe if <50 × 10^9/l
- Should consider investigating aetiology if count <100 × 10^9/l or if platelet count falls by >30%

3.1.2 Aetiology

- Common causes of thrombocytopenia in the ICU include:
  - Sepsis, including disseminated intravascular coagulation (DIC)

- Haemodilution
- Haemofiltration and use of extracorporeal circuits
- Drugs, including:
    - Glycoprotein IIa/IIIb inhibitors
    - Excess alcohol consumption
    - Chemotherapy
- Hypersplenism
- Liver disease
- Post-surgery, e.g. cardio-respiratory bypass
- Macrophage activation syndrome
- Blood-borne viruses, e.g. CMV, HIV, and hepatitis C
- Folate deficiency
- Myelodysplasia
- Uncommon but important causes of thrombocytopenia which may be encountered in the ICU:
    - Thrombotic thrombocytopenia purpura (TTP)
    - Haemolytic uraemic syndrome (HUS)
    - Heparin-induced thrombocytopenia (HIT)
    - Idiopathic thrombocytopenic purpura (ITP)
    - Haemolysis elevated liver enzymes low platelet count (HELLP) syndrome in pregnancy
    - Malaria

3.2 Investigation

- Systematic review of history and systematic examination, including review of drug history.
- Blood film:
    - Blood film is readily available and may be diagnostic
    - Can exclude pseudothrombocytopenia or platelet clumping, and in other cases can help focus differential diagnosis in cases of thrombocytopenia
- Basic tests:
    - B_{12} and folate
    - D-dimer
    - Liver function tests
    - Prothrombin time/activated partial thromboplastin time/fibrinogen
    - Renal function
    - Lactate dehydrogenase
- Also consider:
    - Pregnancy test
    - Blood-borne virus screen
    - Bone marrow aspirate

3.3 Platelet transfusion in the absence of major haemorrhage

- The Joint United Kingdom (UK) Blood Transfusion and Tissue Transplantation Services Professional Advisory Committee (JPAC) have published a transfusion handbook that includes advice on the management of critically ill patients with thrombocytopenia.
- They advise avoidance of antiplatelet agents and NSAIDs in critically ill patients with thrombocytopenia.
- Table 7.2 describes JPACs platelet transfusion recommendations in critically ill patients.

Table 7.2 Indications for platelet transfusion

Indication	Transfusion threshold or target
Non-bleeding patients without severe sepsis or haemostatic abnormalities	Not indicated
Prophylaxis in non-bleeding patients with severe sepsis or haemostatic abnormalities	Threshold $20 \times 10^9/l$
DIC with bleeding	Maintain $>50 \times 10^9/l$
Platelet dysfunction with non-surgically correctable bleeding (e.g. post-cardiopulmonary bypass or potent antiplatelet drugs)	May bleed despite a normal platelet count. Transfusion of one adult therapeutic dose and repeat according to clinical response
Major haemorrhage and massive transfusion	Maintain $>75 \times 10^9/l$ ($>100 \times 10^9/l$ if multiple trauma or trauma to the central nervous system or inner eye)

Adapted from *Handbook of Transfusion Medicine*, 2013, with permission from The Joint UK Blood Transfusion and Tissue Transplantation Service, http://www.transfusionguidelines.org.uk/transfusion-handbook (accessed 18/09/2015). Available under the Open Government Licence v3.0, http://www.nationalarchives.gov.uk/doc/open-government-licence/version/3/

3.4 Thrombocytopenia in the ICU: some specific circumstances

3.4.1 Heparin-induced thrombocytopenia (HIT)

- Rare, accounting for <1% of cases of thrombocytopenia on the ICU.
- HIT is immune mediated.
- HIT usually occurs between days 5 and 10 post-exposure to heparin, but can occur within hours if the patient has had previous recent heparin exposure.
- Platelet count in HIT is typically $50–80 \times 10^9/l$.
- HIT is a prothrombotic state and can manifest with necrotic skin lesions and arterial or venous thrombosis.
- Where HIT is suspected, a pre-test probability score should be calculated e.g. the Warkentin 4-T score(Table 7.3); a low score reliably excludes HIT, a moderate to high score should prompt further investigation:
  - HIT screen should be sent, this generally involves an ELISA test for anti-heparin PF4 antibodies, and a functional test
  - Heparin should be stopped
  - Non-heparin anticoagulation should be commenced, e.g. danaparoid, lepirudin, bivalirudin, or argatroban
- Platelet transfusion is contraindicated in HIT.

3.4.2 Thrombotic thrombocytopenia purpura (TTP)

- TTP is a rare disease with significant mortality and requirement for intensive care admission.
- TTP is a thrombotic microangiopathy (TMA).
- TTP may be associated in some cases with HIV infection, pregnancy, and some drugs (e.g. quinine, clopidogrel, acyclovir).
- TTP has an autoimmune aetiology associated with low levels of ADAMTS-13.
- Clinical manifestations include:
  - Thrombocytopenia

Table 7.3 The Warkentin 4T scoring system for heparin-induced thrombocytopaenia

	Points (0, 1, or 2 for each of four categories: maximum possible score = 8)		
	2	1	0
Thrombocytopenia	>50% platelet fall to nadir ≥20	30–50% platelet fall, or nadir 10–19	<30% platelet fall, or nadir <10
Timing* of onset of platelet fall (or other sequelae of HIT)	Days 5–10, or ≤day 1 with recent heparin (past 30 days)	>Day 10 or timing unclear; or <day 1 with recent heparin (past 31–100 days)	<Day 4 (no recent heparin)
Thrombosis or other sequelae	Proven new thrombosis; skin necrosis; or acute systemic reaction after intravenous UFH bolus	Progressive or recurrent thrombosis; erythematous skin lesions; suspected thrombosis (not proven)	None
Other cause(s) of platelet fall	None evident	Possible	Definite

Pre-test probability score: 6–8 indicates high; 4–5, intermediate; and 0–3, low.
*First day of immunizing heparin exposure considered day 0.
Adapted from *Circulation*, 110, Warkentin TE, 'Heparin-Induced Thrombocytopenia: Diagnosis and Management'.
Copyright (2004) with permission from Wolters Kluwer Health, Inc.

- ■ Microangiopathic haemolytic anaemia (MAHA)
- ■ Microvascular thrombosis and its consequences, e.g.:
  - ▪ Cerebrovascular complications
  - ▪ Cardiac ischaemic involvement; cardiac dysfunction
  - ▪ Renal dysfunction; haematuria
- ● ADAMTS-13 level should be checked if TTP is suspected
- ● Treatment of TTP needs to be prompt to avoid irreversible morbidity and mortality and includes:
  - ■ Management in a specialist centre
  - ■ Plasma exchange
  - ■ Immunosuppressive therapy, e.g. steroids, rituximab
  - ■ Organ support (if required) in ICU
- ● Platelet transfusion is contraindicated in cases of TTP.

3.4.3 Haemolytic uraemic syndrome (HUS)—typical HUS and atypical HUS (aHUS)

- ● HUS is predominantly a renal TMA; previously TTP and HUS were considered to be the same condition.
- ● It is characterized by the following:
  - ■ MAHA
  - ■ Acute kidney injury
  - ■ Thrombocytopenia
- ● Typical HUS is associated with diarrhoea (usually bloody) and infection with shiga toxin-producing pathogens, e.g. *Escherichia coli* 0157.
- ● It is usually more severe at extremes of age and carries a significant mortality.
- ● aHUS can occur sporadically; it can also be familial.

- aHUS is diagnosed in cases where features of HUS are present in the absence of other causes of renal TMA, e.g. typical HUS, TTP, antiphospholipid syndrome, and HIV.
- Management of HUS in adults includes:
  - Supportive therapy in ICU, including organ support, if required
  - Plasma exchange and immunosuppressive agents, e.g. eculizumab

3.5 Some disorders of platelet function

3.5.1 Uraemia/renal failure

- Significant uraemia can lead to impaired platelet function and increased bleeding tendency.
- Renal replacement therapy is effective at improving platelet function.
- Pharmacological agents, such as erythropoietin, desmopressin, and tranexamic acid, also have a role in improving platelet function.

3.5.2 Pharmacological agents

- The use of pharmacological agents, such as aspirin, clopidogrel, and ticagrelor, is widespread in the management of cardiovascular diseases.
- Considerations in the management of patients receiving these agents with significant bleeding is considered in Section 4 of this chapter.

3.5.3 Von Willebrand's disease

- Deficiency of Von Willebrand's factor leading to impaired platelet interaction with vasculature and subsequent increased bleeding tendency.
- Can be familial or acquired.
- Aetiology of acquired disease includes autoimmune, mechanical stress from extracorporeal circuits, and myeloproliferative disorders.
- Desmopressin and antifibrinolytic agents are used in the treatment of acquired Von Willebrand's disease.

3.6 Point of care testing and platelet function

3.6.1 Conventional analysis

- Conventional laboratory platelet counts are quantitative; however, they have the disadvantage of prolonged turnaround time and they give no information regarding platelet function.

3.6.2 Point-of-care systems

- Some point-of-care systems are available (e.g. Platelet Works ® and VerfiyNow ®), which provide indices of platelet function.
- These are of particular promise in the area of cardiac surgery where many patients are on potent antiplatelet medications and the use of extracorporeal circuits is common.

FURTHER READING

Antier N, Quentot JP, Doise JM et al. Mechanisms and etiologies of thrombocytopenia in the intensive care unit: impact of extensive investigations. *Annals of Intensive Care* 2014; 4: 24.

Enriquez JL and Shore-Lesserson. Point of care coagulation testing and transfusion algorithms. *British Journal of Anaesthesia* 2009; 103(BJA/PGA Supplement): i14–22.

Hunt BJ. Bleeding and coagulopathies in critical care. *New England Journal of Medicine* 2014; 370: 847–59.

Van der Linden T, Souweine B, Dupic L et al. Management of thrombocytopenia in the ICU (pregnancy excluded). *Annals of Intensive Care* 2012; 2: 42.

Scully M and Goodship T et al. How I treat thrombotic thrombocytopenia purpura and atypical haemolytic uraemic syndrome. *British Journal of Haematology* 2014; 164(6): 759–66.

Warkentin TE. Heparin-induced thrombocytopenia diagnosis and management. *Circulation* 2004; 110(18): e454–8.

Watson H, Davidson S, Keeling D et al. Guidelines on the diagnosis and management of heparin induced thrombocytopenia: second edition. *British Journal of Haematology* 2012; doi:10.1111/bjh. 12059

4 Coagulopathy

- Coagulopathy is common in ICU patients.
- Coagulopathy is often a marker of illness severity in critically ill patients and is associated with significant morbidity and mortality

4.1 Aetiology and assessment

4.1.1 Aetiology

- Coagulopathy in the ICU is often multifactorial, however common causes include:
  - Disseminated intravascular coagulation (DIC), e.g. due to sepsis
  - Acute coagulopathy of trauma (Section 2)
  - Drugs, e.g.
    - Warfarin
    - Dabigatran
    - Heparins
  - Liver disease
  - Renal disease
  - Hyper-fibrinolysis
  - Vitamin K deficiency
  - Disturbance of systemic physiology, e.g.:
    - Acidosis
    - Low ionized calcium
    - Hypothermia

4.1.2 Investigation and assessment

- Systematic review of history and systematic examination, including review of drug history
- Coagulation screen:
  - Prothrombin time (PT)
  - International normalized ratio (INR) (PT indexed against standard)
  - Activated partial thromboplastin time (APTT)
  - Fibrinogen
- D-dimer
- Full blood count and blood film
- Bleeding time
- B_{12} and folate

4.2 Plasma component transfusion in the absence of major haemorrhage

- In the absence of significant bleeding, most ICU patients with coagulopathy will not require transfusion of plasma components.
- Administration of vitamin K is appropriate if deficiency is believed to underlie the coagulopathy.
- JPAC make several recommendations regarding transfusion of plasma components in their transfusion handbook:
  - Fresh frozen plasma (FFP)
  - Cryoprecipitate
  - Freeze-dried products

4.2.1 Fresh frozen plasma (FFP)

- FFP transfusion is indicated in the context of bleeding and deranged coagulation suspected due to multiple factor deficiency.
- No benefit in patients with liver disease if INR <1.7 (as the 'INR' of FFP is around 1.6).
- Minimum recommended dose is 12–15 ml.kg^{-1}.

4.2.2 Cryoprecipitate

- Cryoprecipitate is a rich source of fibrinogen; it also contains a significant Von Willebrand's component.
- Cryoprecipitate transfusion is indicated in the following situations:
  - Bleeding with acute DIC or liver disease and fibrinogen <1.5 g.l^{-1}
  - Prior to surgery when fibrinogen <1.5 g.l^{-1}
  - In the context of major haemorrhage, should aim to maintain fibrinogen >1.5 g.l^{-1}
- Dose is 2 pooled units for adults

4.2.3 Freeze-dried products

- Freeze-dried preparations are available:
  - Fibrinogen (e.g. RiaSTAP®)
  - Select clotting products (typically II, VII, IX, X) (e.g. prothrombin complex concentrate; Octaplex®)
- Advantages:
  - Easier to store
  - Longer shelf life
  - Smaller volume (if fluid restriction desirable)
  - Quicker to administer
- Disadvantages:
  - Expensive
  - Smaller volume (if volume resuscitation required)
- Licensed indications for freeze-dried products are currently limited.
- Octaplex® has been shown to reverse warfarin effects more quickly than FFP in the context of bleeding.

4.3 Coagulopathy in the ICU: some specific circumstances

4.3.1 Disseminated intravascular coagulation (DIC)

- Defined by International Society of Thrombosis and Hemostasis (ISTH) as 'an acquired syndrome characterized by the intravascular activation of coagulation with loss of localization arising from different causes'.

- Most common cause is sepsis.
- Commonly manifests clinically with bleeding, although can present with microthrombi.
- Laboratory findings include:
  - Hypofibrinoginaemia
  - Prolonged PT and APTT
  - Raised D-dimer
  - Thrombocytopaenia
- Management focuses on identification and treatment of the underlying cause, and transfusion of FFP/platelets if significant bleeding is encountered.
- Unfractionated heparin is used by some practitioners in the presence of thrombotic complications; however, its use is controversial and is not universally accepted.

4.3.2 Coagulopathy due to therapeutic anticoagulants

- ICU patients are frequently on antiplatelet or anticoagulant agents either due to chronic disease or as treatment for an acute insult (e.g. myocardial infarction, pulmonary embolism).
- In the non-bleeding ICU patient reversal of these agents is rarely indicated.
- Reversal may be required in the bleeding or perioperative patient.
- The decision to reverse anticoagulants is made on clinical grounds and risk assessment.
- In some cases stopping the offending agent may be all that is needed.
- Common agents and their reversal strategies are as follows:
  - Antiplatelet agents (e.g. Aspirin, Clopidgrel, Ticagrelor)
    - Platelet transfusion may be required in some cases
  - Vitamin K antagonists (e.g. Warfarin)
    - Vitamin K and FFP may be used—reverses within hours
    - Prothrombin concentrate used if rapid reversal required
  - Novel oral anticoagulants (NOACS) (e.g. Dabigatran, Rivaroxaban)
    - No specific reversal agents available at present—this may change soon
    - Reversal strategies include dialysis, recombinant factor VII, prothrombin concentrate
  - Heparins:
    - Unfractionated heparin (UFH)
      - Very short half life so often nil required
      - Reverses with protamine
    - Low molecular weight heparin (LMWH)
      - Longer half life
      - Partially reverses with protamine
  - Fondaparinux
    - No specific reversal agent
    - Recombinant factor VII used in severe cases

4.3.3 Liver disease

- Impairment of synthetic liver function leads to a reduction in coagulation factors; however, this is often matched by a decrease in the production of endogenous anticoagulants.
- In chronic liver disease particularly, a prothrombotic tendency is thought to exist despite 'abnormal' markers of clotting in routine coagulation screens—in the absence of significant bleeding or thrombocytopaenia, such patients require deep venous thrombosis (DVT) prophylaxis.
- It is reasonable to administer vitamin K to patients with chronic liver disease and abnormal clotting screen.
- Plasma products and platelets should only be administered in the presence of significant bleeding.

4.3.4 Procedures in coagulopathic critically ill patients

- Prophylactic plasma/platelet transfusion in patients with coagulopathy undergoing procedures, such as central venous cannula insertion or arterial line insertion, is often not necessary.
- Current practice is subject to wide variation.
- No consensus approach exists at present.
- A pragmatic approach is required with consideration of risk:benefit ratio, i.e.:
  - How urgent is the procedure? Would more harm be done by waiting for plasma components?
  - Is it possible to compress insertion site externally, if significant bleeding occurs?
  - Could more harm be done if blood products administered? For example, in the context of severe respiratory failure and fluid balance.
  - Use of ultrasound guided/minimally invasive techniques, where possible.
  - Experienced operator should perform such procedures in coagulopathic patients.

4.4 Point-of-care (POC) testing of coagulation

- A variety of POC tests of coagulation are available with results generally available within a maximum of 25 minutes.
- POC tests are used optimally in the context of a protocol or algorithm.

4.4.1 Activated clotting time

- Activated clotting time (ACT) devices are used commonly to measure efficacy and guide titration of unfractionated heparin while using extracorporeal circuits, e.g. haemofiltration, ECMO and cardiopulmonary bypass.

4.4.2 Thromboelastograph (TEG)

- Is an established method of assessing coagulation, which is used in the settings of cardiac anaesthesia, obstetrics, and trauma.
- Describes visco-elastic properties of whole blood, providing information about clot strength, fibrin formation, platelet-fibrin interaction, and fibrinolysis.
- Blood is inserted into two cups heated to 37°C; a pin/torsion wire is inserted into the cup; the cups then rotate in a bidirectional manner; as clot forms, this leads to movement of the pins; the characteristic TEG trace is generated by a transducer, which converts the torsion placed onto the pin into a trace.
- Uses kaolin as an activator to accelerate clotting.
- The Platelet Mapping Assay ® can be added to provide information regarding platelet function.
- A thromboelastograph trace is illustrated in Fig. 7.1.

4.4.3 Rotational thromboelastometry (ROTEM ®)

- Another viscoi-elastic test
- Used in similar settings to TEG
- ROTEM trace is similar to TEG; however, uses optical system, including light-emitting diode, mirror, and camera to generate trace
- Also uses activators to accelerate clotting:
  - Tissue factor in EXTEM(R) cuvette—extrinsic pathway
  - Contact factor in INTEM® cuvette—intrinsic pathway

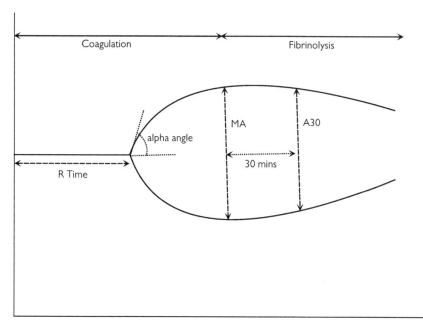

Fig. 7.1 Thromboelastography.

Table 7.4 describes the various variables generated by TEG(R) (with whole blood and kaolin activator) and ROTEM(R) traces and their significance.

Table 7.4 Characteristics of point of care coagulation testing

TEG(R)	ROTEM(R)	Definition	Significance
R (reaction time): 4–8 min	CT (clotting time) INTEM 137–246 s EXTEM 42–74 s	Time until initiation of fibrin formation, taken as a period to 2 mm amplitude on the tracing	Indicates concentration of soluble clotting factors in the plasma
K time: 1–4 min	CFT (clot formation time) INTEM 40–100 s EXTEM 46–148 s	Time period for the amplitude of the tracing to increase from 2 to 20 mm	Measurement of clot kinetics
Alpha angle: 47–74 degrees	Alpha angle INTEM 71–82 degrees EXTEM 63–81 degrees	Angle between a tangent to the tracing at 2 mm amplitude and the horizontal midline	Rapidity of fibrin build up and cross-linking
MA (maximum amplitude): 55–73 mm	MCF (maximum clot firmness) INTEM 52–72 mm	Greatest vertical width achieved by the tracing reflecting maximum clot strength	Number and function of platelets and fibrinogen concentration
CL30	LY30	% reduction in amplitude 30 min after MA	Clot stability and fibrinolysis
CL60	LY60	%reduction of clot firmness 1 hour after MCF	Clot stability and fibrinolysis

Adapted from *Continuing Education in Anaesthesia Critical Care and Pain*, 13, Srivasta and Kelleher, 'Point of care coagulation testing', pp. 12–16. Copyright (2013) with permission from Oxford University Press.

FURTHER READING

Enriquez LJ and Shore-Lesserson L. Point of care coagulation testing and transfusion algorithms. *British Journal of Anaesthesia* 2009; 103(BJA/PGA Supplement): 14–22.

Hunt BJ. Bleeding and coagulopathies in critical care. *New England Journal of Medicine* 2014; 370: 847–59.

Joint UK Blood Transfusion and Tissue Transplantation Service Professional Advisory Committee. Joint UKBTS Joint Professional Advisory Committee, Norwich, UK. *Handbook of Transfusion Medicine*, 2013.

Meybohm P, Zacharowski K and Weber CF et al. Point of care coagulation management in intensive care medicine. *Critical Care* 2013; 17: 218.

Srivasta A and Kelleher A. Point of care coagulation testing. *Continuing Education in Anaesthesia, Critical Care, and Pain* 2013; 13(1): 12–16.

5 Sickle cell disease

5.1 General

5.1.1 Pathology

- Sickle cell disease (SCD) is relatively common in urban areas of the UK, particularly in London.
- It is an inherited disease that is characterized by the presence of the abnormal HbS form of haemoglobin.
- This leads to a form of chronic haemolytic anaemia and recurrent episodes of vaso-occlusion accompanied by acute pain.
- The homozygous SS genotype is most common and is associated with the most aggressive form of disease.
- Heterozygous genotypes, including HbS/beta thalassaemia and HbS/haemoglobin C, can also present with severe disease.

5.1.2 Sickle disease and the intensive care

- Patients with SCD are commonly encountered in the ICU during/as a result of:
    - Perioperative management
    - Vaso-occlusive crisis—usually presenting with acute pain
    - Acute chest crisis
    - Intercurrent illness
- Common precipitants of acute vaso-occlusive crisis in SCD include:
    - Exposure to cold
    - Infection
    - Alcohol intake
    - Stress including surgery
    - Dehydration
    - Menstruation

5.1.3 Management

The mainstays of management of patients presenting to hospital with SCD are:
- Pain control
- Hydration

- Oxygenation
- Specialist multi-disciplinary care
- Transfusion and exchange transfusion
- DVT prophylaxis

5.2 Acute chest crisis

5.2.1 General

- Although acute chest crisis is most commonly found in patients with HbSS, it can present in all genotypes of SCD.
- It is associated with a significant risk of mortality.

5.2.2 Features

- The BCSH ACS guideline defines it as the presence of:
  - Acute illness
  - Fever
  - Respiratory symptoms
  - New pulmonary infiltrate on chest X-ray
- Aetiology includes:
  - Infection
  - Fat embolism
  - Microvascular pulmonary infarction
  - Asthma
  - Atelectasis
- Severe hypoxia is associated with adverse outcome

5.2.3 Management

- Aggressive treatment is required:
  - Specialist multi-disciplinary care in critical care unit
  - Early use of CPAP and NIV should be considered, especially where atelectasis is a significant issue
  - Broncholdilators, if wheeze present
  - Analgesia
  - Treatment with broad-spectrum antibiotics, including atypical +/– antiviral cover
  - Proactive screening for infection
  - Low index of suspicion for PTE and fluid overload—investigate and treat, as appropriate
  - Incentive spirometry and chest physiotherapy
  - Top up +/– exchange transfusion

FURTHER READING

Howard J, Hart N, Roberts-Harewood M et al. Guidelines on the management of acute chest syndrome in sickle cell disease. *British Journal of Haematology* 2015; 169(4): 492–505.

Mak V and Davies SC. The pulmonary physician in critical care, illustrative case 6: acute chest syndrome of sickle cell anaemia. *Thorax* 2003; 58: 726–28.

Vijay V, Cavenagh JD and Yate P. The anaesthetist's role in acute sickle cell crisis. *British Journal of Anaesthesia* 1998; 80: 820–28.

6 Haematological malignancy on the ICU

6.1 General
- Patients admitted to the ICU with haematological malignancy have worse outcomes than the general population.
- In one retrospective study conducted over 5 years in a UK specialist cancer centre, the ICU, hospital and one-year mortality were found to be 34%, 46%, and 59%, respectively (median APACHE II 21; IQR 16-25).
- Multivariate analysis revealed increased mortality to be associated with:
  - Mechanical ventilation (odds ratio 3.0)
  - Greater than two organ failure (odds ratio 5.62)

6.2 Neutropaenic sepsis
6.2.1 Background and definitions
- Neutropaenic sepsis typically refers to the development of fever (often in conjunction with other signs of sepsis) in a patient rendered neutropaenic by anti-cancer treatment.
- For the majority of cytotoxic agents, the nadir of the neutrophil count occurs between days 5 and 7 post-chemotherapy; the incidence of neutropaenia varies significantly with chemotherapy regimen.
- Neutropaenia places the patient at risk of invasive infection:
  - Up to 60% of febrile neutropaenic patients have infection
  - Gram-positive cocci and gram-negative bacilli are the most common organisms
  - Primary fungal infection is uncommon and more likely to occur in patients with prolonged neutropaenia and prolonged broad spectrum antibiotic exposure
- There is some variation in the definition of both neutropaenia and neutropaenic sepsis:
  - The threshold for neutropaenia varies from 0.5 to $1.0 \times 10^9/l$
  - Neutropaenic sepsis is defined as neutropaenia plus a temperature of greater than between 38 and 39°C

6.2.2 Prevention
- Interventions used in some centres to reduce the risk of neutropaenic sepsis include:
  - The use of prophylactic antibiotics (typically a quinolone)
  - The use of granulocyte colony stimulating factor

6.2.3 Investigation
- In addition to the standard infective workup, the potential for opportunistic infection in the neutropaenic sepsis population warrants additional investigation:
  - For patients with respiratory disease, bronchial washings in search of *Pneumocystis jirovecii*, *Cytomegalovirus*, *Mycobacterium* and fungal infection; CT imaging is beneficial
  - For patients with diarrhoeal illness, stool samples for *Cryptosporidium*; consideration of endoscopic biopsy for *Cytomegalovirus*
  - For patients with neurological symptoms, cerebrospinal fluid for toxoplasma and India ink stain (*Cryptococcus*)
  - For skin lesions that appear herpetic in nature, swabs for *Herpes simplex* and *Varicella zoster*

6.2.4 Treatment
- The management of sepsis is discussed in detail in Chapter6, Section 5.
- Reverse barrier nursing and positive pressure isolation are desirable.

- The most commonly used antibiotic regimen for treatment of neutropaenic sepsis is piperacillin/tazobactam with gentamicin; many centres add vancomycin if a central venous catheter is *in situ*.
- Addition of antiviral agent if viral infection suspected, confirmed, or failure for fever to improve within 3 to 5 days of antibiotics.
- Addition of an antifungal agent if fungal infection suspected, confirmed, or failure for fever to improve within 3 to 5 days of antibiotics.
- Consideration of long-term line removal if line infection suspected, confirmed, or failure for fever to improve within 3 to 5 days of antibiotics.

6.3 Tumour lysis syndrome

6.3.1 Background

- Tumour lysis syndrome (TLS) is a metabolic syndrome, caused by the breakdown of malignant cells, characterized by hyperkalaemia, hypocalcaemia, and hyperphosphataemia.
- Lysis of tumour cells leads to:
  - Release of potassium and phosphate into the circulation
  - Phosphate binds to circulating calcium, the resulting calcium phosphate crystalizing in soft tissues, including renal tubules
  - Release of nucleic acids, the metabolism of which causes a rise in plasma uric acid
  - Uric acid crystals are deposited in the renal tubules leading to renal impairment
- The metabolic derangement may result in acute kidney injury, cardiac arrhythmias, seizures, or death.
- Risk factors for TLS include:
  - High tumour load
  - High turnover of tumour cells
  - High tumour sensitivity to chemotherapy agents
  - High LDH
  - Pre-existing renal dysfunction and/or low urine output
- TLS affects between 3% and 6% of patients with high-grade tumours.

6.3.2 Prevention

- Adequate hydration: 3 l per 24 hours of intravenous fluids are recommended.
- Avoidance of other agents which may precipitate uric acid formation (diuretics, alcohol, caffeine).
- Based upon preventing the conversion of nucleic acids to uric acid:
  - Allopurinol:
    - Oral xanthine oxidase inhibitor
  - Rasburicase:
    - Intravenous recombinant urate oxidase preparation

6.3.3 Management

- Maintain adequate hydration and high urine output:
  - Three litres per m^2 body surface area per 24 hours is recommended
  - Aim for 100 ml per hour per m^2 body surface area of urine output
  - Avoid furosemide
- Allopurinol prevents uric acid formation but does not enhance breakdown; it is therefore of little benefit in established TLS.
- Rasburicase catalyses breakdown of uric acid and therefore has a role in the treatment of TLS.
- Alkalinization of the urine is not recommended.
- Electrolyte abnormalities should be managed as standard.
- Renal replacement therapy may be required.

FURTHER READING

Bird GT, Farquhar-Smith P, Wigmore T, Potter M, Gruber PC. Outcomes and prognostic factors in patients with haematological malignancy admitted to a specialist cancer intensive care unit: a 5 yr study. *British Journal of Anaesthesia* 2012; 108(3): 452–9.

Haji-Michael P, Dodgson K, Kaczmarski E, Mutton K. *Guidelines for the Management of Sepsis (Including Neutropenic Sepsis)*. The Christie NHS Foundation Trust Guidelines 2010. Available at http://www.christie.nhs.uk/neutropenic.aspx (accessed December 2015)

Jones GL, Will A, Jackson GH, Webb NJ, Rule S. Guidelines for the management of tumour lysis syndrome in adults and children with haematological malignancies on behalf of the British Committee for Standards in Haematology. *British Journal of Haematology* 2015; 169(5): 661–71.

National Institute for Clinical Excellence. *Neutropenic Sepsis: Prevention and Management of Neutropenic Sepsis in Cancer Patients* 2012. Available at https://www.nice.org.uk/guidance/cg151 (accessed December 2015)

CHAPTER 8

Injury: trauma and environmental

CONTENTS

1 Major trauma

1.1 General

1.1.1 Demographics

- Trauma is the leading cause of death worldwide; it is the leading cause of death in young men in developed nations.
- The disproportionate involvement of young adults leads to a significant impact on families and society.
- Major trauma is defined as an injury severity score (ISS) greater than 15 (scoring systems are outlined in Chapter 12, Section 3.2.3).

1.1.2 Major trauma centres

- There is convincing evidence that centralization of major trauma services to designated major trauma centres leads to a reduction in mortality and improved resource utilization.
- Major trauma centres are typically defined by:
  - Availability of all specialties necessary to manage a seriously injured patient.
  - Presence of a multi-specialty trauma team, which possess the skills to stabilize the seriously injured patient on arrival in the emergency department, available 24 hours per day, and led by a designated consultant.
- Regional major trauma centres rely upon:
  - The presence of pre-hospital triage system to determine which patients require transfer to the regional centre.
  - A pre-hospital care system that can safely transport critically ill patients to the regional centre, bypassing closer hospitals.

1.2 Approach to the seriously injured patient

- Patients suffering major trauma should be managed in a systematic manner utilizing a common framework, e.g. the Advanced Trauma Life Support (ATLS) system developed by the American College of Surgeons.

1.2.1 Primary survey

- The purpose of the primary survey is to identify and address immediately, life-threatening injuries.
- The primary survey follows an A–B–C–D–E approach.
- Airway with cervical spine control
  - In blunt trauma, airway management is undertaken concurrently with cervical spine immobilization.
  - Airway obstruction is a major cause of death in trauma.
  - There should be a low threshold for endotracheal intubation, particularly in the context of altered neurological status, facial or neck injuries, or haemodynamic instability.
  - Endotracheal intubation in the patient who has sustained blunt trauma should be undertaken with manual in-line stabilization.
  - Haemodynamic stability during induction of anaesthesia is important as periods of hypotension are associated with increased mortality in traumatic brain injury.
  - Cervical spine protection classically involves:
    - Cervical hard collar
    - Sand bags
    - Tape
  - The routine use of cervical collars is, however, the subject of debate.
- Breathing
  - Adequacy of oxygenation and ventilation should be assessed.
  - Supplementary oxygen and ventilatory support should be provided, as required.
  - The chest should be examined for evidence of life-threatening injuries impacting on the respiratory system, namely:
    - Tension pneumothorax
    - Massive haemothorax
  - Identification should prompt chest-drain insertion (Box 8.1).
- Circulation with haemorrhage control
  - Two large-bore intravenous cannulae should be inserted.
  - External haemorrhage should be controlled.
  - Evidence of shock in trauma is usually due to bleeding; tension pneumothorax and cardiac tamponade may also be responsible.
  - Point-of-care ultrasound may be used to identify occult haemorrhage (see Section 1.4.3).
  - Haemorrhage occurs:
    - Externally
    - Thoracic cavity
    - Peritoneal cavity
    - Retroperitoneal cavity
    - Pelvis
    - From long bones
  - Initial fluid resuscitation is typically in the form of crystalloid (1–2 litres).
  - Early use of blood products in patients with life-threatening haemorrhage (or if crystalloid resuscitation is ineffective); transfusion of a significant volume of packed red blood cells should prompt concurrent transfusion of plasma components and platelets (see Massive Transfusion—Chapter 7, Section2).

- Disability
  - Assessment of neurological function for evidence of injury to the central nervous system (brain or spinal cord).
- Exposure and environment
  - The patient should be fully exposed in order to identify life-threatening injuries.
  - Hypothermia should be avoided at all costs as it may contribute to coagulopathy.

Box 8.1 Chest-drain insertion

- Identification of insertion site:
  - Between mid and anterior axillary line, posterior to the *pectoralis major* muscle
  - Fourth or fifth intercostal space
  - Insertion over the superior aspect of the rib (thus avoiding the neurovascular bundle on the posterior aspect of the rib)
- Skin preparation:
  - Sterilization of skin with appropriate cleaning solution
  - Infiltration of local anaesthetic, with particular attention to the highly innervated intercostal muscle (this may be combined with intravenous analgesia)
- Insertion
  - Skin incision with a scalpel down to rib
  - Blunt dissection with curved forceps through remaining subcutaneous tissue and intercostal muscle
  - Once the tract enters the pleural space, the forceps are used to guide an intercostal drain into the chest; the drain should be advanced until the last hole is within the chest cavity
  - The drain is attached to an underwater seal and secured to the skin
  - The insertion site is covered with an adhesive dressing

Chest X-ray to confirm position

1.2.2 Secondary survey

- Head to toe examination to identify injuries missed in the primary survey.
- Should involve examination of back, buttocks, and extremities.
- Structured history:
  - Allergies
  - Medications being taken
  - Past medical history
  - Last ate and drank
  - Events surrounding the injury

1.2.3 Tertiary survey

- The process of primary and secondary survey is repeated several times over the following days, in conjunction with review of imaging.
- This minimizes the risk of missed injury.

1.3 Damage control resuscitation

- A concept in acute trauma care which consists of:
    - Permissive hypotension
    - Haemostatic resuscitation
    - Damage-control surgery

1.3.1 Permissive hypotension

- The concept of targeting a lower than normal blood pressure in trauma patients to avoid disruption of clot.
- It has been demonstrated to reduce mortality in a primarily young, urban, male population who have sustained penetrating trauma; the applicability of permissive hypotension to patients with co-morbidities, or those sustaining blunt trauma, or those injured in a non-urban environment is unclear.

1.3.2 Haemostatic resuscitation

- One-third of major trauma patients have a coagulopathy on presentation.
- The coagulopathy of trauma is multifactorial:
    - Loss of clotting factors due to haemorrhage
    - Dilution of clotting factors due to iatrogenic volume replacement
    - Activation of fibrinolysis by tissue injury
    - Shock-related acidosis
    - Hypothermia
- Resuscitation of the trauma patient should aim to correct existing coagulopathy and avoid deterioration in clotting status.
- The management of major haemorrhage and coagulopathy of trauma is discussed in Chapter 7, Section 2.

1.3.3 Damage-control surgery

- If traumatic haemorrhage is associated with significant metabolic derangement (e.g. acidosis or hypothermia), it may be prudent to undertake limited 'damage-control' surgery aimed at the arrest of haemorrhage and prevention of ongoing intra-abdominal soiling.
- If this approach is undertaken, time in the operating theatre is limited to life-saving procedures, the patient is transferred to ICU for restoration of physiological normality, and then returns to theatre in the following days for definitive surgery.

1.4 Diagnostics in trauma

1.4.1 CT imaging

- CT has become the gold standard in major trauma.
- The routine use of non-directed 'pan'-scan is controversial and has not been convincingly demonstrated to improve outcomes.
- Evidence or suspicion of injury to the head, spine, thorax, abdomen, or pelvis should prompt CT imaging.
- Transfer of trauma patients to CT should be undertaken by a suitably qualified team with the same level of monitoring and support found in the resuscitation room.
- Attempts should be made to stabilize the patient prior to transfer; however, resuscitation may be ongoing throughout the scan.

- It may be more appropriate for persistently haemodynamically unstable patients to go to theatre rather than CT.

1.4.2 Plain X-ray

- Plain X-ray of the cervical spine, chest, and pelvis can be undertaken in the resuscitation room, negating the need for transfer to the radiology department.
- The sensitivity of these studies is, however, imperfect and their role is now limited to stable patients, with no evidence of head or torso injury, and a low risk mechanism of injury.
- In major trauma, plain X-ray has largely been replaced by CT scanning.

1.4.3 Ultrasound imaging

- Ultrasound allows rapid, point-of-care imaging, which is free from radiation.
- The Focused Assessment with Sonography in Trauma (FAST) scan has become a standard of care in many centres; FAST involves:
  - Four views:
    - Right upper quadrant (examining the peri-hepatic space—Morrison's pouch)
    - Left upper quadrant (examining the peri-splenic space)
    - Subcostal (examining the pericardium)
    - Suprapubic (examining the pouch of Douglas)
  - The examination focuses on the presence of fluid in dependent areas of the abdomen (which in the trauma patient is assumed to be blood); the classic FAST scan does not examine the solid organs.
  - Examination of the pericardium allows identification of pericardial effusion, which, in the haemodynamically unstable patient, may be assumed to be tamponade.
- A number of extended versions of FAST exist; ultrasound may also be used to:
  - Conduct more extensive echocardiographic assessment of the heart and estimation of volume status
  - Examination of the pleural space for presence of pneumothorax or effusion
  - Examination of the great vessels for evidence of dissection or rupture
  - Examination of the abdominal viscera

FURTHER READING

American College of Surgeons Committee on Trauma. *Advanced Trauma Life Support Student Course Manual*. American College of Surgeons. Chicago, 2012.

Bickell WH, Wall Jr MJ, Pepe PE, et al. Immediate versus delayed fluid resuscitation for hypotensive patients with penetrating torso injuries. *New England Journal of Medicine* 1994; 331(17): 1105–9.

Brohi K, Parr T, Coats T. Regional trauma systems. *Interim Guidance for Commissioners*. London, Royal College of Surgeons of England, 2009.

Shakur H, Roberts I, Bautista R, Caballero J, Coats T. Effects of tranexamic acid on death, vascular occlusive events, and blood transfusion in trauma patients with significant haemorrhage (CRASH-2): a randomised, placebo-controlled trial. *Lancet* 2010; 376(9734): 23–32.

Spahn DR, Bouillon B, Cerny V, et al. Management of bleeding and coagulopathy following major trauma: an updated European guideline. *Critical Care* 2013; 17(2): R76.

2 Spinal cord injury

2.1 Overview of spinal cord injury

2.1.1 Aetiology

- Car accidents, motor bike, and bicycle: 45%
- Falls: domestic 20%; industrial: 5%
- Sporting: 12%
- Diving: 8%
- Bleeding/abscess/surgery: 9%
- Gunshot/stab wounds: 1%

2.1.2 Epidemiology of spinal cord injury

- Suspect in all severe trauma and head injury.
- Suspect in any surgical procedure with potential for ischaemia to the cord (e.g. aortic cross clamp).
- Increased risk in the presence of pre-existing abnormalities, e.g.:
  - Degenerative diseases
  - Canal stenosis
  - Ankylosing spondylitis
  - Previous spinal fractures
  - Osteomyelitis
  - Rheumatoid arthritis
  - Spinal tumours
- The cervical spine is most commonly affected region (55% of adult injuries); C4–6 is the most mobile region.
- Most spinal injuries occur in young males (>80% age 15–35 years).
- Alcohol often a contributing factor.
- Isolated spinal cord injury is associated with:
  - Hospital survival rates >90%
  - Severe permanent disability
- Distribution of spinal cord injury (SCI) levels:
  - 60% cervical injury (C4–6 predominates as the most mobile region)
  - 30% thoracic

2.2 Mechanisms of spinal cord injury

- The mechanisms underlying spinal cord injury may be divided into traumatic and non-traumatic.

2.2.1 Non-traumatic spinal cord injury

- Non-traumatic mechanisms account for approximately one-third of SCI.
- More common in older patients and females.
- Unlike traumatic injuries, in which cervical pathology predominates, the incidence of non-traumatic injury is distributed equally throughout the cervical, thoracic, and lumber/sacral regions.
- 40% of lesions are complete; 60% incomplete.
- 75% result in paraplegia; 25% in quadriplegia.
- Aetiologies include:
  - Spinal canal tumours (primary and secondary)

- Spinal cord tumours (e.g. astrocytoma, ependymoma)
- Spinal cord infections (of posterior spine, anterior spine, epidural space, subdural space, or cord)
- Myelitis (Consider Tuberculosis, HIV, *Human T-Lymphotrophic Virus 1, Herpes Simplex Virus* (HSV) 1, HSV2, *Varicella Zoster Virus, Cytomegalovirus* lymphoma)
- Vascular malformations or injury:
  - Aortic surgery—hypotension, arterial infarct, embolism, venous infarct
  - Arteriovenous malformations
- Nutritional deficits:
  - Vitamin B12 deficiency (subacute combined degeneration of the cord)
  - Vitamin E deficiency
- Multiple sclerosis (including transverse myelitis)
- Motor neurone disease
- Acute and chronic demyelinating inflammatory demyelinating polyneuropathies
- Paraneoplastic
- Toxic
- Radiation injury

2.2.2 Traumatic spinal cord injury

- Account for approximately two-thirds of SCI.
- Typically in the younger, male population.
- Affect the more mobile sections of the spine: 1/2 cervical, 2/5 thoracic, 1/10 lumbosacral.
- 90% incomplete; 10% complete.
- 50% paraplegia; 50% quadriplegia.
- Mechanisms of injury:
  - Flexion:
    - Usually affecting the cervical region
    - Common in motor vehicle accidents, domestic falls
    - Associated bilateral dislocation and associated ligamentous damage
  - Rotation:
    - Commonly in cervical or lower thoracic and lumbar region
    - Typically motor vehicle passengers wearing lap belts or sustaining side impacts
    - Associated with:
      - Unilateral fracture-dislocation
      - Posterior ligamentous damage
      - Vertebral body fractures
      - Frequently combined with flexion injuries
  - Extension:
    - Usually elderly with osteoarthritis or spondylosis changes
    - Minor bony damage with intervertebral discs and spinal cord stretch
    - Associated with central cord syndrome
  - Compression:
    - Common in cervical or lumbar injuries
    - Vertebral body burst fractures into spinal cord
    - Frequently minor neurological damage
  - Direct:
    - High-energy or incisive direct blow to vertebral column

   ▪ Gunshot or knife wounds

   ▪ May result in Brown–Sequard syndrome

2.2.3 Classification of spinal cord injury

See Box 8.2.

Box 8.2 American Spinal Injury Association (ASIA) Standard Classification

Scale of SCI

A = Complete: no motor or sensory
B = Incomplete: sensory but no motor
C = Incomplete: motor function < grade 3
D = Incomplete: motor function > grade 3
E = Normal: motor and sensory function

Adapted from *ASIA Learning Center Materials* – International Standards for Neurological Classification of SCI (ISNCSCI) Exam, American Spinal Injury Association (ASIA) Standard Classification, 2015

- Complete injury:
  - Loss of all conscious motor and sensory function below the level of the lesion
  - Often associated with complete or near complete spinal cord transection
- Incomplete injury:
  - Preservation of some motor and/or sensory function
- Subtypes of incomplete injury:
  - Anterior cord syndrome:
    - Often due to injury to anterior two-thirds of cord from:
      - Anterior spinal artery injury
      - Vertebral body injury
    - Variable loss of motor and pinprick sensation
    - Preserved light touch, proprioception, deep pressure sense
    - Poor muscle recovery prognosis
  - Posterior cord syndrome:
    - Uncommon
    - Loss of light touch, proprioception, deep pressure sense, pain, and temperature sense
    - Variable motor preservation
    - Poor functional recovery due to proprioceptive loss
  - Central cord syndrome:
    - In cervical SCI mostly (associated with hyper-extension)
    - Motor weakness more in arms than legs with sacral sparing
    - Good prognosis
    - Recovery sequence: lower limbs, bladder and bowel, proximal upper limbs, distal upper limbs
  - Cruciate paralysis:
    - Associated with C1–C2 or cervico-medullary injury
    - Upper limb weakness with minimal lower limb weakness
    - 25% have respiratory compromise
    - Good prognosis

- Brown-Sèquard syndrome:
    - Hemisection syndrome with:
        - Ipsilateral loss of all sensation above lesion
        - Ipsilateral flaccid paralysis below lesion
        - Ipsilateral loss of vibration and proprioception below lesion
        - Contralateral loss of pain and temperature sense
- Cauda equina lesion:
    - Lower motor neurone lesion of cauda equina
    - Flaccid lower limbs
    - Atonic bladder and bowel
    - Absent sacral reflexes
    - Variable sensation loss
- Conus medullaris syndrome:
    - Conus medullaris lies at L1 level and supplies L4–S1 segments
    - Associated with an L1–L2 injury
    - Mixed picture:
        - Upper motor neurone (conus)
        - Lower motor neurone (nerve root)
        - Preserved sacral reflexes in higher injury

2.3 Pathophysiology of acute spinal cord injury

2.3.1 Neuromuscular system complications

- Acute issues:
    - Primary injury to the cord:
        - Avulsion or transection (tearing/shearing)
        - Axonal injury
        - Intraparenchymal haemorrhage
        - Ischaemia
    - Secondary injury to the cord:
        - Cellular hypoxia
        - Ischaemia
        - Cord oedema
    - 'Spinal shock' with flaccid paralysis and loss of muscle reflexes below injury level
    - Level or degree of injury may progress during first week of injury ('ascending level'):
        - This may be reversible or irreversible
        - May compromise respiratory, autonomic, or brainstem function, depending on initial injury level
- Chronic issues:
    - Spasticity in lower muscle groups may occur at resolution of spinal shock
    - Uncontrolled myoclonus can occur and contribute to autonomic dysreflexia
        - Consider use of benzodiazepines or baclofen;
    - Joint complications, contracture management, limb orthotics, and heterotopic ossification need to be considered as part of long-term complications.
    - Neurological level determines possible long-term function:
        - C1–2: ventilator-dependent, head and shoulder movement

- C3: short periods of unaided ventilation possible
- C3,4,5: ('diaphragm alive'): possible unaided ventilation
- C5: deltoid, biceps—elbow flexion
- C6: wrist extension
- C7: triceps, extensor digitorium—elbow and finger extension
- C8: finger extension
- T1: fine hand movements
- T2–12: intercostals intact, full upper extremity control; wheel-chair mobility
- T6–12: better core abdominal muscle function; effective cough
- T12–L3: short-distance ambulation with callipers or crutches
- L3: quadriceps for knee extension
- L4–5: foot inversion and full knee flexion
- S3: full hip control with normal gait
- S2–5: varying degrees of bladder, bowel, and sexual dysfunction

2.3.2 Airway and respiratory complications

- Acute issues:
  - Airway related:
    - If intubation is required:
      - Unopposed vagal stimulus at intubation may result in extreme bradycardia or asystolic arrest; consider pre-treatment with atropine at intubation.
      - In-line manual stabilization may impede laryngoscopy view.
      - Retropharyngeal haematoma from cervical injury may impede laryngoscopy.
      - Nasal intubation risk with mid-facial or base-of-skull fracture.
    - Depolarizing neuromuscular blockade (suxamethonium) has high risk at Day 3 to 2 years post-injury; risk of bradycardia, hyperkalaemia, arrhythmia, and cardiac arrest.
    - Surgical tracheostomy may be preferable to percutaneous dilational tracheostomy in ventilator-dependent cervical SCI patients with recent cervical fixation surgery.
  - Oxygenation and ventilatory management:
    - Cervico-thoracic spinally injured patients often have complex ventilation management in the acute phase.
    - Aim for normoxia and normocapnia in acute phase.
    - Serial bedside spirometry (on admission and once per shift):
      - Can determine deteriorating ventilatory function
        - Forced Vital Capacity (FVC) <1,000 ml (or <12–15 ml/kg)—high risk of ventilatory failure requiring intubation
        - FVC 1,000–1,500 ml—shift-by-shift assessment required for potential intubation for ventilator support
      - Can determine success of extubation in high-spinal patients
      - Normal Vital Capacity (VC): 50–70 ml/kg
        - Acute quadriplegics, expect only 25–30%
    - Cough deficiencies:
      - T12 or higher have poor cough
      - Sputum management more difficult with higher levels
      - Assistive cough devices and regular intensive physiotherapy
    - Ventilation and positional support for recurrent atelectasis:
      - Supine lying

- Use of 'sigh breath' (1–2 Synchronized Intermittent Mandatory Ventilation (SIMV), 300 ml above Vt breaths per minute)
        - Consider high tidal volume (up to 20 ml/kg) to prevent atelectasis
        - Edgerton turning bed for position changes without log-rolling
        - Manual hyperinflation
        - Mechanical insufflation-exsufflation
        - Non-invasive ventilation
    - Diaphragmatic pacing:
        - May be needed in high cervical spinal injury patients
- Chronic issues:
    - Airway management:
        - Tracheostomy may be:
            - Permanent
            - Temporary
            - Converted to a mini-tracheostomy for secretion management
        - Potential risk of intubation complicated subglottic stenosis post-tracheostomy decannulation.
        - Repeat tracheostomy for a critically unwell chronically spinally injured patient may be technically difficult and requires discussion with an airway surgeon.
    - Ventilatory management
        - C1–3 level injury: likely permanent mechanical ventilation.
        - May need to consider continuous or intermittent positive pressure ventilation via non-invasive ventilation or tracheostomy.
        - Older spinal patients may have associated central and obstructive sleep apnoea problems.
        - Consider the development of a syrinx at the injury level in patients with worsening neurology or worsening respiratory performance complications; MRI is the investigation of choice.

2.3.3 Cardiovascular and autonomic nervous system complications

- Acute issues:
    - Evidence exists for improved neurological recovery in patients resuscitated to MAP>85 mmHg for 7 days post-initial injury.
    - There may be an initial transient hypertensive phase (from catecholamine surge).
    - Injuries above T1 cause sympathetic paralysis below the injury through loss of cardio-accelerator fibres T1–T4.
    - Procedures that increase vagal tone may therefore trigger asystole due to unopposed vagal stimulation:
        - Airway suction
        - Intubation:
            - Consider pre-treatment with atropine
    - Neurogenic shock describes the hypotension associated with an acute SCI above T6; it relates to spinal cord hypo-activity below the level of the injury, loss of reflexes, and loss of sympathetic outflow to the heart; it is more pronounced at higher levels; it may last day to weeks.
    - Care must be taken, however, not to dismiss hypotension as neurogenic:
        - In patients with injury above T6, relative tachycardia suggests another underlying cause of shock (e.g. blood loss).
        - Hypotension in a patient with SCI injury at or below T6 is most likely another cause of shock.

- Other autonomic features of high SCI include:
    - Hypothermia due to inability to effectively vasoconstrict
    - Paralytic ileus
    - Faecal incontinence
    - Priapism in males
    - Urinary retention
- Autonomic dysreflexia (AD):
    - AD is a medical emergency of hypertensive crisis, often after a period of spinal shock has resolved.
    - Exaggerated reflexive response causing hypertension (+/– bradycardia) in response to a strong stimulus below the level of injury.
    - Patients with SCI above sympathetic outflow (T6–T8) are at risk; present in approximately 50–85% of these patients.
    - Occurs due to intact sensory afferent pathways triggering sympathetic activity in preganglionic sympathetic neurones below injury level; accompanied by incomplete inhibitory signal to region due to loss of descending inhibitory fibres.
    - Results in:
        - Regional vasoconstriction:
            – Splanchnic and gastrointestinal vasculature
        - High peripheral vascular resistance and blood pressure
        - Reflexive bradycardia from brainstem
    - Symptoms and signs (above lesion):
        - Hypertension >20–40 mmHg above normal—with risks of hypertensive crisis
        - Headache and anxiety
        - Flushing
        - Sweating
        - Sympathetic symptoms below level of injury
    - Recognition of AD should prompt search for precipitant:
        - Urinary retention
        - Faecal impaction
        - Painful stimulus below the level of the lesion
    - Medication:
        - Consider use of agents with rapid onset and off-set:
            – Glyceryl trinitrate
            – Hydralazine
            – Nifedipine

2.3.4 Gastrointestinal complications

- Acute issues:
    - Dysphagia may occur after a high-cervical injury and its associated anterior spinal fixation surgery.
    - Tracheostomy, halothoracic braces, and cervical collars contribute to dysphagia.
    - Gall bladder function may be impaired with injury levels above T10.
    - Paralytic ileus is common after SCI, particularly injury at the cervical and thoracic level:
        - Occurs in first 3–5 days due to autonomic dysfunction
        - Management may include:
            – Nasogastric decompression
            – Use of pro-kinetics

      – Regular bowel regimen
- Feed enterally once bowel sounds present.
- Acute gastritis, pancreatitis, and peptic ulceration may occur in acute phase:
  - Gastric ulceration may be prevented by effective resuscitation, PPI, H2RB, and early enteral feeding.
- SCI above conus medullaris (T12) results in a spastic anal sphincter.
- Anal tone is intact in incomplete injury.
- Chronic issues:
  - Diagnosing an acute abdomen in an SCI patient requires a high level of suspicion:
    - Signs may include shoulder tip pain, changes in bowel habit, abdominal distension.
  - Effective management of constipation and abdominal distension of neurogenic bowel through regular bowel regimen reduces respiratory complications:
    - Example regimen:
      - Day 1: start once feeding commences
      - Day 2: commence nocturnal aperients:
        - Senna tablets 2–4 or Movicol Sachet X 1
      - Day 3: continue nocturnal bowel aperients
      - Day 4: commence morning suppositories: bisocodyl (high rectal, left side-lying)—dwell time 20–30 minutes
    - Faecal diversion may be required for hygiene and social issues
  - Haemorrhoids occur in more than half of SCI patients at 5 years.

2.3.5 Genito-urinary complications

- Acute issues:
  - Urinary retention
  - Priapism
- Chronic issues:
  - May need to consider suprapubic catheter in long-term.
  - Long-term spinal patients are often colonized by multi-resistant organisms in the urinary tract.
  - Urinary tract infection is a common long-term complication.

2.3.6 Integumentary complications

- The spinal patient is at high risk of pressure sores; these should, however, be entirely preventable.

2.3.7 Haematological complications

- Acute issues:
  - High risk of deep vein thrombosis and pulmonary embolism:
    - Vascular pooling
    - Decreased mobility
  - Risk may be mediated by:
    - Low molecular weight heparin in the acute phase; warfarin when enteral feeding established.
    - Mechanical devices:
      - Thromboembolic deterrent (TED) stockings
      - Calf compressors
      - Calf stimulators

▪ Inferior vena cava filter may be justified in settings of complex coagulation and bleeding problems.

2.3.8 Psychological, vocational, and social considerations

- Acute issues:
    - Sexual and relationship difficulties.
    - Concomitant neurological injury from traumatic brain injury.
    - Pre-existent mental health or substance-abuse issues.
    - Fertility and reproduction.
- Chronic issues:
    - Complete alteration in vocational capacity.
    - Advance care planning and legal instruments.
    - Palliation concerns, including self-cessation of ventilation.
    - Death after spinal cord injury may be a coronial referral even many years after injury.

2.4 Principles of management phases of spinal cord injury

Spinal cord injured patients are managed by inter-professional teams within established trauma and rehabilitation systems.

2.4.1 On-scene management

- Up to 25% of additional SCI may occur during on-scene management.
- Appropriate spinal protection administered at the scene within the protocols of advanced trauma life-support.
- Patients who should be considered at risk of unstable spinal injuries include:
    - Multi-trauma victim, particularly if a 'high-energy' injury has been sustained (e.g. fall from height, high-speed deceleration)
    - Unconscious patient
    - Any person with complaints related to the spine
- Extrication and transport may place the spinal cord at risk of secondary injury.

2.4.2 Transportation

- Cervical spine immobilization by:
    - Hard collar with:
        - Manual in-line stabilization or
        - Sandbags and head tape
- Thoracolumbar spine immobilization options:
    - Hard 'spine board'
    - Scoop stretcher
    - Whole body 'bean-bag' mattress
    - Semi-rigid brace.
- Patient transport positioning:
    - Secured to transport vehicle to:
        - Enable fully immobilized spine in a neutral position
        - Enable airway management in event of vomiting or respiratory complications

2.4.3 Airway management

- Endotracheal intubation should be undertaken if:
    - Glasgow coma score ≤8 or aspiration risk

- Confused, uncooperative, or combative
- Inadequate oxygenation or ventilation
- Decreased central drive
- Higher level spinal injury with loss of:
  - Phrenic nerve C3–C5
  - Intercostal nerves T1–T12
- Long-distance transport to definitive care
- In the patient with potential spinal injury, endotracheal intubation should be undertaken with in-line manual stabilization of cervical spine:
  - May increase difficulty of laryngoscopy
  - Unopposed vagal tone in high SCI may result in bradycardia or asystole on induction of anaesthesia or laryngoscopy

2.4.4 Imaging modalities

Radiological assessment varies between centres; options include:
- Plain X-ray
  - Full vertebral column:
    - Anteroposteriorand lateral views
    - Cervical oblique views, if cervical injuries suspected
    - Cranio-cervical ('peg' views)
    - Cervico-thoracic junction (swimmer's view)—C1–C7/T1 junction needed
  - Important features of cervical spine X-rays:
    - Spinous processes of C2–T1 intact, aligned, and evenly spaced
    - Vertebral bony contour intact
    - Lateral edges of cervical spine aligned
    - The width of the normal prevertebral soft tissue should be:
      - <1/3 vertebral body width above C4
      - <100% of the vertebral body width below C4
      - Paravertebral soft tissue in excess of these parameters may represent haematoma and associated fracture
- Computed tomography (CT)
  - Better delineation of extent and displacement of fractures than plain X-ray
  - Often occurs at same time as CT brain or CT trauma series
  - Limited sensitivity for soft tissue injury and spinal cord injury in the absence of bony injury
- Magnetic resonance imaging (MRI)
  - In addition to assessment of bony integrity, the MRI provides information regarding:
    - Integrity of ligamentous structures
    - Intervertebral discs
    - Intrinsic spinal cord impairment (e.g. oedema, haemorrhage)
    - Additional pathology (e.g. pathological fracture)
  - Usually performed prior to surgery, if logistics allow
  - Benefits:
    - High sensitivity for:
      - Fractures
      - Spinal cord injury
      - Nerve plexus injury
      - Disc injury
      - Soft tissue and ligamentous injuries

- Pitfalls:
  - Length of the imaging time in a remote location, unsuitable for physiologically unstable patients
  - Need for MRI compatible equipment

2.4.5 Clearance of spinal column for ongoing care

- 'Clearing the spine' requires demonstration of a stable spinal column at cervical, thoracic and lumbar levels.
- This may be done clinically, radiologically, or after specialist surgical intervention or opinion.
- The management or immobilization of each element of the spine must be specifically documented and communicated to ensure safe patient care.
- Clearing the spine at the earliest opportunity is desirable as it:
  - Allows removal of the collar, thereby enhancing venous drainage from the head and allowing access to the neck for line and tracheostomy placement.
  - Allows greater mobilization in the bed, greater ease of nursing care, reduced risk of pressure injury from collar, and immobility.

2.4.5.1 Methods of spine clearance

- Clinical clearance:
  - May occur if there is:
    - Intact judgement (no head injury/intoxication/depressed level of consciousness)
    - No distracting injury
    - Neurologically intact
  - And if examination reveals:
    - No point tenderness
    - No deformity/bony step
    - Pain free, normal active range of movement
  - For many patients in the intensive care, these criteria will not be met and a radiological approach may be necessary.
- Radiological clearance:
  - Local policies vary; follow local procedure and ensure documentation.
  - A fine-slice CT of spine in the patient with low suspicion of spinal injury may be sufficient to 'clear the spine' and remove spinal precautions.
  - If doubt exists due to clinical state, or the CT appears to demonstrate abnormalities, MRI imaging is necessary.

2.4.5.2 Methods of spinal protection before formal clearance or fixation

- Turning and positioning:
  - Head-holding (+/− ETT) on turning (uncleared C-spine)
  - Log-roll procedure with up to 5–6 team members (uncleared thoracolumbar spine)
  - Side-lying positioning with wedge supports
  - Edgerton tilting spinal bed
- Cervical spine protection:
  - Without cervical spinal collar
    - In-line manual stabilization during procedures or orthotic manipulations
    - Head blocks
    - Strapping

- Sand-bags
- Traction tongs
- With cervical spinal collar
  - Philadelphia collar (expected clearance <24–48 hours)
  - Aspen collar (expected clearance >48 hours)
  - Miami J collar
- Thoracolumbar spine protection
  - Bed remains flat or in reverse Trendelenburg—as directed and documented by trauma, orthopaedic, or spinal surgical team
  - Bracing is uncommon, yet possible

2.4.6 Surgical interventions

- Interventions include:
  - Neural decompression:
    - May requires anterior or posterior approach, depending on injury mechanism
  - Spinal stabilization:
    - Three-column theory (spine is unstable if 2 out of 3 columns are disrupted):
      - Anterior column: anterior vertebral body, anterior longitudinal ligament, anterior annulus fibrosus
      - Middle column: posterior vertebral body, posterior longitudinal ligament, posterior annulus fibrosus
      - Posterior column: pedicles, laminae, infraspinal and supraspinal ligament
  - External orthosis:
    - Bony injury may heal with orthotic management if no ligamentous injury
    - External orthosis may be required to further stabilize internally reduced fractures
    - Options include:
      - Head traction
      - Halothoracic brace (for injuries from occiput to C2)
      - Cervical collar:
        - Philadelphia (for injuries from C3 to C7)
        - Miami J (for injuries from occiput to C2)
      - Cervicothoracic orthosis (for injuries from T1 to T3)
      - Thoracolumbosacral orthosis (for injuries from T4 to L2)
      - Lumbosacral orthotic (+/– spica) (for injuries below L3)
- Timing of surgery:
  - Controversial area; however, early decompression and stabilization may:
    - Prevent further secondary injury
    - Reduce pain and deformity
    - Enable earlier rehabilitation

2.4.7 Medical therapies

- Steroid therapy in acute spinal injury:
  - Likely limited additional neurological recovery at expense of steroid-related superinfection and metabolic effects.
  - Not recommended in patients with concomitant traumatic brain injury.
- Regenerative spinal medicine:
  - A complex field with no current broad clinical application outside clinical trials.

2.4.8 Longer term care of acute and chronic spinal cord injured patients

- Broader issues that need to be considered are:
  - Advanced care planning
  - Psychological support
  - Sleep management
  - Relationship management, including sexual and reproductive issues
  - Ventilation weaning
  - Tracheostomy decannulation
  - Social and vocational rehabilitation with functional and mobility aids:
    - Orthotics
    - Wheelchairs
    - Seating
    - Communication tools
    - Transportation

FURTHER READING

Campagnolo DI, Kirschblum S (ed.). *Spinal Cord Medicine*, 2nd edn. Philadelphia, USA, 2011. Lippincott, Williams, and Wilkin.

Canadian CT Head and C-Spine (CCC) Study Group. Canadian C-Spine Rule study for alert and stable trauma patients: I. Background and rationale. *Canadian Journal of Emergency Medicine*, 2004; 4(2): 84–90.

Cooper DJ, Ackland, HM. Clearing the cervical spine in unconscious head injured patients—the evidence. Critical Care and Resuscitation 2005; 7(3): 181–4.

Hoffman JR, Wolfson AB, Todd K, Mower WR. Selective cervical spine radiography in blunt trauma: methodology of the National Emergency X-Radiography Utilization Study (NEXUS). *Annals of Emergency Medicine* 1998; 32(4): 461–9.

Patel, M, Humble SS, Cullinane, DC, et al. (EAST group). Cervical spine collar clearance in the obtunded adult blunt trauma patient: A systematic review and practice management guideline from the Eastern Association for the Surgery of Trauma. *Journal of Trauma and Acute Care Surgery* 2015; 78(2) 430–41.

Kirschblum SC, Burns SP, Biering-Sorenson F, et al. International standards for neurological classification of spinal cord injury (Revised 2011). *Journal of Spinal Cord Medicine* 2011; Nov; 34(6): 535–46.

3 Burns

3.1 Classification and assessment

3.1.1 Mechanism

- Heat (dry or wet)
- Cold
- Electrical
- Chemical

3.1.2 Thickness

- **Superficial epidermal**: dry, red burn involving the epidermis only. Does not blister. May be painful. Heals completely without scarring.

- **Superficial dermal** (partial thickness): pale pink burn, which blisters within a few hours of injury. Involves the epidermis and upper layers of the dermis. Usually extremely painful.
- **Mid-dermal** (partial thickness): a darker red burn that involves the epidermis, dermis, and some of the more superficial adnexal structures (e.g. sweat glands and piloerector apparatus). May be painful.
- **Deep dermal** (partial thickness): blotchy red burn with absent capillary refill. Sensation is reduced. Epidermis and most of the dermis, including adnexal structures, are involved. Large, early blisters are common.
- **Full thickness**: white, waxy appearance; no sensation. Epidermis, dermis, and all adnexal structures involved. No blisters. No potential for spontaneous healing.

3.1.3 Area

- Accurate estimation of area is important in terms of management and prognosis.
- Area may be estimated using one of three methods:
  - 'The rule of nines'
    - The skin is divided into areas, each representing 9% of body surface:
      - Head and face (front and back)
      - Each arm (front and back)
      - Front of each leg
      - Back of each leg
      - Front of chest
      - Back of chest
      - Front of abdomen
      - Back of abdomen including buttocks
      - The groin represents 1%
  - Lund–Browder chart
  - The area of the patient's palm represents 1% of body surface

3.2 Initial management

- Severe burns often occur in the context of major trauma; initial care should follow a systematic ATLS approach and burns should not distract from the management of more immediately life-threatening injuries.
- Specific considerations in the patient with burns include:
  - Airway
  - Breathing
  - Circulation and fluid management
  - Disability and pain relief
  - Referral to a specialist burns centre

3.2.1 Airway

- An assessment for evidence of airway burns should be made:
  - Facial burns
  - Singed nasal hairs
  - Hoarse voice
  - Stridor
  - Carbonaceous sputum.
- Evidence (or suspicion) of airway involvement should prompt early tracheal intubation before airway oedema develops.

- An uncut endotracheal tube should be used to allow for facial swelling.
- In cases of severe facial swelling, the endotracheal tube may require securing by inter-dental wiring.
- Patients with established airway oedema may require an awake fibre optic intubation or awake tracheostomy under local anaesthesia.

3.2.2 Breathing

- Respiratory dysfunction in the burns' patient can arise for several reasons:
  - Smoke inhalation (see Chapter 1, Section 7):
    - Direct lung injury and impaired gas exchange
    - Carbon monoxide poisoning and impaired oxygen carriage
    - Cyanide poisoning and impaired oxygen utilization
  - Circumferential thoracic burns lead to restriction of ventilation

3.2.3 Circulation and fluid management

- Fluid loss from burns is considerable and adequate fluid replacement is essential.
- Hypovolaemia secondary to burns does not, however, occur immediately and shock early in presentation should prompt the search for an alternative cause.
- Intravenous fluid replacement is necessary in patients with burns affecting greater than 15% of body surface area, or greater than 10% if concurrent inhalational injury.
- The Parkland Formula is classically used to calculate required fluid replacement:
  - 4 ml.kg^{-1} for every% body surface area affected over the first 24 hours
  - The 24 hours starts at the time of injury, not time of presentation or calculation
  - The first half of calculated fluid is given in the first 8 hours; the remaining fluid over 16 hours
  - Hartmann's solution is preferred
  - Any fluid already given should be deducted from the calculated volume
- Whilst formulae are useful as a guide, they should be used in conjunction with clinical judgement and other markers of adequacy of fluid resuscitation, such as urine output, lactate and base excess.
- After the first 24 hours, nutritional intake is increased and fluid replacement of insensible losses (ml.h^{-1}) is calculated as: (25+% body surface burn) $\times$ m^2 BSA.

3.2.4 Disability and pain relief

- Superficial and partial thickness burns are painful.
- Adequate analgesia in the form of opiates plus adjunctive agents is required.

3.2.5 Referral to a specialist burn centre

- The decision to refer to a specialist burn centre will be dependent upon the local availability of burns and plastic surgical expertise.
- In the UK, the National Network for Burn Care designate hospitals as:
  - Burn facilities—standard plastic surgical input can provide inpatient care for non-complex burn patients.
  - Burn units—offer a specific burn ward and are able to manage moderately complex burns.
  - Burn centres—offer burn-specific ward and critical care areas; have immediate access to burns theatres. Can cater for the most complex burn patients.

- Comprehensive guidance regarding referral criteria can be found in the UK National Network for Burn Care's 'National Burn Care Referral Guidance'.
- All patients with >40% body surface area burns or >25% surface area with concurrent inhalational injury should be managed in a *burn centre*.
- Patients with between 10% and 40% body surface are burns should be managed in a *burn unit*.
- Patients with between 3% and 10% body surface are burns should be managed in a *burn facility*.
- The following patients should also be *referred* to specialist burn services:
  - All full thickness burns
  - All circumferential burns
  - Burn not healed in 2 weeks
  - Any burn in which a non-accidental mechanism is suspected (for specialist assessment within 24 hours)
- In addition, the following circumstances should be *discussed* with a specialist burn service:
  - Burns to hands, feet, perineum, genitalia, or face
  - Chemical, electrical, or friction burns
  - Cold injuries
  - Where there is concern that comorbidities will impact upon burn treatment or healing

3.3 Ongoing management

3.3.1 Cardiovascular support

- Shock in burn patients is multifactorial:
  - Fluid leak leads to hypovolaemia
  - The inflammatory response may cause vasodilation and cardiac dysfunction
  - Secondary sepsis is common
- Invasive haemodynamic monitoring, careful fluid management, and the use of pharmacological haemodynamic support may be necessary.

3.3.2 Respiratory support

- Lung protective ventilation.
- Early bronchoscopy for assessment of lower airway burns and bronchial toilet.
- Nebulized heparin is believed to have an anti-inflammatory effect and may have a survival benefit in those with inhalational injury.

3.3.3 Infection

- Severely burned patients are at high risk of infection.
- Identification of sepsis may be problematic as it may be masked by the burn-induced systemic inflammatory response.
- Early excision and skin grafting are believed to reduce the risk of infection.
- Silver dressings have antimicrobial properties.
- The use of prophylactic antibiotics is controversial and of unproved benefit.

3.3.4 Nutrition

- Severe burns are associated with a profound hypermetabolic state with significant protein wasting; this peaks at between 7 and 10 days post-injury.
- Inadequate nutritional support impairs wound healing and increases the risk of infection.
- Nutritional supplementation with glutamine appears to improve wound healing and decrease mortality.

FURTHER READING

Bishop S, Maguire S. Anaesthesia and intensive care for major burns. *Continuing Education in Anaesthesia, Critical Care and Pain* 2012; 12(3): 118–22.

National Network for Burn Care, *National Burn Care Referral Guidance*, 2012. Available at http://www.britishburnassociation.org/referral-guidance (accessed December 2015)

Snell JA, Loh N, Mahambrey T, Shokrollahi K. Clinical review: the critical care management of the burn patient. *Critical Care* 2013; 17(5): 241.

4 Drowning

4.1 General

4.1.1 Definitions

- The International Liaison Committee on Resuscitation (ILCOR) has defined drowning as a 'primary respiratory impairment from submersion/immersion in a liquid medium'.
    - Submersion—the airway goes below the surface
    - Immersion—water splashes over the face

4.1.2 Mechanisms

- Initial response to submersion or immersion is breath holding.
- Within around a minute, the desire to breath cannot be resisted and water is inhaled.
- Laryngospasm may protect the lower airways initially, however, as cerebral hypoxia ensues, laryngospasm resides and water enters the lungs.
- Hypoxia ensues and subsequent loss of consciousness and respiratory arrest.
- Bradycardic pulseless electrical activity precedes asystole and death.

4.1.3 Pathophysiology of drowning lung injury

- Water within the alveoli leads to:
    - Surfactant dysfunction
- The creation of an osmotic gradient across the alveolar membrane leads to:
    - Increased permeability of the membrane
    - Fluid and electrolyte shift
    - Widespread alveolar membrane-capillary damage
- This manifests as an ARDS like picture of:
    - Atelectasis
    - Pulmonary oedema
    - Impaired gas exchange
    - Decreased compliance
- Whilst the trans-alveolar membrane osmotic gradient created by fresh water and salt water differs, the pathophysiological process is the same.
- Microorganisms and chemical irritants (e.g. chlorine) may contribute to the lung injury.

4.2 Initial management

4.2.1 Pre-hospital

- Advanced airway support and cardiopulmonary resuscitation cannot be delivered in the water.
- The aim is to deliver the patient safely to land and provide care.

- To provide effective management:
  - Place in supine position
  - Head and body should be at same elevation
  - Follow ABC (not CAB) format of resuscitation
  - Five initial rescue breaths
  - Regurgitation of stomach contents is very common if CPR is required

4.2.2 Hospital management

- The location of hospital management will be dependent upon clinical findings.
- Patients requiring only low F_iO_2 respiratory support, and with no haemodynamic compromise, may be discharged home or managed in a ward environment.
- The need for high concentrations of oxygen to maintain adequate SpO_2 or the presence of shock is associated with far higher mortality and these patients should be managed in a high-dependency or intensive care unit.

4.3 Treatment in intensive care

4.3.1 Respiratory system

- Essentially, standard ARDS management (as discussed in Chapter 1, Section 6).
- The recovery from drowning-related ARDS tends to be more rapid than other insults; consider relatively early weaning of ventilated patients (from 24 hours onwards).
- Prophylactic antibiotics are not necessary; pneumonia post-drowning is uncommon and tends to evolve later (after 48 hours); following resolution of pulmonary oedema.
- No evidence to support the routine use of glucocorticoids.
- Therapeutic bronchoscopy is only rarely indicated.
- In severe cases consider ECMO.
- Partial liquid ventilation, inhaled nitric oxide, and artificial surfactant are under investigation.

4.3.2 Circulatory system

- Hypoxia, hypothermia, and acid–base disturbance may contribute to cardiac dysfunction; arrhythmia may be encountered.
- Rewarming of the hypothermic patient may lead to additional haemodynamic instability.
- Fluid resuscitation is often required in the early stages; invasive haemodynamic monitoring should guide cardiovascular management in later stages.

4.3.3 Neurological system

- The hypoxia associated with drowning can lead to brain injury and associated cerebral oedema; recommendations relating to the neurological sequelae of drowning are extrapolated from the management of other forms of hypoxic brain injury (e.g. cardiac arrest).
- Careful temperature management is key: hyperthermia is neurologically harmful; hypothermia may provide a degree of neuro-protection.
- Drowning victims who are hypothermic on presentation should not therefore be allowed to 'over-shoot' and become hyperthermic on rewarming. Rather temperature should be actively managed and maintained in the mildly hypothermic range in the early stages of admission.

4.3.4 Other complications

- Sepsis is more common after 48 hours.
- Renal failure and metabolic acidosis usually correctable by intravenous fluids.
- The majority of patients do not aspirate significant amounts of water, therefore, efforts to expel water by abdominal thrusts or positioning are usually futile.

4.4 Outcome

- Predictors of outcome include:
  - Administration of early basic and advanced life support
  - Hypothermia during drowning (may be neuroprotective)
  - Short duration of submersion

FURTHER READING

Carter E, Sinclair R. Drowning. Continuing Education in Anaesthesia, Critical Care & Pain 2011; 11 (6): 210–213.

Idris A, Berg R, Bierens J, et al. Recommended Guidelines for Uniform Reporting of Data From Drowning The "Utstein Style". *Circulation* 2003; 108(20): 2565–74.

Spizlman D, Bierens JLM, Handley AJ, Orlowski J. Current concepts in drowning. *New England Journal of Medicine* 2012; 366: 22.

5 Heatstroke and heat-related illnesses

Heat-related illnesses are expected to increase if global temperatures continue to rise. This section focuses on the extreme case of hyperthermia as a primary or secondary illness.

5.1 Thermoregulation

5.1.1 Temperature control

- Body temperature is controlled when temperate-sensitive neurones in the skin and internal organs communicate with the anterior and ventromedial hypothalamus eliciting efferent responses that modify body temperature.

5.1.2 Thermoregulatory responses

- Responses include:
  - Higher cognitive:
    - Reduce activity
    - Move to cooler area
  - Peripheral vasodilatation to facilitate conductive heat loss from the circulation to the environment; large changes in cardiac output can occur to allow enhanced heat exchange in the periphery.
  - Sweat production.
  - The opposite occurs as a response to hypothermia and shivering is a further physiological response to increase muscle tone and metabolic activity.
- Four physical processes are available to facilitate heat loss, as outlined in Table 8.1.

5.2 Definitions in heat-related illness

5.2.1 Spectrum of disease

- Heat-related illnesses occur on a continuum from mild to severe.
- Hyperthermia occurs when the body's physiological mechanisms to control temperature are overcome by illness, medication, exertion, or environmental heat.

5.2.2 Mild heat-related illness

- The following are syndromes associated with mild heat injury:

Table 8.1 Physical processes in thermoregulation and temperature management

Mechanism	Description	Example
Conduction	Transfer of heat energy from a warm to cold surface from two solids in contact	Heat transfer between skin and clothing
Convection	Transfer of heat from a solid state body to a body in a different state	Heat loss from warm skin to colder air
Evaporation	Heat loss via phase state change from liquid to gaseous state	Sweat loss as water vapour
Radiation	Transfer of heat using electromagnetic (predominantly infrared) radiation	Heating from sunlight

- Heat oedema—peripheral oedema as a result of hyperthermia caused by orthostatic pressure, standing, and cutaneous vasodilatation. Usually benign and resolves on cooling.
- Heat syncope—transient loss of consciousness associated with hyperthermia-associated vasodilation; usually managed by removal from heat source, passive cooling, and oral and/or intravenous fluids.
- Heat exhaustion—nausea vomiting and fatigue secondary to salt and water loss in sweat; core temperature may not be elevated and no tissue damage occurs.

5.2.3 Severe heat-related illness

- Cellular damage and significant physiological disturbance occur when body temperatures reach 40°C.
- Heatstroke—a core body temperature of more than 40°C with associated central nervous system dysfunction i.e. encephalopathy.
- Exertional heat stroke—resulting from strenuous exercise in a hot environment in an otherwise healthy individual.
- Classic heat stroke—occurring in an ill patient without strenuous activity secondary to illness or medication.

5.2.4 Temperature measurement

- Temperature measurement is, therefore, necessary to define heatstroke:
  - Core temperature is measured via the oesophageal or ideally rectal route—considered gold standard
  - Peripheral temperature (axilla, skin, tympanic) may underestimate core temperature

5.3 Medications associated with hyperthermia

Medications may induce hyperthermia by increasing metabolic rate or demand and/or impairing the normal thermoregulatory processes.

5.3.1 Recreational drugs

- 3,4-Methylenedioxymethamphetamine (sMDMA)
- Cocaine
- Amphetamines

5.3.2 Cardioactive and vasoactive medications

- Beta blockers

- Alpha adrenergics
- Anticholinergics
- Calcium-channel antagonists

5.3.3 Neuroleptic medications

- Antipsychotics
- Phenothiazines
- Tricyclic anti-depressants
- Benzodiazepines
- Selective serotonin reuptake inhibitors

5.3.4 Others

- Diuretics
- Laxatives
- Thyroid agonists
- Antihistamines

5.4 Consequences of hyperthermia

5.4.1 Cardiovascular

- Diversion of blood to peripheries in an attempt to cool leads to a reduction in the perfusion of other organs:
  - Reduced splanchnic blood flow with relative visceral ischaemia; translocation of gut bacteria and SIRS response.
  - Reduced cerebral perfusion contributes to CNS depression.
- Direct thermal injury:
  - To endothelium leads to activation of the clotting system and disseminated intravascular coagulation.
- Vasodilation occurs in an attempt to regulate temperature and as a consequence of the SIRS response: may result in hypotension.

5.4.2 Renal

- Fluid and electrolyte disturbance secondary to sweating
- Rhabdomyolysis
- Acute kidney injury

5.4.3 Haematological

- Disseminated intravascular coagulation

5.4.4 Neurological

- Altered mental state
- Possibility of permanent neurological injury in survivors

5.5 Cooling methods

- A core temperature of less than 39°C should be sought

5.5.1 Passive cooling

- Use in the pre-hospital setting until other methods available

- Move patient to cooler area
- Loosen clothing and insulate patient from the warm ground

5.5.2 Cold water immersion (CWI)

- Optimum field treatment
- Rapid conductive heat loss due to the high thermal conductivity of water
- Enhanced by ice-cold water
- Impractical in the critically ill patient
- Cooling rate 0.2°C/minute

5.5.3 Evaporative cooling

- Second line if CWI is unavailable or impractical
- Spray water over the skin to provide interface with environmental air
- Provide cool air over the patient
- Cooling rate 0.04 to 0.08°C/minute

5.5.4 Other modalities

- Ice packs to groins, axilla
- Cold intravenous fluids (4°C):
    - Unsuitable as monotherapy—initiate while preparing other methods
- Active temperature management systems—e.g. intravascular cooling systems
- Extracorporeal circuits—renal replacement therapy, ECMO, and cardiopulmonary bypass will contribute to normalisation in temperature
- Body cavity lavage—relatively understudied as a cooling, rather than warming, strategy

5.6 Pharmacotherapy

5.6.1 Antipyretics

- Theoretical benefit in inhibition of prostaglandins and reduction in hypothalamic set point
- Examples include paracetamol, ibuprofen, aspirin
- No benefit in cooling or outcome demonstrated in heatstroke
- Not recommended

5.6.2 Dantrolene

- Theoretical benefit in inhibiting calcium release from sarcoplasmic reticulum and preventing muscle rigidity and heat production
- Presently indicated to treat malignant hyperthermia and neuroleptic malignant syndrome
- No benefit in cooling or outcome demonstrated in a randomized controlled trial in heatstroke patients
- Not recommended

FURTHER READING

Lipman GS, Eifling, KP, Ellis MA, Gaudio, FG, Otten WM, Grissom CK. Wilderness Medical Society Practice Guidelines for the Prevention and Treatment of Heat-Related Illness. *Wilderness and Environmental Medicine* 2013; 24: 351–61.

Walter E, Venn R, Stevenson T. Exertional heat stroke–the athlete's nemesis. *Journal of the Intensive Care Society* 2012; 13(4): 304–8.

6 Hypothermia

6.1 Definitions

- Accidental hypothermia: an involuntary reduction in core body temperature to <35°C.
- Primary hypothermia: excessive cold in a healthy person in a cold environment.
- Secondary hypothermia: excessive cold in an ill person, even in a warm environment.

6.2 Staging

- Hypothermia may be staged in terms of temperature:
  - Mild 35–32°C
  - Moderate: 32–28°C
  - Severe: <28°C
- Or by clinical features using the Swiss Staging System:
  - Stage 1: conscious and shivering
  - Stage 2: impaired consciousness, no shivering
  - Stage 3: unconscious
  - Stage 4: not breathing (may be in ventricular fibrillation or asystole)
  - Stage 5: death
- Differentiation between stage 4 and 5 is difficult in the early stages of resuscitation and, unless clear evidence of death (e.g. rigor mortis) is present, a prolonged resuscitation attempt may be necessary to demonstrate lack of reversibility.

6.3 Consequences of hypothermia

- The primary concerns in the hypothermic patient are cardiac.

6.3.1 Cardiac instability

- Cardiac dysfunction more common at lower temperatures:
  - Arrhythmias—bradycardia and atrial fibrillation are common and not prognostic, ventricular arrhythmias confer poor prognosis
  - J waves on ECG
  - Hypovolaemia may occur due to cold diuresis
  - Hypotension is common during rewarming due to vasodilation
  - VF and then asystolic cardiac arrest may be the consequence of extreme hypothermia (<28°C)
  - Rescue collapse—cardiac arrest following rescue or extrication
  - Increased myocardial work (secondary to vasoconstriction and increased viscosity of blood)

6.3.2 Haematological

- Coagulopathy
- Increased risk of thrombosis

6.3.3 Neurology

- Altered neurological state
- Neurological assessment, including pupillary reflexes cannot be reliably undertaken until rewarmed
- Neuro-protective effect

6.3.4 Respiratory

- Decrease in metabolic rate reduces oxygen requirements and carbon dioxide production

6.4 Management principles

6.4.1 Fluids

- Considerable amounts may be required due to cold diuresis
- No specific fluids are thought to be superior
- Warm fluid to 38–42°C to prevent further heat loss
- Be cautious with vasopressors as arrhythmias are more common in hypothermic patients

6.4.2 Avoidance of cardiovascular instability

- Avoid unnecessary movement
- Care on insertion of central venous catheters (may precipitate arrhythmia)
- Judicious fluids (to replace fluid lost during diuresis)
- Reduce dose pressors, including in cardiac arrest (due to altered drug metabolism)

6.4.3 Rewarming

- The use of a rewarming strategy depends on the desired rate of rewarming and the justification of the risk of the particular method based on the likelihood of death without a high rewarming rate.
- Rewarming strategies include:
  - Simple interventions (warm environment, warm drinks, physical activity)—these can raise temperature at around 1°C/hour but require the patient to be conscious and cooperative.
  - Active external warming may be undertaken using forced air warmers; warmed intravenous fluids provide a minimally invasive means of rewarming.
  - Peritoneal dialysis and haemodialysis techniques have been described for rewarming; these probably allow more rapid rewarming than the less invasive techniques described (1–4°C/hour) but their role is uncertain.
  - In centres with extracorporeal capabilities, extracorporeal membrane oxygenation (ECMO) or cardiopulmonary bypass (CPB) offer a rapid means of temperature correction; a veno-arterial ECMO and CPB have the added advantage of supporting the circulation during cardiac arrest and therefore can maintain perfusion whilst the patient is rewarmed and spontaneous circulation restored.
- Afterdrop is a phenomenon that occurs when redistributed cooler blood causes a further fall in temperature after rewarming.

FURTHER READING

Brown DJA, Brugger H, Boyd J, Paal, P. Current concepts in accidental hypothermia. *New England Journal of Medicine* 2012; 366: 22.

Durrer B, Brugger H, Syme D. The medical on-site treatment of hypothermia: ICAR-MEDCOM recommendation. *High Altitude Medicine and Biology* 2003; 4(1): 99–103.

Toxicology

CONTENTS

1 General principles

1.1 Background
- Poisoning is common and accounts for 5–10% of all medical admissions.
- It is usually intentional but rarely fatal (mortality in UK from poisoning is less than 0.5%).
- The list of agents with potential to poison is huge but the general principles of management are the same.

1.2 Approach to toxicological emergencies
- There are five facets to the management of any toxicological emergency:
  - Resuscitation and reversal of life-threatening physiological derangement
  - Identification of agent and quantification of exposure
  - Drug manipulation to limit absorption and enhance removal
  - Specific antidotes
  - General supportive care

1.3 Specialist advice
- Early specialist advice is essential.
- The UK has a National Poisons Information Service—this provides up to date online advice via the website [www.toxbase.org] and is also available to discuss complicated/severe cases via telephone 24 hours a day.

1.4 Resuscitation and reversal of life-threatening derangement
- Initial stabilization of the poisoned patient may require the following:
  - Airway patency and protection
  - Provision of supplemental oxygen, if required
  - Implementation of mechanical ventilation, if required
  - Intravenous access
  - Management of life-threatening arrhythmias

- Control of life-threatening hyper- or hypotension
- Cessation of seizures
- Correction of life-threatening metabolic derangement
- Control of body temperature

1.5 Identification of agent and quantification of exposure

1.5.1 History

- The toxin:
  - If tablets:
    - Number
    - Strength
    - Duration over which taken
  - If non-pharmaceutical toxin (e.g. agricultural chemicals):
    - Mode of exposure (ingestion, inhalation, etc.)
    - Exact nature of poison (containers and packaging are useful)
    - Duration of exposure
    - First-aid measures undertaken
- Factors that may impact upon metabolism of the toxin:
  - Prescription and non-prescription medications
  - Alcohol use
  - Chronic liver or renal dysfunction
- Current symptoms (with particular reference to the symptoms common to the toxidromes described in Section 2 of this chapter).

1.5.2 Investigation

- Investigation (Table 9.1) is directed at:
  - Identification and quantification of the toxin
  - Identification of factors that will impact upon toxin clearance
  - Assessment of physiological derangements associated with the toxin

Table 9.1 Investigation of poisoning

Investigation	Significance	Calculation
Urinalysis	Rapid urine toxicology screens are widely available; cannot differentiate between drugs responsible for current presentation and other recently ingested drugs	
Biochemistry	Renal or hepatic impairment: • Will alter clearance of toxins • May represent significant adverse effect of toxin	
Arterial blood gas	Acid base state is altered by a number of toxins	
Anion gap (AG)	AG is elevated by presence of unmeasured anions in plasma; a feature of poisoning by a number of agents: ethanol, methanol, ethylene glycol, metformin, cyanide, isoniazid, salicylates	$(Na^+ + K^+) - (Cl^- + HCO_3^-)$ Normal 10–14 mmol.l^{-1}

Osmolar gap (OG)	OG is elevated by presence of unmeasured osmotically active particles in plasma, commonly seen in alcohol toxicity: ethanol, methanol and ethylene glycol	Measured osmolality – calculated osmolality $(2Na^+ + K^+ + urea + glucose)$ Normal <10 mOsm.l^{-1}
ECG	Arrhythmia and conduction defects are common feature of many toxins	
Plasma drug levels	Beneficial in only a small number of drugs: paracetamol, salicylates, iron. digoxin, lithium, and some anti-epileptic drugs	

1.6 Limitation of absorption

- Gut decontamination incorporates a range of techniques aimed at limiting absorption of poison from the gut.

1.6.1 Induced emesis

- This practice of induced emesis is historical and no longer used.

1.6.2 Gastric lavage

- Gastric lavage involves irrigation of the stomach and proximal bowel by repeated injection and aspiration of water via a nasogastric tube.
- It is only beneficial within 1 hour of ingestion and of limited value even at this.
- It should not be attempted if corrosive agents have been ingested.

1.6.3 Activated charcoal (AC)

- The most commonly employed form of gut decontamination.
- A porous substance with large surface area, it binds the majority of ingested toxins (with the exception of heavy metals, strong acids/alkali, cyanide, and alcohols), preventing systemic absorption.
- It should be administered within 1 hour of ingestion.
- The therapeutic window is, however, extended in those drugs:
  - That slow gastric emptying (opiates, tricyclic anti-depressants).
  - That exhibit entero-hepatic recirculation (e.g. carbamazepine, theophylline, digoxin, quinine, and phenobarbital) in which AC may be effective for up to 4 hours post-ingestion.
- Repeated doses of AC may be of use in the case of sustained release preparation drugs with entero-hepatic recirculation, e.g. theophylline.

1.6.4 Whole bowel irrigation

- Non-absorbable polyethylene glycol is infused down a nasogastric tube causing rapid expulsion of gut contents as liquid stool.
- This technique may be employed for those agents not absorbed by AC or in those with non-absorbable but potentially dangerous objects in their gut (e.g. 'body-packers').

1.7 Enhanced elimination

1.7.1 Forced alkaline diuresis

- The elimination of acidic drugs with low pKa may be enhanced by forced alkaline diuresis.
- This technique requires infusion of intravenous sodium bicarbonate, often in combination with a loop diuretic, with a view to increasing urinary pH to around 7.5.

- The acidic drug molecules, which are normally filtered at the glomerulus and then reabsorbed, convert to the ionic form within the abnormally alkaline conditions of the tubule and are, therefore, not reabsorbed by tubular cells.
- Forced alkaline diuresis is classically used in aspirin poisoning but may also have a role with methotrexate and phenobarbital.
- Hypokalaemia is a recognized complication.

1.7.2 Renal replacement therapy

- In severe toxicity, extracorporeal techniques may be required to enhance drug elimination.
- Renal replacement therapy—either haemofiltration or haemodialysis—will assist elimination of many drugs; however, it is most effective for molecules that are:
  - Small (MW<500 Da)
  - Water soluble
  - Low protein binding
  - Small volume of distribution
- Very high replacement rates (50–100 ml/kg) may be required in the management of poisoning.

1.7.3 Haemoperfusion

- Haemoperfusion, in which a charcoal cartridge replaces the dialysis membrane within the extracorporeal circuit.
- It is more effective at removing larger molecules (1000–1500 Da).
- It is an expensive technique, with limited availability and with no evidence of superiority to more conventional techniques.
- It has a theoretical advantage in poisoning with theophylline, carbamazepine, verapamil, phenobarbital, and paraquat.

2 The toxidromes

2.1 Features, causative agents, and management principles associated with the toxidromes

- Many of the agents subject to accidental or deliberate overdose manifest with similar signs and symptoms.
- These are classified into toxidromes (Table 9.2).

Table 9.2 The toxidromes

	Features	Causative agents	Management principles
Cholinergic	Confusion, decreased conscious state, salivation, bronchorrhoea, bronchospasm, bradycardia, emesis, incontinence, abdominal cramps, sweating, hypotension	Organophosphates, some fungi	Anti-cholinergic—atropine Anticholinesterase reactivator—pralidoxime Benzodiazepines

Anti-cholinergic	Tachycardia, hypotension, confusion, coma, dry skin, fever, flushing, ileus, urinary retention	Antihistamines Anti-depressants Anti-Parkinsonian Anti-psychotics Atropine	Supportive
Opioid	Coma, pinpoint pupils, respiratory depression, bradycardia, hypotension	Opioids	Opioid receptor antagonism—naloxone
Hypno-sedative	Ataxia, central nervous system depression, coma, nystagmus, hypotension, hypothermia	Benzodiazepines Barbituates Anti-depressants Alcohols Gamma-hydroxy-butyric acid	Supportive
Serotonin syndrome	Altered mental status, autonomic dysfunction, neuromuscular hyper-activity	Anti-depressants Amphetamines Ecstasy	Benzodiazepines Serotonin antagonist – cyproheptadine
Sympathomimetic	Delusions, paranoia, tachycardia, hypertension, hyperreflexia, diaphoresis, piloerection	Amphetamines Cocaine Sympathetic agents (e.g. pseudoephedrine, salbutamol)	Benzodiazepines

3 Specific toxins

3.1 Paracetamol

3.1.1 Pharmacology and toxicity

- Paracetamol is metabolized primarily by a phase 2 reaction to sulphate and glucuronide metabolites.
- A small amount is metabolized via the cytochrome P450 system to the toxic metabolite N-acetyl-benzoquinone-imine (NAPQI).
- Under normal circumstances NAPQI is detoxified by being bound to glutathione, the compound is then renally excreted.
- In overdose, the phase 2 metabolism to sulphate and glucuronide is overwhelmed.
- Metabolism via the P450 system increases and NAPQI production rises.
- If NAPQI production exceeds available glutathione, hepatic NAPQI levels rise and toxicity ensues.
- The degree of toxicity is proportional to the magnitude of overdose; the situation may, however, be exacerbated by:
    - Pre-existing glutathione depletion (a feature of eating disorders, chronic alcoholism, cystic fibrosis, and HIV)
    - Pharmacological induction of the cytochrome P450 system (e.g. phenytoin, rifampicin, and carbamazepine)

3.1.2 Presentation and assessment

- Initial symptoms are typically absent or vague (nausea, vomiting, and sweating).
- As hepatotoxicity progresses (24–72 hours) right upper quadrant pain may develop, the liver function tests become abnormal, and synthetic hepatic function deteriorates, as reflected by an increase in the international normalized ratio (INR).

- Elevation in plasma lactate may occur for two reasons:
  - Very high paracetamol levels can impair mitochondrial function leading to anaerobic respiration
  - As a consequence of hepatic failure
- Kidney injury is common, and occasionally the predominant feature (mechanism is unclear but may represent direct renal toxicity or a hepatorenal-like syndrome).
- If hepatic injury progresses, fulminant liver failure, with jaundice, encephalopathy, coagulopathy, hypoglycaemia, and multi-organ failure may follow.

3.1.3 Management

- Management should follow the general approach to poisoning outlined in Section 1.2.
- AC is indicated if presentation occurs within 1 hour of ingestion.
- The specific antidote is n-acetylcysteine (NAC), its initiation is guided by the plasma paracetamol level on presentation, referenced against a widely available nomogram (Fig. 9.1).
  - Those with a time-referenced plasma level above the 'treatment line' should be commenced on the NAC regime.
  - Levels are only helpful if the entire overdose was taken at the same time; staggered overdoses should be treated with the antidote regime regardless of plasma level at presentation.
  - Previously two treatment nomograms existed in the UK with a second nomogram specifically aimed at patients identified to be at 'high risk' of hepatic injury secondary to paracetamol overdose; however, this system was simplified to a single nomogram in 2012.

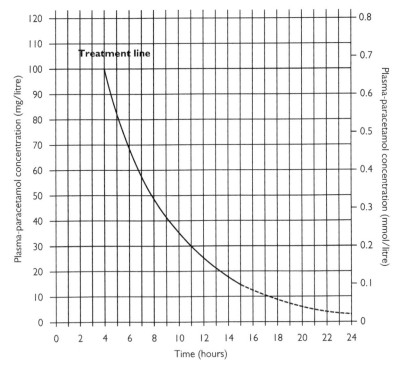

Figure 9.1 Paracetamol overdose nomogram.

Reproduced from *Drug Safety Update*, 6, 2:A1, Medicines and Healthcare products Regulatory Agency (MHRA), 'Treating paracetamol overdose with intravenous acetylcysteine: new guidance', Copyright 2012, with permission from MRHA.

- NAC is believed to reduce the risk of paracetamol toxicity by providing a reservoir of sulfhy-dryl groups, which bind NAPQI, and by stimulating production of glutathione.
- Side-effects include rash, angioedema, and bronchospasm. These reactions are not a contra-indication to NAC use and can be ameliorated by slowing the rate of infusion and administra-tion of antihistamine.
- Best outcomes are achieved if NAC is administered within 10 hours of ingestion but it is con-sidered effective for several days.
- In the context of paracetamol toxicity, referral to a specialist liver centre is recommended (Kings College Hospital Liver Guidelines) in the presence of:
  - Acidosis (pH<7.3 after fluid resuscitation) or
  - Prothrombin time >100 s (INR>6.5) and creatinine >300 mmol.l^{-1} and grade 3–4 encephalopathy
- Liver transplant may offer the only hope of survival in fulminant liver failure; serious psychiatric disorder is, however, a contra-indication to transplant.

3.2 Salicylates

3.2.1 Pharmacology and toxicity

- Aspirin is rapidly converted to salicylic acid.
- At toxic levels this activates the:
  - Chemoreceptor trigger zone (leading to nausea and vomiting)
  - Respiratory centre (with resultant respiratory alkalosis)
- Higher plasma levels lead to uncoupling of cellular respiration and subsequent lactic acidosis.

3.2.2 Presentation and assessment

- Features include:
  - Fever
  - Tinnitus
  - Hypoglycaemia
  - Vertigo
  - Visual disturbance
  - Coagulopathy
  - Pulmonary oedema

3.2.3 Management

- AC and supportive treatment are the mainstays of initial management.
- Forced alkaline diuresis (to maintain blood pH 7.40–7.50 and urinary pH 6.0–7.0) and hae-modialysis (as described in Section 1.7) are indicated for cases with very high plasma levels (>750 mg/l) or life-threatening features.

3.3 Tricyclic anti-depressants

Tricyclic anti-depressants (TCA) are the leading cause of death from overdose in those who arrive at hospital alive; they account for 50% of ICU poisoning admissions.

3.3.1 Pharmacology and toxicity

- The features of TCA toxicity occur via two mechanisms:
  - Cholinergic antagonism (the anti-cholinergic toxidrome)
  - Sodium channel blockade

Table 9.3 Features of tricyclic anti-depressant overdose

Cardiovascular	Tachycardia
	Arrhythmia (occur primarily due to slowing of phase 0 depolarization)
	(likelihood significantly increased when QRS duration >100 ms)
	Hypotension
Neurological	Dilated pupils and blurred vision
	Decreased level of consciousness
	Seizures (likelihood significantly increased when QRS duration >160 ms)
Respiratory	Respiratory depression
Gastrointestinal	Dry mouth
	Prolonged gastric transit
Other	Warm dry skin
	Urinary retention

3.3.2 Presentation and assessment

- Virtually every system is affected (Table 9.3); however, cardiovascular and neurological effects are most significant.
- Key investigations are the ECG and the arterial blood gas (both QRS duration and arterial pH are prognostic markers and guides to management).
- All patients with a history of TCA overdose require observation of ECG (with both continuous monitoring and serial 12 lead ECG) and of conscious state.

3.3.3 Management

- Absorption of TCA may be reduced by AC—repeated doses are warranted as TCA slows gastric transit.
- Intubation may be required for low conscious state.
- In those patients with features of severe toxicity (acidosis, hypotension, QRS>100 ms or arrhythmias), attempts should be made to manipulate the pH:
  - Increasing the pH (usually to >7.45) has the theoretical advantage of reducing the available ionized free drug.
  - This alkalosis may be achieved by means of hyperventilation in the mechanically ventilated patient or by administration of intravenous sodium bicarbonate solution.
  - The latter intervention might also be beneficial as the high sodium load may overcome sodium channel blockade.
- If unstable arrhythmia occurs: sodium bicarbonate, magnesium, and, if required, lidocaine can be used.
- Lipid emulsion has be used in severe haemodynamic instability.
- If seizure—bendodiazepines should be used rather than phenytoin; barbiturates are second line.

3.4 Serotonergic agents

3.4.1 Pharmacology and toxicity

- The serotonin syndrome is a consequence of hyper-stimulation of serotonin receptors and is a dose-dependent reaction to a host of both medicinal and recreational agents (Table 9.4).

3.4.2 Features and assessment

- Serotonin syndrome (Table 9.5) classically presents as the triad of:
  - Altered mentation
  - Autonomic dysfunction
  - Neuromuscular hyper-reactivity

Table 9.4 Agents implicated in the serotonin syndrome

Inhibition of serotonin reuptake	Selective serotonin reuptake inhibitors, tricyclic anti-depressants, tramadol, pethidine, St. John's Wort
Increase in serotonin release	Amphetamines, ecstasy
Partial serotonin agonists	LSD, buspirone

Table 9.5 Features of serotonin syndrome

Altered mentation	Agitation, confusion (rarely seizures)
Autonomic dysfunction	Nausea, diaphoresis, tachycardia, tremor, diarrhoea, fever
Neuromuscular hyper-reactivity	Hyper-reflexia, clonus, (rarely progresses to rhabdomyolysis, hyperkalaemia, AKI, DIC)

3.4.3 Management

- Management of serotonin syndrome involves withdrawal of precipitant, AC for early presentations and supportive therapy.
- Supportive care involves rehydration, temperature control, control of hypertension/hypotension, DIC, sepsis, and rhabdomyolysis.
- Benzodiazepines are the first-line agents for management of agitation, autonomic dysfunction, and neuromuscular hyper-reactivity; benzodiazepines alone are usually sufficient for minor cases.
- Limitation of opioids (e.g. fentanyl), as these can increase serotonin release.
- More severe poisoning may require general anaesthesia and muscle relaxants.
- The serotonin antagonist cyproheptadine is recommended for severe poisoning and, whilst no high-level evidence for its use is available, numerous case studies report good outcomes.

3.5 Neuroleptic malignant syndrome

3.5.1 Pharmacology and toxicity

- Neuroleptic malignant syndrome (NMS) is an idiosyncratic reaction to anti-psychotic agents.
- Blockade of dopaminergic signalling leads, in genetically predisposed individuals, to the triad of:
  - Rigidity
  - Fever
  - Autonomic instability
- NMS occurs most commonly secondary to anti-psychotic agents; however, other drugs that exhibit dopamine antagonism (e.g. metoclopramide) may also be implicated. NMS in response to rapid withdrawal of dopamine agonists (e.g. levodopa) has also been reported.

3.5.2 Features and assessment

- In addition to the triad described in Section 3.5.1, affected individuals may exhibit confusion, drowsiness, diaphoresis, and elevation of plasma creatinine kinase and white cell count.
- May be confused with serotonin syndrome; however, both the mortality risk and the treatment options are significantly different and, therefore, differentiation is important (Table 9.6).

Table 9.6 Comparison of neuroleptic malignant syndrome and serotonin syndrome

	Serotonin Syndrome	Neuroleptic Malignant Syndrome
Relationship to dose	Dose-dependent	Idiosyncratic
Onset	Rapid (within 24 hours)	Slow (days to weeks)
Neuromuscular findings	Hyper-reactivity, increased reflexes	Muscular rigidity, reduced reflexes
Laboratory findings	Abnormalities uncommon	Elevated white cell count and creatinine kinase common
Caused by	Increased serotonergic activity	Antagonism of dopaminergic pathways
Management	Benzodiazepines, Cyproheptadine	Bromocriptine, Dantrolene
Resolution	Rapid (hours)	Slow (days to weeks)
Mortality	<1%	Up to 10%

3.5.3 Management

- Withdrawal of offending agent and supportive care.
- Active cooling should be undertaken and benzodiazepines may be useful for agitation.
- Specific agents are:
  - The muscle relaxant *dantrolene* (which acts by inhibiting excitation–contraction coupling in skeletal muscle)
  - Dopamine agonist *bromocriptine*
  - Efficacy has not, however, been clearly demonstrated

3.6 Alcohols

Poisoning with alcohols (ethanol, methanol, or ethylene glycol) produces a classical and unique biochemical picture.

3.6.1 Pharmacology and toxicity

- This CNS depressant effect is common to all alcohols and can lead to hypothermia, aspiration, and increases risk of trauma.
- Some alcohols also have secondary, toxic effects:
  - Methanol, when metabolized to formic acid:
    - Impedes mitochondrial function (causing metabolic acidosis)
    - Exerts direct toxicity on the optic nerve (causing visual impairment)
    - Approximately 10 ml of pure methanol may result in permanent blindness; the fatal dose is around 30 ml
  - Ethylene glycol is metabolized to glycoaldehyde, glycolate, and oxalate; these lead to:
    - Cerebral oedema
    - Metabolic acidosis
    - Renal failure

3.6.2 Features and assessment

- Initial presentation is one of decreased conscious state, ataxia, dysarthria, and vomiting.
- All alcohols are osmotically active. The presence of an osmolar gap (Table 9.1), particularly in the context of low conscious state, raises the possibility of alcohol ingestion.
- Classically, alcohol poisoning also causes a raised anion gap metabolic acidosis secondary to:
  - Plasma dilution (for all forms of alcohol)
  - Increase in the anions formic acid (methanol) or glycolate and oxalate (ethylene glycol)

3.6.3 Management

- The management of known or suspected alcohol ingestion includes gastric lavage (activated charcoal has no role) and supportive care.
- The secondary toxic effects of ethylene glycol and methanol can be mitigated by blocking the metabolic pathway that converts the alcohol into toxic products.
- The key enzyme in metabolism of alcohols is alcohol dehydrogenase:
  - Alcohol dehydrogenase has a far greater affinity for ethanol than other alcohols.
  - Administration of ethanol to patients at risk of methanol or ethylene glycol toxicity, therefore, prevents the production of toxic metabolites.
  - Administration and dosing of ethanol is, however, problematic.
  - As a result, the alcohol dehydrogenase inhibitor fomepizole, is a preferred alternative, if available.

3.7 Cyanide

Cyanide poisoning is uncommon however it is a frequent examination topic.

3.7.1 Pharmacology and toxicity

- Cyanide is contained in some insecticides and in the smoke from burning plastics.
- The possibility of cyanide toxicity should be considered in anyone presenting with smoke inhalation.
- Cyanide is a metabolite of the anti-hypertensive sodium nitroprusside: prolonged use at high doses may lead to iatrogenic cyanide toxicity.
- Cyanide reversibly binds to, and inhibits, cytochrome oxidase within the mitochondria.
- The resultant disruption of electron transport chain function blocks aerobic respiration; ATP is produced only by anaerobic means and a cytotoxic hypoxia ensues.

3.7.2 Features and assessment

- Clinical features are vague:
  - Confusion
  - Seizures; dyspnoea
  - Tachypnoea
  - Coma
- The classical biochemical picture is of unexplained lactic acidosis and high $ScvO_2$ (venous hyperoxia): a reflection of the anaerobic cellular metabolism, despite adequate oxygen delivery.

3.7.3 Management

- Care must be taken by healthcare professionals not to become contaminated as cyanide may be absorbed via the skin.
- Gastric lavage is indicated in the context of cyanide ingestion.

- Antidotes:
  - Amyl nitrate
    - Converts haemoglobin to methaemoglobin (metHb) (the iron atom being converted from the ferrous Fe^{2+} to the ferric Fe^{3+} state).
    - Cyanide has a higher affinity for metHb than for cytochrome oxidase and, therefore, preferentially binds to the former.
    - MetHb has, however, no oxygen-binding capacity and high levels may result in failure of oxygen delivery.
    - Amyl nitrate therapy should be titrated to a metHb of 20–30%.
    - The methaemoglobinaemia may itself be treated with methylene blue.
  - Hydroxocobalamin (vitamin B12a)
    - Binds cyanide to form cyanocobalamin, which is excreted in the urine.
    - A large dose is required; however, it has no apparent adverse effects.
    - Hydroxocobalamin is used on a routine basis by some centres for victims of smoke inhalation, regardless of whether there is evidence of cyanide exposure.
  - Sodium thiosulphate
    - Binds cyanide to form thiocyanate, which is excreted in the urine.
    - The reaction is slow and sodium thiosulphate cannot, therefore, be used in isolation.
  - Dicobalt edetate (EDTA)
    - The cobalt ions bind cyanide in a similar manner to iron.
    - It may have a faster onset of action than other cyanide antidotes; however, the relative toxicity of cobalt-containing compounds limits the use of EDTA to severe cases.
    - The co-administration of glucose may reduce the risk of EDTA toxicity.

3.8 Carbon monoxide

3.8.1 Pharmacology and toxicity

- Carbon monoxide (CO), produced by the incomplete combustion of carbon, binds to haemoglobin with an affinity around 200 times greater than that of oxygen.
- This causes a left shift in the oxy-haemoglobin dissociation curve and impaired tissue oxygen delivery.
- CO also binds to cytochrome oxidase, in a similar manner to cyanide, resulting in uncoupling of cellular respiration.
- It probably also has a direct neurotoxic effect, particularly in cases of chronic exposure.

3.8.2 Features and assessment

- Symptoms are primarily neurological in nature and range from mild confusion to coma.
- The classical cherry red appearance of the skin is uncommon; cyanosis is more frequent.
- Levels of carboxyhaemoglobin (COHb) are routinely measured by blood gas analysers.
- The level associated with symptoms varies between individuals and is dependent upon the chronicity of exposure:
  - Cigarette smokers frequently have COHb levels of 10%
  - Levels over 40% are generally accepted to represent a life-threatening exposure
  - Levels over 60% are commonly lethal

3.8.3 Management

- Management of CO toxicity is aimed at replacing the CO bound to Hb with oxygen.

- The half-life of CO in plasma is:
  - 4 hours whilst breathing room air
  - 1 hour with 100% oxygen
  - 25 minutes when breathing 100% oxygen at 3 atmospheres pressure in a hyperbaric chamber
- There is no evidence that hyperbaric therapy improves neurological outcomes or survival, and the logistics of transfer to, and management in, a hyperbaric chamber makes this an unrealistic option under most circumstances.
- Oxygen therapy is continued until COHb levels fall below 5%.

3.9 Paraquat

3.9.1 Pharmacology and toxicity

- Paraquat is contained in pesticides.
- Availability is limited to commercial agriculture in the UK; however, it is freely available else-where in the world.
- The lethal dose is low (ingestion of 15–20 ml of 20% solution has a mortality of 75%).
- The onset of action is fast (peak plasma concentration is reached at 30 minutes to 2 hours).

3.9.2 Presentation and assessment

- Initial presentation is with:
  - Abdominal pain
  - Vomiting
  - Local corrosive effects (mouth, pharynx, and oesophagus)
- Typically followed by:
  - Dypnoea: a consequence of non-cardiac pulmonary oedema, which quickly progresses to irreversible pulmonary fibrosis.
  - Cardiac, renal, and hepatic dysfunction also feature.

3.9.3 Management

- AC may reduce absorption.
- Minimize oxygen exposure: high levels of oxygen are thought to accelerate the fibrotic process.
- Cyclophosphamide and methylprednisolone have both been suggested as a means of reducing the pulmonary inflammatory response.
- Palliative care may, however, be the most appropriate approach.

3.10 Iron toxicity

3.10.1 Pharmacology and toxicity

- Acute iron toxicity primarily relates to inadvertent ingestion by children.
- The degree of toxicity relates to the mass of elemental iron ingested: ferrous sulphate and ferrous fumarate tablets carry a higher risk of toxicity than other preparations.
- Ingestion of greater than 60 mg/kg of elemental iron is associated with serious toxicity and risk of death.
- Iron toxicity has a number of effects at a sub-cellular level; free radical production impacts upon mitochondrial function and impairs the Kreb's cycle.

3.10.2 Features and assessment

- Clinical manifestations include:
  - Gastrointestinal (occurs in the first 6 hours post-ingestion):
    - Direct mucosal injury leads to abdominal pain, vomiting, diarrhoea, and haematemesis.

- Early gastrointestinal symptoms are commonly followed by a latent phase of around 24 hours during which the patient is largely asymptomatic.
- In patients with severe toxicity this is followed by multi-organ involvement:
  - Hypovolaemia (from GI bleeding and fluid misdistribution)
  - Myocardial dysfunction (due to direct cardiac toxicity)
  - Vasodilation
  - Iron-induced mitochondrial dysfunction may impair oxygen utilization
  - Iron inhibition of prothrombin induces coagulopathy
  - Hepatotoxicity is common due to the high iron levels within the portal circulation and the high metabolic activity of the liver. This may progress to hepatic necrosis over a period of days.
- Specific investigation includes:
  - Serum iron levels—the timing of ingestion and the impact of modified release preparations must be considered during interpretation. A serum iron of greater than 500 µg per decilitre is associated with serious toxicity. Total iron binding capacity is of no value.
  - Blood gas analysis—typically demonstrates a raised anion gap metabolic acidosis.
  - Plain abdominal X-ray may demonstrate iron tablets in the GI tract which may prompt GI decontamination.

3.10.3 Management

- Supportive therapy.
- GI decontamination:
  - Minimal absorption with AC
  - Whole bowel irrigation is the only effective technique
- Deferoxamine is the antidote of choice:
  - Chelating agent that binds ferric iron to form ferrioxamine, a water-soluble compound excreted by the kidneys.
  - It should be given early as it only chelates free iron within the plasma; tissue-bound iron is inaccessible.
  - Associated with hypotension and the risk of ARDS.
- Extracorporeal elimination is of limited benefit as only free iron is removed.

3.11 Beta blockers and calcium channel antagonists

3.11.1 Pharmacology and toxicity

- Beta blockers are a class of cardiovascular agent with variable pharmacokinetics and pharmacodynamics; the unifying feature is the blockage of beta-adrenergic receptors.
- Beta blockers vary in their beta-adrenergic selectivity (in terms of β_1 and β_2 activity).
- Of particular note are propranolol (a non-selective beta blocker, which, unlike others in class, crosses the blood–brain barrier and exerts a CNS effect), labetalol (which exerts alpha-adrenergic antagonism), and sotalol (which blocks potassium channels in addition to beta blockade).
- Calcium channel antagonists are cardiovascular agents broadly divided into:
  - Dihydropyridines:
    - Exert their effect primarily on the vasculature, reducing systemic vascular resistance; minimal effect upon the myocardium.
    - E.g. amlodipine, nifedipine, lercandipine.
    - In overdose, however, the vascular selectivity of dihydropyridines is lost and myocardial toxicity may arise.

- Non-dihydropyridines:
    - Exert their effect primarily upon the myocardium, reducing heart rate, contractile force, and myocardial oxygen consumption; less vascular activity than dihydropyridines.
    - E.g. verapamil, diltiazem.

3.11.2 Presentation and assessment

- Toxicity relating to beta blockers and calcium channel antagonist relates to the cardiovascular effects:
    - Hypotension
    - Bradycardia
    - Cardiac failure
    - Beta blockers may cause hypoglycaemia; calcium channel antagonists may cause hyperglycaemia
- Be aware of the delayed effects of modified-release preparations.
- Assessment of adequacy of cardiac output allows determination of severity of overdose to be quantified e.g.:
    - Clinical features of a low cardiac output state (decreased level of consciousness, syncope, kidney injury)
    - Cardiac output monitoring
    - Plasma lactate
    - Central venous oxygen saturation
    - Assessment of cardiovascular status is further discussed in Chapter 1, Section 2.

3.11.3 Management

- Standard means of increasing cardiac output may be attempted but, in the context of beta blocker or calcium channel antagonist toxicity, these may prove of limited benefit:
    - Fluids
    - Atropine for bradycardia
    - Catecholamines, e.g. dobutamine, noradrenaline, adrenaline
    - Electrical pacing
    - Calcium chloride infusion (particularly for calcium channel antagonists)
- Improvement in cardiac performance may be better achieved by manipulation of metabolic pathways:
    - Glucagon was the traditional agent of choice:
        - Large doses of glucagon (50 µg/kg) increase intracellular cAMP concentrations via an adrenergic independent mechanism
        - Positive inotropic effect but often short-lived
    - Increasingly high dose insulin therapy (HDIT) is used as an alternative to glucagon.
    - A typical HDIT regimen might consist of:
        - 1 unit/kg intravenous bolus
        - 0.5–1.0 unit/kg/hour infusion, titrated to cardiovascular effect (doses of up to 10 unit/kg/hour have been reported)
        - Concurrent administration of 10–20% dextrose solution and regular blood glucose monitoring to ensure euglycaemia
        - Concurrent administration of potassium and regular monitoring to ensure normokalaemia

- Refractory shock may require veno-arterial extracorporeal membrane oxygenation as a bridge to recovery.

3.12 Digoxin

3.12.1 Pharmacology and toxicity

- Digoxin is a cardiac glycoside derived from digitalis; it exerts its cardiac effects by:
  - Anti-muscarinic activity leading to a slowing of atrio-ventricular conduction.
  - Blockade of the sodium–potassium ATP-ase pump in the cardiac membrane; the resultant increase in intracellular sodium leads to increased influx of calcium via the sodium–calcium pump; the increase in intracellular calcium has a positive inotropic effect.
- Digoxin has a narrow therapeutic index; small rises in plasma concentrations may lead to toxicity.
- A number of commonly used drugs interact with the pharmacokinetics of digoxin and may serve to increase plasma concentrations, e.g.:
  - Amoxicillin
  - Clarithromycin
  - Amiodarone
  - Quinine
- Excretion is primarily renal and therefore kidney injury may impact upon clearance.
- Hypomagnesaemia, hypokalaemia, hypernatraemia, and hypercalcaemia all potentiate the effects of digoxin, again potentially contributing to toxicity.

3.12.2 Presentation and assessment

- The presentation of digoxin toxicity is dependent upon the speed at which levels have risen:
  - Acute toxicity (e.g. deliberate ingestion of large quantity of tablets) typically results in bradycardia and hypotension.
  - Chronic toxicity (e.g. accumulation of digoxin over several weeks due to impaired renal function or drug interaction) tends to present with a more insidious onset and less specific signs.
- Digoxin toxicity may produce a variety of ECG abnormalities, common findings include:
  - AV block
  - Paroxysmal tachycardia with AV block
  - Sinus bradycardia
  - Ventricular tachycardia
- Initial investigation should focus upon:
  - Plasma digoxin levels (6 hours post-acute overdose provides a more accurate reflection of digoxin load than earlier measurement)(normal range 0.8–2.0 ng.ml^{-1})
  - Potassium and magnesium levels (hypokalaemia and hypomagnesaemia may potentiate toxicity; hyperkalaemia may be a feature of digoxin toxicity)

3.12.3 Management

- AC, if presentation within 2 hours of acute ingestion.
- Correction of electrolyte disturbance.
- Atropine for bradycardia.
- Digoxin-specific antibody fragments bind free digoxin in the plasma, creating a concentration gradient down which tissue digoxin will move; indications for antibody fragments are:
  - Ingestion of more than 10 mg of digoxin
  - Acute ingestion with a serum steady state level >10 ng.ml^{-1}

- Chronic ingestion with a serum steady state level >6 ng.ml^{-1}
- Any arrhythmia, not responding to more conservative measures
- Serum potassium greater than 5.5 mmol.l^{-1} secondary to acute digoxin overdose
- Each vial of digoxin-specific antibody fragments (digoxin-Fab) binds 0.5 mg of digoxin.
- Pacing is of little benefit.
- Extracorporeal removal of digoxin is ineffective due to a large volume of distribution and high protein binding.

3.13 Lithium

3.13.1 Pharmacology and toxicity

- Lithium is a mood stabilizing agent used in the treatment of bipolar disorder.
- The mechanism of action is unclear but is believed to relate to modification of neurological signalling pathways.
- Lithium is a monovalent cation that is rapidly absorbed and widely distributed to all body compartments; it is not protein bound.
- Lithium is not metabolized but rather is excreted unchanged by the kidney; concurrent use of diuretics or drugs acting upon the renin–angiotensin–aldosterone axis may impact upon clearance.
- Three distinct patterns of lithium poisoning are described:
  - Acute: large exposure to a lithium naive individual
  - Acute on chronic: large acute exposure in an individual who has been loaded with lithium previously
  - Chronic: gradual accumulation of lithium levels over time, usually due to renal dysfunction or drug interactions
- The plasma lithium level associated with toxicity is dependent upon the chronicity of exposure.

3.13.2 Presentation and assessment

- Features of lithium toxicity include:
  - Neurological:
    - Ataxia
    - Dysarthria
    - Dysarthria
    - Tremor
    - Seizures
    - Reduced level of consciousness
  - Gastrointestinal:
    - Nausea and vomiting
    - Diarrhoea
  - Renal:
    - Polyuria
    - Acute kidney injury
    - Nephrogenic diabetes insipidus is a common side-effect, even within therapeutic range

3.13.3 Management

- AC has no role: it does not absorb lithium.
- Whole bowel irrigation may reduce absorption and has a role in the ingestion of sustained-release preparations.

- Haemodialysis effectively clears lithium; it should be instituted in any individual with severe features of lithium toxicity (e.g. seizures, altered conscious state) or in whom intrinsic clearance is impaired (namely renal failure).
- Hyponatraemia impedes renal clearance of lithium and should, therefore, be avoided.

3.14 Propofol infusion syndrome

3.14.1 Pharmacology and toxicity

- Propofol infusion syndrome is a rare but life-threatening complication of propofol use in intensive care.
- It is associated with prolonged (>48 hours) infusion of high dose (4 mg.kg.h^{-1}) propofol.
- The pathophysiology is believed to occur at a mitochondrial level, with inhibition of the respiratory chain and impaired oxygen utilization.
- It appears to be more common in children, although probably occurs in adults also; the relatively non-specific features make it difficult to determine the true incidence.

3.14.2 Presentation and assessment

- Feature include:
    - Metabolic acidosis
    - Rhabdomyolysis
    - Bradyarrhythmias
    - Progressive myocardial dysfunction

3.14.3 Management

- Treatment is largely supportive
- Propofol should be ceased
- Extracorporeal removal of propofol has been proposed as a means of enhancing clearance

3.15 The trans-urethral resection of prostate (TURP) syndrome

3.15.1 Pharmacology and toxicity

- The trans-urethral resection of prostate (TURP) syndrome relates to the intra-operative absorption of hypotonic, glycine-based irrigation fluid through open venous sinuses.
- The irrigation solution is hypo-osmolar (~220 mosmol.kg^{-1}, in comparison to plasma osmolarity of 280–300 mosmol.kg^{-1}); glycine is a neurotransmitter.
- Whilst originally described, and most commonly associated with, the TURP procedure, other operations requiring glycine irrigation (such as endoscopic endometrial resection) also carry the risk.
- Risk factors include:
    - Pressure of irrigation fluid
    - Duration of exposure
    - Extent of resection
    - Smoking

3.15.2 Presentation and assessment

- Up to 8% of patients undergoing TURP will display evidence of mild TURP syndrome; severe TURP syndrome is far less common but has been reported to have a mortality of up to 25%.
- Clinical features include those related to:
    - Volume overload:
        - Increase in total circulating volume leads to hypertension, bradycardia, and chest pain.
        - Pulmonary oedema leads to respiratory symptoms.

- Changes in plasma sodium content and plasma osmolality:
  - Affects neural membrane excitability resulting in a constellation of neurological symptoms; ranges from restlessness through to seizures and coma.
  - Hyponatraemia alone is less problematic than hyponatraemia combined with plasma hypo-osmolality.
- Glycine:
  - Glycine is an inhibitory neurotransmitter that contributes to the neurological sequelae of the TURP syndrome.

3.15.3 Management

- Largely supportive: airway protections, benzodiazepines for seizures, consideration of invasive haemodynamic monitoring
- Diuretics may be used for volume overload
- Sodium correction should follow similar principles to those outlined in Chapter 3, Section 3.1; rapid correction should be avoided; hypertonic saline should be reserved for life-threatening neurological symptoms

FURTHER READING

Decker BS, Goldfarb DS, Dargan PI, et al. Extracorporeal treatment for lithium poisoning: Systematic review and recommendations from the EXTRIP workgroup. *Clinical Journal of the American Society of Nephrology* 2015; 10: 875–87.

Jelic T. Emergency department management of calcium-channel blocker, beta blocker, and digoxin toxicity. *Emergency Medicine Practice* 2014; 162: 1–19

Lavonas EJ. Management of the Critically Poisoned Patient. In: Yealy DM, Callaway C, eds. Emergency Department Critical Care: Oxford University Press, 2013.

Lheureux PE, Zahir S, Gris M, Derrey A-S, Penaloza A. Bench-to-bedside review: hyperinsulinaemia/euglycaemia therapy in the management of overdose of calcium-channel blockers. *Critical Care* 2006; 10(3): 212.

Kam P, Cardone D. Propofol infusion syndrome. *Anaesthesia* 2007; 62: 690–701.

Medicines and Healthcare Product Regulatory Authority (MHRA). Treating paracetamol overdose with intravenous acetylcystine: new guidance. September 2012. https://www.gov.uk/drug-safety-update/treating-paracetamol-overdose-with-intravenous-acetylcysteine-new-guidance

O'Donnell AM, Foo IT. Anaesthesia for transurethral resection of the prostate. *Continuing Education in Anaesthesia, Critical Care & Pain* 2009; 9: 92–6.

Roberts RJ, Barletta JF, Fong JJ, et al. Incidence of propofol-related infusion syndrome in critically ill adults: a prospective, multicenter study. *Critical Care* 2009; 13: R169.

Shah AD, Wood DM, Dargan PI. Understanding lactic acidosis in paracetamol (acetaminophen) poisoning. *British Journal of Clinical Pharmacology* 2011; 71: 20–8.

Shepherd G, Klein-Schwartz W. High-dose insulin therapy for calcium-channel blocker overdose. *Annals of Pharmacotherapy* 2005; 39(5): 923–30.

Timmer RT, Sands JM. Lithium intoxication. *Journal of the American Society of Nephrology* 1999; 10: 666–74.

Ward C, Sair M. Oral poisoning: an update. *Continuing Education in Anaesthesia, Critical Care & Pain* 2010; 10: 6–11.

Obstetrics

CONTENTS

- This chapter highlights principles and concepts around the management of a woman of re-productive age with consideration given to complications of conception, pregnancy, and the peripartum period.
- Care of the critically unwell pregnant woman is often clinically, logistically, and psychosocially challenging, and necessitates high levels of team performance.
- In all cases, women of reproductive age should be assessed for pregnancy; careful consideration of the well-being and goals of care for the mother and unborn child must be achieved through early and proactive engagement of specialized perinatal, obstetric, neonatal, and maternal health services.

1 Normal phases of pregnancy and birth

1.1 Anatomical and physiological changes of pregnancy relevant to intensive care

1.1.1 Airway

- Airway management in a pregnant patient should be considered potentially difficult due to:
  - Oedema and capillary engorgement of upper airway (particularly in the latter stages of labour and in pre-eclampsia)
  - Enlarged breasts may impede manipulation of the laryngoscope
  - Higher risk of uncontrolled epistaxis with nasal route (due to engorged mucosa)
  - Higher point of thoracic kyphosis
  - Higher risk of gastro-oesophageal reflux:
    - Decreased gastro-oesophageal junction tone
    - Stomach compression from gravid uterus
    - Reduced gastric emptying from opiates, pain
    - Normalizes 24–48 hours postpartum

1.1.2 Respiratory

- 60% increase in oxygen consumption and carbon dioxide production (up to 100% during labour).
- Progesterone increases sensitivity to CO_2 of respiratory centre.
- Tidal volume increases by 40%.
- Minute ventilation has increased by 45% by the second trimester.
- Respiratory rate minimally increases (15%).
- Chronic respiratory alkalosis at third trimester:
  - P_aCO_2 <4kPa
- Progesterone-induced bronchodilation:
  - Reduced lower airway resistance
- Reduced respiratory compliance:
  - Thoracic diameter increases with resultant reduced chest wall compliance
  - Elevation of diaphragm in second and third trimester
  - Reduced vital capacity and inspiratory residual volume
  - Reduced FEV1
  - Reduced lung transfer factor
  - 10–15% reduction in Functional Residual Capacity:
    - Reduced residual volume
    - Earlier hypoxia in intubation

1.1.3 Cardiovascular

- Hormone-induced vasodilation and 15% reduction in systemic vascular resistance.
- Increased cardiac output to maximum of 40% at 20–28 weeks (further 20% increase in labour).
- Sufficient arterial pressure for utero-placental perfusion maintained by:
  - Early pregnancy (6–8 weeks): increased stroke volume (35%) via increased end diastolic volume and ventricular mass
  - Later pregnancy, cardiac output increased by relative tachycardia (+15%)
- Normal clinical features may include:
  - Displaced apex beat
  - Gallop rhythm
  - Flow murmur
  - Left axis deviation on ECG
- Aorto-caval compression from gravid uterus leading to impaired venous return and decreased cardiac output when supine:
  - Occurs more in late second and third trimester
  - Asymptomatic:
    - Engorged epidural venous system (epidural catheter risk)
  - Symptomatic—left-sided uterine displacement:
    - Left tilt, right hip wedge, or left lateral decubitus

1.1.4 Haematological and immunological

- Maximum haematological changes around 30 weeks.
- Expanded red cell volume (15% increase).
- Haemoglobin oxygenation saturation curve shift to right.
- 50% increase in plasma volume.
- Dilutional anaemia and lower haematocrit.

- Relative hypercoagulable state to enable uteroplacental separation:
  - 10 times venous thromboembolism (VTE) risk when pregnant
  - 25 times VTE risk peripartum
- Usual leucocytosis of pregnancy (~14,000 per ml):
- Increased platelet production, but normal measures due to higher rates of destruction.
- Higher rates of asymptomatic bacteriuria.
- Relatively immunotolerant due to foetal antigens.

1.1.5 Pharmacological considerations

- Choices of pharmacological approaches in the pregnant woman are influenced by:
  - Altered volume of distribution
  - Potential for teratogenicity
  - Potential for neonatal injury in breast-feeding

1.2 High-risk pregnancy

1.2.1 Risk factors

- Increasing average maternal age, increasing incidence of co-morbidities amongst the obstetric population, and the increase in assisted conception has led to a significant increase in the number of pregnancies considered to be 'high-risk'.
- Factors associated with high-risk pregnancy are outlined in Table 10.1.

Table 10.1 Factors associated with high-risk pregnancy

Age	• Higher maternal age
Medical conditions	• Obesity
	• Chronic hypertension
	• Maternal cardiac disease (valvular, congenital, cardiomyopathy)
	• Diabetes mellitus
	• Immunological disease +/− immunosuppression
Obstetric conditions	• Assisted conception
	• Previous ectopic pregnancy
	• Multiple pregnancy
Psychosocial circumstances	• Domestic violence
	• Drug or alcohol misuse
	• Psychiatric illness

1.2.2 Approach to the high-risk obstetric patient

- High-risk pregnancies should be managed in an appropriate, high volume, centre with the availability of obstetric, anaesthetic, and neonatal expertise, and with access to any necessary support services.
- Adult intensive care may have a role to play in providing critical care at any point in pregnancy or the peripartum period.

FURTHER READING

Tan EK, Tan EL. Alterations in physiology and anatomy during pregnancy. *Best practice & research. Clinical Obstetrics & Gynaecology* 2013; 27(6): 791–802.

2 Approach to the pregnant and peripartum woman in intensive care

2.1 General considerations

2.1.1 Epidemiology

- Critical care admission will be required in up to 13.5 per 1,000 deliveries.
- Admissions are due to a combination of both pregnancy-related pathologies (e.g. haemorrhage or eclampsia) and non-pregnancy-related complications.

2.1.2 Organizational considerations

- Early engagement and liaison with obstetric, midwifery, and neonatal services.
- As a general rule, maternal life and stability takes priority over foetal wellbeing.
- Foetal monitoring may be carried out by continuous cardiotocography (CTG) or intermittent assessment, as guided by obstetrics.
- Evidence for management of the critically ill pregnant woman is limited, as most landmark intensive care medicine trials have excluded pregnant women.

2.1.3 Specific clinical considerations

- Consider ventilation in a semi-recumbent position as much as possible; mechanical ventilation should be adjusted to maintain low P_aCO_2 (P_aCO_2 within normal range will lead to foetal acidosis).
- Difficulties with vascular access may be encountered due to maternal weight-gain.
- All vasopressor agents impact upon umbilical blood flow; noradrenaline is an acceptable agent for continuous infusion and is not associated with adverse foetal outcomes; phenylephrine is the vasopressor of choice for standard perioperative care (e.g. Caesarean section) as it is associated with better cord pH.

2.1.4 Diagnostic considerations

- Minimize radiological interventions with high-dose radiation exposure (e.g. CT, radionucleotide imaging).
- Seek advice regarding dose reduction of unavoidable imaging and timing of imaging in relation to gestational age/organogenesis.
- Utilize maternal abdominal radiation shielding.
- Maximize use of ultrasound imaging.
- Ensure risks and benefits are clearly explained to mother and next of kin.

2.2 Foetal assessment

- Mechanisms of foetal assessment include:

2.2.1 Clinical

- Foetal size and position.
- Foetal heart rate (intermittent auscultation with Pinard stethoscope or electronic aid).

2.2.2 Non-invasive investigation

- CTG (intermittent or continuous).
- 2D and Doppler ultrasound for assessment of foetus and placenta.

2.2.3 Invasive investigation

- Amniotic fluid assessment.
- Foetal scalp blood sampling (intra-partum).

2.3 Labour and birth on the intensive care unit

2.3.1 Tocolysis

- Tocolysis provides a means of suppressing pre-term labour and delaying birth.
- Indications:
  - Pre-term labour (24–34 weeks):
    - To facilitate transfer to definitive specialist centre
    - To allow time for maternal steroid administration (to assist foetal lung maturation)
- Contra-indications:
  - Antepartum haemorrhage
  - Sepsis (in particular chorioamnionitis)
  - Advanced cervical dilatation
  - Non-reassuring CTG
  - Placental insufficiency
  - Pre-eclampsia
  - Maternal contra-indication to tocolytic agents
- Available agents:
  - Nifedipine
  - Salbutamol
  - Atosiban (oxytocin receptor antagonist)

2.3.2 Labour in the intensive care unit

- Vaginal delivery in the intensive care department is challenging and potentially difficult.
- If, in the rare event this occurs, it should be undertaken with adequate obstetric and midwifery support in parallel to the critical care teams.

2.3.3 Breast-feeding

- Breast-feeding should be attempted and offered to all live-born survivors of critically ill mothers, to be in line with the WHO recommendations.
- Breast-feeding may be contra-indicated due to the maternal condition or therapy.
- Breast pumps may have a role.
- Management of unwanted lactation can be controlled with oestrogen preparations.
- Mastitis may complicate the management of a critically ill parturient.

FURTHER READING

Cornthwaite K, Edwards S, Siassakos D. Reducing risk in maternity by optimising teamwork and leadership: an evidence-based approach to save mothers and babies. *Best Practice & Research Clinical Obstetrics & Gynaecology* 2013; 27(4): 571–81.

Francis S, Yentis S. Antenatal anaesthetic assessment of the pregnant woman. *Anaesthesia & Intensive Care Medicine* 2004; 5(7): 218–21.

---

3 Peripartum collapse and maternal death

3.1 Maternal cardiac arrest

3.1.1 General

- Occurs in around 1 in 30,000 pregnancies.
- Increasing incidence with increasing age and presence of co-morbidities.

- Frequently a reversible aetiology:
  - Haemorrhage
  - Amniotic fluid embolus
  - Thromboembolism
  - Local anaesthetic toxicity
  - Hypermagnesaemia
  - Cardiomyopathy related

3.1.2 Peripartum resuscitation

- Advanced life-support algorithms.
- Early intubation.
- Manual displacement of the uterus to the left (insertion of wedge is no longer advocated by the UK Resuscitation Council).
- Preparation for peri-mortem Caesarean section.

3.1.3 Peri-mortem Caesarean section

- Should be commenced at 4 minutes into the cardiac arrest.
- All pregnancies over 20 weeks.
- May save the baby; primary rationale is however to save maternal life: relieves aorto-caval compression thereby enhancing venous return.

FURTHER READING

Maternal collapse in pregnancy and the puerperium (Green top guideline number 56). Royal College of Obstetricians and Gynaecologists, London 2011 http://www.rcog.org.uk/files/rcog-corp/GTG56.pdf

UK Resuscitation Council. Cardiac arrest in special circumstances. In: *Advanced Life Support*, 6th edn. UK, 2012.

3.2 Maternal death—statistics

3.2.1 Reducing risk through audits and confidential enquiries

- Mothers and Babies: Reducing Risk through Audits and Confidential Enquiries in the UK (MBR-RACE) (previously called the UK Confidential Enquiry into Maternal Deaths) is a national report examining deaths in pregnancy or the first 6 weeks postpartum.
- The report was published in 2014 and covers the years 2009–12.
- The maternal mortality rate in the UK for this period was 10 per 100,000 women giving birth.

3.2.2 Causes of death

- Causes of death are divided into:
  - Direct—those deaths directly related to the pregnancy, delivery, or a pathological process precipitated by pregnancy.
  - Indirect—deaths not directly related to the pregnancy.
- The most common causes of death in the UK maternal population over this period are outlined in Table 10.2.

Table 10.2 Direct and indirect causes of maternal death in the UK 2009–12

Direct		Indirect	
Thrombosis and thromboembolism	10.7%	Cardiac disease	22.2%
Genital tract sepsis	4.9%	Indirect neurological causes	12.9%
Haemorrhage	4.5%	Psychiatric causes	6.6%
Pre-eclampsia and eclampsia	3.7%	Indirect malignancies	1.2%
Amniotic fluid embolism	3.3%	Other indirect causes	25.1%
Anaesthesia	1.7%		

Data from the *Confidential Enquiry into Maternal Death*, 2014, Knight M et al, 'Saving Lives, Improving Mothers' Care Lessons learned to inform future maternity care from the UK and Ireland Confidential Enquiries into Maternal Deaths and Morbidity 2009-2012'.

3.2.3 Risk factors for maternal death

- Social disadvantage
- Minority ethnic groups
- Late booking or poor attendance
- Delayed pregnancy
- Obesity
- Domestic violence
- Substance abuse
- Suboptimal clinical care
- Lack of inter-professional and/or inter-agency communications

3.3 Management of perinatal death

3.3.1 Maternal death

- Principles and jurisdictional procedures around end-of-life care and brain-death diagnosis should be followed in cases involving pregnant women.
- Maternal brain-death may raise ethical and clinical questions around:
  - Period of support of the brain-dead mother for foetal viability and delivery
  - Clinical and legal decision-making around the medico-legal status of mother and unborn child
  - Posthumous-assisted reproduction
- Methods of withdrawal of cardio-respiratory supports in a palliative care setting need to be carefully considered with the family.

3.3.2 Neonatal death

- Surviving members of the neonate's family, in the immediate, early, and later phases, should be consider and offered supports, including:
  - Opportunity to view or care for deceased child
  - Bereavement supports (maternal and paternal focus)
  - Access to clinical or professional photography, handprints, or keepsakes
  - Counselling and support for future pregnancies
  - Neonatal and paediatric death support services
  - Social work support
  - Pastoral care and religious supports

- General practitioner engagement
- Remembrance and anniversary activities and support

3.3.3 Organ and tissue donation

- Family-sensitive clinical care and communication regarding the logistics of organ and tissue donation and foetal delivery need to be prioritized.
- Precedent exists for neonatal organ and tissue donation.
- These issues must be sensitively explored with a highly informed and engaged clinical and donation team.

FURTHER READING

Knight M, Kenyon S, Brocklehurst P, Neilson J, Shakespeare J, Kurinczuk J. Saving lives, improving mothers' care lessons learned to inform future maternity care from the UK and Ireland Confidential Enquiries into Maternal Deaths and Morbidity 2009–12, 2014. Available at https://www.npeu.ox.ac.uk/downloads/files/mbrrace-uk/reports/Saving%20Lives%20Improving%20Mothers%20Care%20report%202014%20Full.pdf (accessed December 2015)

4 Pregnancy-induced hypertension and related disorders

4.1 Pregnancy-induced hypertension

4.1.1 Definition and severity

- Occurs in up to 17% of pregnant women.
- New onset hypertension, occurring after 20 weeks pregnancy, in the absence of significant proteinuria.
- 'Significant' proteinuria defined as:
  - Urinary urea: creatinine ratio >30 mg.mmol^{-1}
  - 300 mg protein in a 24-hour urine collection
- Severity of hypertension:
  - Mild (140/90–149/99 mmHg)
  - Moderate (150/100–159/109 mmHg)
  - Severe (≥160/110 mmHg)

4.1.2 Management

- Patients diagnosed with PIH should undergo more frequent follow-up.
- Blood pressure of >160/110 mmHg should be treated:
  - First line: oral labetalol
  - Other agents: methyldopa, nifedipine

4.1.3 Significance

- Up to 50% of patients diagnosed with PIH will progress to pre-eclampsia (i.e. will develop significant proteinuria or evidence of end-organ failure).
- Extremes of blood pressure, even in the absence of proteinuria, carry the risk of stroke.

4.2 Pre-eclampsia and eclampsia

4.2.1 Definition and severity

- A pregnancy-specific syndrome that occurs in up to 10% of pregnancies

- New hypertension after 20 weeks gestation with significant proteinuria.
- Severe pre-eclampsia:
    - BP >160/110 mmHg
    - +/− symptoms
    - +/− haematological or biochemical complications
    - +/− previous eclamptic fit

4.2.2 Risk factors

- Risk factors for pre-eclampsia include:
    - First pregnancy
    - Advanced maternal age
    - Family history
    - Past history of pre-eclampsia
    - Factors which increase placental mass:
        - Obesity
        - Diabetes mellitus
        - Multiparity

4.2.3 Pathophysiology

- Absolute or relative placental ischaemia leads to diffuse systemic endothelial activation.
- Possibly secondary to incomplete invasion of the foetal trophoblast into the spiral arteries; this leads to an immune maladaptation.
- As a consequence numerous pathological changes occur:
    - Increased sensitivity to vasoconstrictor agents
    - Decreased production of vasodilators (e.g. nitric oxide)
    - Platelet activation
    - Activation of the clotting cascade
    - Increased capillary permeability
- This manifests as:
    - Vasoconstriction
    - Fluid extravasation
    - Proteinuria
    - Oedema (peripheral, pulmonary, cerebral)
    - Decreased intravascular volume
    - Decreased organ perfusion

4.2.4 Clinical and biochemical features of severe pre-eclampsia

- Symptoms:
    - General malaise
    - Headache, altered cognition
    - Visual impairment, central scotoma
    - Dyspnoea, chest pain
    - Abdominal pain (especially right upper quadrant)
    - Peripheral oedema
    - Oliguria
    - Bruising
- Clinical findings:
    - Hypertension (>160/110 mmHg)

- Tissue oedema
- Renal impairment:
    - Proteinuria (>2 g/24 hours)
    - Oliguria (<500 ml/24 hours)
    - Creatinine (>2x normal)
- Hepatic impairment:
    - Raised bilirubin
    - Transaminitis
- Neurological impairment:
    - Hyperreflexia
    - Clonus
    - Seizures
    - Central scotoma
- Haematological impairment:
    - Thrombocytopaenia
    - Haemolysis

4.2.5 Eclampsia

- Convulsive disorder associated with pre-eclampsia.
- Seizures can occur up to 2 weeks after delivery.

4.2.6 HELLP syndrome

- Haemolysis, elevated liver enzymes, and low platelets as evidenced by:
    - Microangiopathic haemolysis
    - Hepatic dysfunction
    - Thrombocytopaenia (without DIC)
- A life-threatening extension of the spectrum of pre-eclampsia/eclampsia (1% maternal mortality).
- Occurrence rate: pre-eclampsia (10%) and eclampsia (30–50%).
- May occur in the last trimester or peripartum period.
- Laboratory findings:
    - Full blood count:
        - Anaemia; thrombocytopaenia (<100 x $10.ml^{-6}$); reticulocytosis
    - Peripheral blood film:
        - Microangiopathic haemolytic anaemia (MAHA)
        - Schistocytes/fragments
        - Helmet cells
    - Haemolysis testing:
        - Direct antigen test (DAT) negative
        - Elevated serum LDH (>600 $units.l^{-1}$)
        - Reduced haptoglobin
        - Elevated plasma-free haemoglobin
    - Liver function
        - Elevated bilirubin (raised unconjugated fraction)
        - Aspartate aminotransferase (AST) >70 $units.l^{-1}$.
- Differential diagnosis
    - Acute fatty liver of pregnancy (AFLP):
        - Usually more severe signs of hepatic and renal failure

- Thrombotic thrombocytopaenic purpura (TTP)—haemolytic uraemic syndrome (HUS) spectrum:
  - Fever and more pre-dominant neurological symptoms
  - Associated infective prodrome in HUS
  - Often more severe thrombocytopaenia (<20 x 10^9/l)
  - May persist >48 hours after delivery
- Systemic lupus erythematosus (SLE):
  - Check anti-double stranded-DNA levels (high) and complement levels (low)
- Potential sequelae
  - Pre-eclampsia and eclampsia may result in:
    - Intracranial haemorrhage
    - Liver rupture
    - Placental abruption
    - Disseminated intravascular coagulation
    - Heart failure

4.3 Treatment of severe pre-eclampsia or eclampsia

4.3.1 Principles of management

- Early delivery
- Control blood pressure
- Prevent seizures

4.3.2 Early delivery

- Administration of steroids for foetal lung maturity, if pre-term delivery expected.

4.3.3 Anti-hypertensives

- The aim is to prevent intracranial haemorrhage, heart failure, or placental abruption, whilst maintaining uterine perfusion.
- Patients tend to be inappropriately vasoconstricted and intravascularly deplete: concurrent volume replacement may be necessary; caution necessary as tissue oedema is a major problem.
- The mainstays of treatment are:
  - Hydralazine
    - Long history of use
    - Oral or intravenous
    - Causes reflex tachycardia
  - Labetalol
    - Non-selective beta blocker with some alpha antagonism
    - Oral or intravenous
  - Nifedipine
    - Oral only
    - Causes uterine relaxation
- Other options include:
  - Sodium nitroprusside (risk of foetal cyanide toxicity with prolonged use)
  - Glyceryl trinitrate
  - Methyldopa

4.3.4 Seizure prevention and treatment

- Magnesium sulphate:

- Indicated in cases of severe pre-eclampsia to prevent the development of seizures.
- The Magpie trial demonstrated a lower incidence of seizures and a trend towards lower maternal mortality when administered to patients with pre-eclampsia.
- Initial load: 4 g intravenous magnesium sulphate over 5 minutes.
- Continuing infusion: 1 g magnesium sulphate per hour for 24 hours.
- Monitoring:
  - Clinical:
    - Signs of respiratory depression
    - Reflexes—absence suggests toxicity
    - Measure serum magnesium if signs of overdose
  - Biochemical:
    - Aim Mg^{2+} levels between 2.5 and 3.5 mmol.l^{-1}
- Benzodiazepines and anti-epileptic drugs are best avoided but may be necessary in the case of recurrent seizures or when magnesium is contraindicated.

4.3.5 Coagulation disorder

- Significant bleeding unlikely at platelet count $>100 \times 10^{-6}$.
- Avoid platelet therapy, if possible.
- Manage life-threatening coagulopathy with coagulation factors (FFP, cryoprecipitate).
- Thrombocytopaenia may be improved by corticosteroids (10 mg iv dexamethasone b.d.).
- Consider plasma exchange for refractory haemolysis and thrombocytopaenia.
- Clinical, haematological, and biochemical monitoring until maternal recovery.

FURTHER READING

Clarke SD, Nelson-Piercy C. Pre-eclampsia and HELLP syndrome. *Anaesthesia & Intensive Care Medicine* 2005; 6(3): 96–100.

Cottam S, Sizer E. Laboratory tests in hepatic and renal failure. *Anaesthesia & Intensive Care Medicine* 2006; 7(2): 46–8.

The Magpie Trial Collaborative Group. Do women with pre-eclampsia, and their babies, benefit from magnesium sulphate? The Magpie Trial: a randomised placebo-controlled trial. *Lancet* 2002; 359(9321): 1877–90.

National Collaborating Centre for Women's and Children's Health. Hypertension in pregnancy: the management of hypertensive disorders during pregnancy, National Collaborating Centre for Women's and Children's Health (UK) London: RCOG Press; 2010 Aug. 2010.

National Institute for Health and Care Excellence. *Hypertension in pregnancy overview*, 2015. Accessed 9 July 2015. Available from: http://pathways.nice.org.uk/pathways/hypertension-in-pregnancy – path=view%3A/pathways/hypertension-in-pregnancy/hypertension-in-pregnancy-overview.xml&content=view-index

---

5 Obstetric haemorrhage

5.1 Ectopic pregnancy

5.1.1 General

- The gravid uterus is a highly vascular organ that receives around 15% of cardiac output at term; haemorrhage can be massive.

- Implantation of pregnancy outwith the uterus; the majority lie in the Fallopian tube.
- Occurs in up to 20 in 1,000 pregnancies.
- Risk factors for ectopic pregnancy:
  - Previous ectopic pregnancy
  - Previous disease or surgery to Fallopian tubes:
    - Pelvic inflammatory disease.
  - Smoker
  - Intra-uterine contraceptive device

5.1.2 Presentation

- Typically presents with:
  - Abdominal, pelvic, or shoulder tip pain
  - Vaginal bleeding
- Positive pregnancy test.
- Ultrasound confirmation of ectopic implantation.

5.1.3 Management

- The majority of cases of ectopic pregnancy requiring intensive care input will be haemo-dynamically unstable and warrant surgical control.
- Methotrexate offers a conservative, tube sparing, management option in haemodynamically stable patients.

5.2 Antepartum haemorrhage

5.2.1 Placental abruption

- Separation of the placenta from the uterus leading to significant bleeding and compromising foetal blood supply.
- Features:
  - Severe abdominal pain
  - 'Woody' quality to the uterus on palpation
  - Vaginal bleeding
  - Foetal compromise/death
- Management:
  - Resuscitation and delivery

5.2.2 Placenta praevia

- Insertion of the placenta into the lower uterine segment; potential for massive haemorrhage, particularly during delivery.
- Severity graded by position:
  - I.   Placenta is in lower segment, but the lower edge does not reach the internal orifice of the cervix uteri (internal os)
  - II. Lower edge of placenta reaches internal os, but does not cover it
  - III. Placenta covers internal os partially
  - IV. Placenta covers internal os completely
- Features:
  - Typically presents with painless vaginal bleeding after 20 weeks gestation
- Management:
  - Resuscitation

- Ultrasound evaluation of placental position
- Careful delivery

5.3 Postpartum haemorrhage

5.3.1 General

- Postpartum haemorrhage (PPH) is estimated to affect between 1 and 5% of deliveries.
- PPH is divided into:
  - Primary: occurring within the first 24 hours following delivery
  - Secondary: occurring between 24 hours and 6 weeks
- PPH is quantified by the Royal College of Obstetricians and Gynaecologists as:
  - Minor (500–1,000 ml)
  - Major:
    - Major (moderate) (1,000–2,000 ml)
    - Major (severe) (>2,000 ml)

5.3.2 Aetiology

- PPH is the consequence of:
  - Tone (and tissue)
    - Uterine atony is the most common cause of PPH
    - Associated with retained products of conception, prolonged labour, multiparity, macrosomia
  - Trauma
    - Tears to uterus, cervix, or vagina
    - More common following instrumental delivery
  - Thrombus (or more precisely, inability to form thrombus)
    - Coagulopathy or thrombocytopaenia
    - Associated with pre-eclampsia, or inadequate resuscitation from earlier haemorrhage

5.3.3 Management

- Urgent team-based maternal and foetal resuscitation:
  - Large-calibre vascular access
  - Haemodynamic monitoring
  - Prepare for massive transfusion
- Haemorrhage control:
  - Urgent delivery of retained products in operating theatre
  - Fundal massage
  - Bimanual uterine compression and examination under anaesthesia
- Uterotonic therapy:
  - Fundal massage
  - Oxytocics:
    - Intravenous oxytocin (5 U iv bolus or 10–20 U/l rapid infusion)
    - Intra-uterine/intramuscular prostaglandin F2 alpha
- Extended therapies:
  - External aortic compression (above umbilicus)
  - Uterine arterial angio-embolization
  - Internal iliac arterial ligation
  - Hysterectomy

6 Amniotic fluid embolus

6.1 General
6.1.1 Epidemiology

- Rare: 1 in 100,000 labours.
- Catastrophic: mortality rate >90% in some series; many survivors are left with neurological injury.

6.1.2 Pathophysiology

- Significant volume of amniotic fluid enters the maternal circulation via open veins in the cervix or placental bed.
- Profound inflammatory response:
  - Pulmonary vasospasm leads to acute cor pulmonale and cardiovascular collapse (within first 15–30 minutes)
  - Ventilation/perfusion (V–Q)mismatch and non-cardiogenic pulmonary oedema causes profound hypoxia
  - Left ventricular failure may be a delayed feature
  - Disseminated intravascular coagulation is a common sequelae of the systemic inflammatory response

6.1.3 Risk factors

- Precipitous labour
- Advanced maternal age
- Instrumental delivery
- Placenta praevia
- Placental abruption
- Grand multiparity (>5)
- Foetal distress
- Eclampsia
- Medical induction

6.2 Clinical approach
6.2.1 Clinical features

- May present as peripartum cardiac arrest
- Conscious patients may complain of chest pain, dyspnoea
- Cardiogenic shock with right ventricular strain on echocardiography
- Hypoxia
- DIC

6.2.2 Management

- There is no specific treatment; management is supportive.
- Cardiovascular:
  - Advanced life-support protocols
  - Invasive monitoring
  - Pharmacological support
  - Early consideration of ECMO

- Respiratory:
    - Mechanical ventilation with high PEEP
- Haematological:
    - Management of DIC

FURTHER READING

Scrutton M. Obstetric emergencies. *Anaesthesia & Intensive Care Medicine* 2005; 6(3): 100–5.

---

7 Incidental critical illness in pregnancy

7.1 Sepsis

7.1.1 General

- The diagnosis of sepsis may be problematic in pregnancy due to the difficulty differentiating normal physiological changes (e.g. tachycardia, tachypnoea, leucocytosis) from signs of sepsis.
- The Royal College of Obstetricians and Gynaecologists identify the following as risk factors for life-threatening sepsis in pregnancy:
    - Obesity
    - Impaired glucose tolerance/diabetes
    - Impaired immunity/immunosuppressant medication
    - Anaemia
    - Vaginal discharge
    - History of pelvic infection
    - History of group B streptococcal infection
    - Amniocentesis and other invasive procedures
    - Cervical cerclage
    - Prolonged spontaneous rupture of membranes
    - Group A Streptococcal infection in close contacts/family members

7.1.2 Sources of sepsis

- Antepartum:
    - Pyelonephritis
    - Chorioamnionitis
    - Septic abortion
    - Necrotizing fasciitis
    - Septic thrombophlebitis
- Postpartum:
    - Caesarean wound infections
    - Episiotomy infections
    - Mastitis
    - Deep vein thrombosis
    - Pneumonia
- *Escherichia coli* and *Group A Streptococcus* are the organisms most commonly associated with death in the maternal population.
- Mixed Gram-positive and Gram-negative organisms are, however, common, particularly in chorioamnionitis.

7.1.3 Management

- The use of an early warning scoring system, adapted to account for normal changes in maternal physiology, is recommended.
- Sepsis should be managed in the standard fashion, including suitable microbiological samples, early antibiotics, appropriate haemodynamic resuscitation, and, where necessary, source control.
- Empirical antibiotics should be broad-spectrum and provide both Gram-positive and Gram-negative cover; consideration should be given to an agent that suppresses exotoxin production (e.g. clindamycin).

7.1.4 Antibiotics in pregnancy

- As with all drugs in pregnancy, antibiotics should only be administered if maternal benefit outweighs the risk to the foetus. Clinicians should refer to a current formulary prior to prescribing in pregnancy.
- Safety data are often limited, particularly with newer antibiotics, and therefore manufacturers are usually reluctant to provide complete reassurance regarding use of antibiotics in pregnancy.
- Beta lactams are generally considered safe and usually first line in pregnant patients. The manufacturer of anti-pseudomonas penicillin piperacillin advises avoidance unless benefits are judged to outweigh risks; the manufacturer of meropenem provides similar advice on the basis of lack of data; imipenem with cilastatin has been shown in animal models to be teratogenic.
- Tetracyclines may impact upon skeletal development in the first trimester and cause discoloration of teeth; also associated with maternal hepatotoxicity in higher doses. Tetracyclines should, therefore, be avoided in pregnancy.
- Aminoglycosides carry a theoretical risk of ototoxicity and nephrotoxicity in the foetus if used in the second or third trimester; whilst the risk with aminoglycosides in common use (e.g. gentamicin) is very low, these should be avoided unless no suitable alternative.
- Macrolides are not known to be harmful in pregnancy; the manufacturers of the more modern macrolides (clarithromycin and azithromycin) recommend avoiding unless the benefits outweigh the risks.
- Clindamycin is not known to be harmful in the second or third trimesters.
- Trimethoprim is a folate antagonist and is, therefore, teratogenic in the first trimester; it is associated with methaemoglobinaemia and haemolysis in the third trimester. The use of trimethoprim (and combination drugs containing trimethoprim e.g. **co-trimoxazole**) must, therefore, be avoided in pregnancy.
- Quinolones have been shown to cause arthropathy in animal studies and should be avoided in pregnancy.
- The manufacturer of metronidazole recommends avoidance of high dose regimens.

FURTHER READING

Joint Formulary Committee. *British National Formulary*. 70th ed. London: BMJ Group and Pharmaceutical Press; 2015.

7.2 Cardiac complications

- Cardiac disease is the most common cause of maternal death in the UK.
- Pregnancy and labour places significant demand on the cardiovascular system leading to decompensation of existing cardiac disease.
- Pregnancy is associated with *de novo* cardiac failure: peripartum cardiomyopathy.

7.2.1 Non-pregnancy-related cardiac disease

- In the UK, pregnant patients with existing cardiac disease are becoming more common:
  - Increasing maternal age
  - Increasing number of patients with congenital cardiac anomalies surviving to adulthood
  - Rheumatic disease in patients originating in other countries
- Conditions encountered which may impact upon pregnancy and delivery include:
  - Ischaemic heart disease and myocardial infarction
    - In those patients with risk factors: increasing age, smoker, diabetes, obesity, family history
  - Aortic dissection:
    - Most common in the context of Marfan's syndrome; may occur in non-Marfan patients with systemic hypertension
  - Valvular disease:
    - May be secondary to rheumatic disease
    - Mitral stenosis can cause pulmonary oedema during labour due to increased cardiac output through a fixed valve
    - Aortic stenosis may produce profound hypotension with loss of afterload (e.g. spinal anaesthesia)
  - Pulmonary hypertension:
    - Carries a particularly high risk of death
    - Careful management in an appropriate tertiary centre

7.2.2 Peripartum cardiomyopathy

- A dilated cardiomyopathy occurring in the peripartum period, not attributable to another pathological process.
- Rare, but associated with a significant risk of death; survivors are frequently left with severe heart failure necessitating transplant.
- Believed to be an immunologically driven process; viruses may play a role.

7.2.3 Management of cardiac disease in pregnancy

- In general, the management of cardiac disease in pregnancy is similar to management in non-pregnant patients.
- Specific considerations:
  - Multi-disciplinary management in an appropriate tertiary centre
  - Careful planning by obstetrics, anaesthetics, and cardiology with a view to mitigating the cardiovascular stresses of pregnancy and labour
  - Optimization of underlying cardiac disease
  - Avoidance of ACE inhibitors, angiotensin II receptor blockers, thrombolysis

FURTHER READING

Burt CC, Durbridge J. Management of cardiac disease in pregnancy. *Continuing Education in Anaesthesia, Critical Care & Pain* 2009; 9(2): 44–47.

Calderwood C, Nelson-Piercy C. Medical disorders complicating pregnancy. *Anaesthesia & Intensive Care Medicine* 2004; 5(8): 256–63.

Elkayam U. Clinical characteristics of peripartum cardiomyopathy in the United States: diagnosis, prognosis, and management. *Journal of the American College of Cardiology* 2011; 58(7): 659–70.

Royal College of Obstetricians and Gynaecologists. Sepsis in Pregnancy, Bacterial (Green-top Guideline No. 64a). Royal College of Obstetricians and Gynaecologists, London, 2012. https://www.rcog.org.uk/en/guidelines-research-services/guidelines/gtg64a/ (Accessed December 2015).

Royal College of Obstetricians and Gynaecologists. Sepsis following Pregnancy, Bacterial (Green-top Guideline No. 64b). Royal College of Obstetricians and Gynaecologists, London, 2012. https://www.rcog.org.uk/en/guidelines-research-services/guidelines/gtg64b/ (Accessed December 2015).

8 Trauma in pregnancy

8.1 Primary survey

8.1.1 Airway
- Consider early intubation and plan for a difficult airway.

8.1.2 Breathing
- Risk of early and profound hypoxaemia:
    - Consider early nasogastric intubation for gastric decompression
    - Consider higher insertion point for thoracocentesis
    - Difficult intracranial pressure management with impaired ventilation after traumatic brain injury

8.1.3 Circulation
- Under-recognized extent of haemorrhage due to physiological changes.
- Small changes in tachycardia and hypotension may represent significant haemorrhage.
- Uteroplacental circulation:
    - Maintained by early and aggressive volume expansion
    - Target high-normal venous pressures
    - Early transfusion to maintain foetal oxygen delivery
- Aortocaval compression: difficult to manage in potential spinal and pelvic injuries.
- Consider amniotic fluid embolism.

8.1.4 Foeto-maternal haemorrhage
- Can occur in 30% of trauma cases.
- Rhesus-negative mothers need anti-D immunoglobulin, as risk of sensitization for future pregnancies.

8.1.5 Trauma imaging
- Prioritize diagnosis of maternal injury over foetal radiation dose.
- Focused assessment with sonography in trauma (FAST) offers a radiation-free alternative to X-ray or CT but may be difficult to interpret in the pregnant abdomen.
- If X-ray or CT is used, utilize shielding and reduced dose imaging protocols.

8.2 Secondary survey considerations

8.2.1 Chest and abdomen
- May have atypical injury patterns due to gravid uterus

8.2.2 Pelvic injuries

- Difficulty with pelvic binder: early surgical stabilization.
- Risk of:
    - Foetal injury
    - Placental abruption
    - Uterine injury

CHAPTER 11

Dying, death, organ, and tissue donation

CONTENTS

The ability of intensive care medicine to support failing organs, even when death is inevitable, creates a number of unique challenges and opportunities. Concepts such as brain death, organ donation, and withdrawal of life-sustaining treatment exist almost exclusively within the intensive care unit. An understanding of the ethical, legal, and practical issues surrounding end-of-life care is key to intensive care practice.

1 Recognition of dying

1.1 Process of dying

- Death is a process, not an event.
- Each individual will undergo elements of death that can be considered in these categories:
  - Biological death
  - Medical death
  - Legal death
  - Religious or spiritual death or transition
  - Social death
- Each society and person will place various weights on each of these elements, with some components being non-negotiable.
- It is incumbent upon the clinician to understand and cater for each element for each individual in their care within their context.

1.2 Features of the dying process

It is often difficult to recognize the commencement of the dying process however, these may provide indicators to consider the diagnosis of 'dying':

- Recurrent admissions to hospital within the preceding month
- Involvement of palliative care services
- Dependence on hospital-based care
- Dependence on community-based nursing-home care
- Failure to recover from illness, despite maximal available medical therapy

- Physically frail appearance
- Cachexia
- Reduced mobility
- Reduced self-care
- Reduced oral intake
- Mottled skin
- Cool peripheries
- Cheyne–Stokes periodic breathing
- Reduced mentation or cognition
- Patient or family statements of 'having had enough'

FURTHER READING

Sleeman KE, Collis E. Caring for a dying patient in hospital. *British Medical Journal* 2013; 346: 2174.

---

2 Care of the dying

2.1 Palliative care

2.1.1 Principles

- The care of the dying is based on the principles of relieving symptoms without accelerating or impeding the natural processes; this approach is codified by the World Health Organization and national organizations.
- Palliation, or relief of symptoms, applies to all clinical scenarios, with the level of intensity of palliation ranging from nil to full-scale.
- Palliation can be applied in parallel to therapeutic or curative clinical processes but may, eventually, become the sole focus of clinical care.
- When care with curative intent ceases, palliative care continues.

2.1.2 Managing transition

- The transition from curative and palliative care to palliative care alone is a process, not an event, and requires careful communication, planning, and implementation.
- It is important to ensure that discrepancies between requested and actual palliative care practices are minimized.
- End-of-life care (EOLC) is a subset of the palliative care skill-set, which an intensivist must develop.

2.2 Principles of palliation

2.2.1 Alleviate suffering

- Physical
- Psychological
- Social
- Spiritual or existential
- Cease ongoing therapies that are not contributing comfort

2.2.2 Cease unnecessary interventions

- Change to a minimally invasive management model:
  - Remove invasive lines not required for comfort care

- Intravenous or subcutaneous fluids
- Oxygen delivery systems
- Antibiotics
- Blood tests
- Blood product infusions
- Feeding sources
- Blood tests
- Physiological monitoring
- Provision of a subcutaneous catheter for medication routes
- Engagement of palliative care services.

2.2.3 Common symptoms

- Pain
- Dyspnoea
- Nausea
- Cognitive disturbance:
  - Primary disease
  - Medication side-effects
- Dry mouth
- Terminal secretions

2.3 Methods of palliation

2.3.1 Physical relief

- Heat or cold packs
- Body positioning
- Massage
- Mouth care
- Eye care

2.3.2 Pharmacological

- Intermittent dosing for interval symptoms
- Infusional (intravenous or subcutaneous)
  - Based on previous dosages and breakthrough doses

2.3.3 Social

- Request for all important persons to visit
- Easing of ICU visitation restrictions
- Pet visitation
- Facilitate attendance of remote family and friends
- Empowerment of family in nursing of patient

2.3.4 Spiritual

- Appropriate rituals and clerical process arranged in timely fashion.

2.4 Relationship with palliative care

2.4.1 Similarities and shared dialogue

- There are many similarities with palliative care medicine and intensive care medicine in managing this important process.

- A shared dialogue on individual cases and a working relationship between departments in an institution help to facilitate best-practice palliation and EOLC.

2.4.2 Advantages of engagement with palliative care

- Provision of expertise in managing difficult palliation problems
- Assistance in managing family and friends of dying patient
- Provision of resources not normally available to an intensive care
- Provision of a palliative care bed for palliative patients prior to their EOLC period
- Ongoing monitoring of best-practice of palliative care provided in the intensive care department
- Provision of alternative supports for dying patients on the ward who are not deemed appropriate for intensive care management

2.4.3 Intensive care unit palliative care practice

- Decisions about how to deliver palliative care and EOLC in intensive care depend upon these factors:
  - Expected longevity of patient survival
  - Ability to provide an intensive care resource for palliation
  - Level of invasiveness of therapy deemed acceptable by healthcare team and family
  - Environment for palliation able to be provided that is deemed acceptable
  - Risk of transfer to another care environment for palliation
  - Staff, patient, and family relationships

FURTHER READING

Jones D, Moran J, Winters B, Welch J. The rapid response system and end-of-life care. *Current Opinion in Critical Care* 2013; 19(6): 616–23.

Psirides AJ, Sturland S. Withdrawal of active treatment in intensive care: what is stopped-comparison between belief and practice. *Critical Care and Resuscitation* 2009; 11(3): 210–4.

---

3 Withdrawal of cardio-respiratory support

Withdrawal of cardio-respiratory support can be achieved in many ways to allow a person a natural death. Clinical scenarios vary, and ethical and lawful practice must guide clinical practice.

3.1 Principles

3.1.1 Consensus

- Consensus that this is to occur on medical grounds.
- Agreement to proceed with the family.
- Aim not to provide prolonged invasive futile therapy whilst reasonably waiting for other family members to arrive.

3.1.2 Communication

- Explanation to family of expected changes within dying person.
- Empowerment of the family to assist in EOLC:
  - Family to advocate for appropriate symptom relief

- Ongoing nursing care provided by the family, as appropriate
- Engagement of appropriate religious and spiritual figures

3.2 Practicalities

3.2.1 Setting

- Palliative procedures are in place prior to withdrawal of cardio-respiratory support.
- Bed space is prepared to allow family maximal private and dignified access to the dying person.

3.2.2 Cessation of interventions

- Cessation of non-essential medicines and investigation
- Cessation of non-essential monitoring
- Removal of:
  - Mechanical ventilation:
    - Immediate cessation or one-way weaning
  - Artificial airways:
    - Endotracheal tubes
    - Tracheostomy
  - Feeding tubes
  - Central vascular lines
- Cessation of oxygen delivery
- Cessation of vasopressor and inotropic supports:
  - Immediate cessation or one-way weaning

3.2.3 Palliative care measures

- Transition to palliative care regimen
- Initiation of symptom relief
- Continuation of medicines or procedures that relieve distress:
  - Urinary catheter
  - Opiates
  - Anxiolytics
- Maintenance of clear communication between family and healthcare staff

---

FURTHER READING

Walton L, Bell D. The ethics of hastening death during terminal weaning. *Current Opinion in Critical Care* 2013; 19(6): 636–41.

---

4 Death

4.1 Diagnosis of death

- With advances in medical technology, the modern diagnosis of death has evolved.
- A standardized method of diagnosing death is required in each jurisdiction and must be followed.
- Death of an individual can be described when there is:
  - Loss of capacity for consciousness
  - Loss of capacity for ventilation

- As such three modes of the diagnosis of death exist in the current medical paradigm:
  - Somatic death
  - Circulatory death
  - Neurological death

4.1.1 Somatic death

- Historical diagnosis of death based on visual signs:
  - Associated with decomposition, rigor mortis, or decapitation

4.1.2 Circulatory death

- Death of the individual as diagnosed by healthcare staff
- Recognized as irrevocable death of the individual
- Defined as occurring after 2–5 minutes of cessation of circulation
- Requires demonstration of:
  - Cessation of circulation
  - Absence of ventilation
  - Absence of brain function and brain stem reflexes
  - Absence of movement

4.2 Neurological (brain) death

4.2.1 Definition

- There is no internationally uniform diagnostic process for brain death.
- Diagnosis of brain death must be made according to local guidelines and legislation; in the UK a consensus statement of the Royal Colleges from 1976 has been accepted as the standard definition (Box 11.1); no statute exists.

4.2.2 Process

All brain death must have the features of:
  - Pre-conditions for diagnosis of brain death
  - A period of pre-test observation
  - Appropriate physiological support for testing
  - Clinical examination:
    - Irreversible coma
    - Absence of brain-stem reflexes
    - Apnoea
  - Examination process:
    - Requires more than one experienced clinician
  - Radiological confirmation:
    - Gold standards:
      - Four-vessel cerebral angiography
      - Radionuclide testing
    - Currently not accepted:
      - CT cerebral angiography
      - MRI cerebral angiography
      - Electro-encephalogram
  - Failure of diagnosis of brain death:
    - Need for repeated testing to diagnose brain death

– Away from the context of potential organ donation

– In the context of potential organ donation

☐ Evidence of catastrophic neurological injury to enable withdrawal of cardio-respiratory supports

Box 11.1 Brainstem death in the UK

- Preconditions
  - ☐ Cause of coma must be established—structural and irreversible
  - ☐ Reversible causes must be absent, i.e.
    - – Hypothermia
    - – Drugs (sedatives, neuromuscular blocking agents)
    - – Circulatory failure (MAP<60 mmHg)
    - – Metabolic (urea, sodium, glucose, magnesium, ammonia)
  - ☐ Must be able to test cranial nerve reflexes (one ear, one eye)
- Personnel
  - ☐ Two doctors
    - – Both of at least 5 years standing
    - – At least one consultant
    - – Both competent at the procedure
    - – Neither from the transplant team
    - – Both must undertake the tests—there is no minimum time interval between tests
- **Absence of cranial nerves**
  - ☐ Fixed dilated pupils
  - ☐ Absent corneal reflex
  - ☐ No facial motor response to painful stimuli in both central (supraorbital) and peripheral (limb) areas
  - ☐ Absent oculo-vestibular reflex (ear canal checked for obstruction, then 50 ml ice-water, injected into ear over 1 minute, whilst observing for eye movement)
  - ☐ Absent gag reflex (to posterior pharyngeal stimulation)
  - ☐ Absent cough reflex (to tracheal stimulation)
- If cranial nerve reflexes absent, proceed to apnoea test:
  - ☐ Pre-oxygenate for >5 minutes
  - ☐ Reduce minute volume to achieve P_aCO2 >6.0 kPa and pH <7.4
  - ☐ Baseline blood gas
  - ☐ Disconnect from ventilator for 5 minutes (oxygenate with either catheter in endotracheal tube or via Waters' circuit)
  - ☐ After 5 minutes, confirm P_aCO_2 increased by >0.5 kPa.
  - ☐ If no breathing observed, loss of respiratory drive is confirmed

Death is *confirmed* after the *second* test; *time of death* is however recorded as *first* test.

4.2.3 Family support

- Managing the family's non-acceptance of the diagnosis:
  - ■ Explanation of the process and explore misunderstandings
  - ■ Invitation for family members to observe the process of brain-death testing
  - ■ Arrange additional confirmatory testing to demonstrate the diagnosis
  - ■ Agreement to withdraw cardio-respiratory supports on brain-dead patient as there has been a catastrophic neurological injury
  - ■ Engagement of medico-legal supports, if possible (rare)

FURTHER READING

Eelco F, Widjicks M. Brain death testing: accepted fact but no global consensus in diagnostic criteria. *Neurology* 2002; 58: 20–5.

Gardiner D, Shemie S, Manara A, Opdam H. International perspective on the diagnosis of death. *British Journal of Anaesthesia* 2012; 108(Suppl 1): i14–28.

Simpson P. A Code of Practice for the Diagnosis and Confirmation of Death. London, Academy of Royal Medical Colleges, 2008.

4.3 Aftercare of the deceased

4.3.1 Management of the person and family

- The provision of aftercare for a family is an extension of the pre-mortem family management.
- Items that may be considered as routine matters for discussion for a family who are recently bereaved are:
  - Offering of condolence
  - Provision of accurate and complete post-mortem documentation
    - Limits family distress and administrative errors
  - Offer of post-mortem examination
  - Assistance with coronial processes
  - Explanation of death certification process
  - Management of the body after death
  - Viewing of the body
  - Religious rituals to be completed
  - Organization of funeral services
  - Discussion of any post-mortem donation processes (tissue or eye donation)
  - Referral to bereavement services
  - Ongoing social work support for financial, administrative and practical matters

4.3.2 Management of the healthcare staff

- Care of the healthcare staff is part of the intensivist's role
- In some circumstances, it may be necessary to offer staff the following:
  - Debriefing opportunities
  - Feedback on practice
  - Opportunities for quality improvement process
  - Referral for psychological support and follow-up

5 Organ donation

- Organ and tissue donation practice associated with intensive care medicine continues to evolve due to expansion of indications for transplantation, organ preservation techniques, and quality and safety management processes.
- Donation is based on the concept of altruism and is achieved through a request for donation in the appropriate clinical setting with adequate, balanced information to enable an enduring decision that fits the patient and family.
- The proactive and early engagement of donation services is increasingly seen and can be a part of ethical intensive care practice; family management is a key factor in the donation process, which can sometimes extend EOLC processes for over 48 hours.

- If consensus regarding death or withdrawal of cardio-respiratory support has not been achieved, donation should not be raised.

There are two deceased donor organ donation pathways: donation after brain death (DBD) and donation after circulatory death (DCD).

5.1 Donor organs

5.1.1 Potential donor organs

- Heart
- Lungs
- Liver
- Kidneys
- Pancreas
- Intestine
- Multi-visceral
- Limbs

5.1.2 Ischaemia time

- The time from cessation of circulation to cold-perfusion of organs is the 'warm ischaemia time' (WIT).
- The time from cold-perfusion to implantation with perfusion is the 'cold-ischaemia time' (CIT).
- All attempts are made to minimize each of these periods to improve transplanted graft function.
- Future strategies may include *ex vivo* organ resuscitation and evaluation to minimize these effects.

5.2 Considerations in organ donation

5.2.1 Factors associated with assessment for donation

- Each person who is considered for donation (potential donor) is evaluated against strict criteria, with subset criteria for each organ and tissue.
- An organ donated may be considered to fit the standard criteria for donation or an extended criteria donation (ECD).
- ECD donation has a potential added risk to the recipient, should the recipient consent to implantation.
- These issues are managed by the organ and tissue donation service; the intensivist's role is to assist the donation service as much as practicable in preparing for donation, after the appropriate level of assent/consent for this process to commence from the family or senior next-of-kin.

5.2.2 Considerations relating to the potential donor and suitability of organs

- Age
- Current illness and diagnostic uncertainties
- Current physiological state
- Current organ function evaluation
- Non-communicable disease profile:
  - Previous and active malignancy
  - Hypertension
  - Diabetes mellitus
  - Hypercholesterolaemia
  - Smoking
  - Alcohol

- Vascular disease risk factors
- Oncological risk
- Communicable disease:
  - Current uncontrolled sepsis
  - Recent remote travel
  - High-risk behaviours
  - Hepatitis B and C viruses, Human Immunodeficiency Virus
  - Tuberculosis, syphilis
  - *Herpes Simplex Virus, Cytomegalovirus, Epstein Barr Virus, Varicella Zoster Virus*
  - *Human Herpes Virus 6 and 8, Human T Lymphotropic Viruses 1 & 2*
  - *JC virus, BK virus*
  - Toxoplasma
  - Creutzfeld–Jakob disease
- Immunological matching:
  - Blood group
  - Pre-existent antibodies
  - Major Histocompatibility Complex matching
- Some evaluations of a potential donor require further imaging or testing (bronchoscopy, echo-cardiography, CT imaging), which require specific consent from the family, with appropriate follow-up of abnormal results.
- Previous absolute contra-indications, such as HIV infection or previous malignancy, may be relative contra-indications with evolution of medical care and donation programmes.

5.2.3 Considerations relating to the potential recipient

- Position on transplant waiting-list
- Immunological matching
- Acceptance of offer based on organ-allocation protocols
- Acceptance of risk of standard versus extended criteria organ
- Logistics of receipt of organ

5.2.4 Systematic and logistics issues

- Time for assessment and offering of potential organs and tissues
- Cessation of donation process based on:
  - Medical unsuitability
  - Failure of potential donor physiological support
  - Logistic reasons
  - Withdrawal of family consent
- Coronial cases:
  - Requires prior consent from coroner to undertake donation
- Time-frames for donation:
  - Ability of organ procurement operation to be performed
  - Consideration of transfer of potential donor to another hospital to facilitate donation within a pre-ordained protocol
- Management of deterioration of potential donor in pre-donation phase

5.2.5 Family considerations

- Inclusion of EOLC rituals before, during, and after donation

- Some families raise the possibility of organ and tissue donation prior to consensus to palliate:
  - Defer donation discussions to an appropriate time after active treatment course has been completed.
- Family-centred management of donation processes:
  - Explanation of time-frames involved in donation process.
  - EOLC is not targeted at meeting time-frames of donation after circulatory death.
- Deterioration of a brain-dead donor:
  - Possible change to a donation after circulatory death process with family consent, if logistically feasible.
  - Physiological support may fail and preclude donation.
- Consent for pre-mortem interventions:
  - Consent for pre-circulatory arrest interventions to clarify donation risk.
  - Bolus of heparin in DCD for organ preservation at time of terminal apnoea.

5.2.6 Physiological support of the potential multi-organ and tissue donor

- Donation considerations may commence around the time of commencement of EOLC.
- End-of-life practices continue with usual bedside practice and incorporate the parallel donation processes of donation informed consent, medical suitability assessment, donation operations, and aftercare.
- The engagement of the organ and tissue donation services throughout this process assists staff and families to manage the complex emotional, clinical, and logistic issues of a donation process over the subsequent hours to days.
- The physiological support of a potential organ and tissue donor requires consent from the family.
- Physiological support is achieved to enable timely assessment of medical suitability and support to facilitate potential donation outcomes.

5.3 Donation after brain death (DBD)

- A brain-dead individual has a complex physiological state that needs consideration and management.
- Brain death causes complex cardiovascular, neurohumoral, inflammatory, and coagulation responses, which need to be managed if donation after brain death is to occur.

5.3.1 General

- Whilst preparation for donation is ongoing, the following aspects of care should be continued:
  - Aseptic techniques
  - Nutrition
  - Endotracheal suctioning
  - Physiotherapy
  - Antibiotics

5.3.2 Cardiovascular

- Brain-stem death is associated with a massive catecholamine surge, typically resulting in profound hypertension and arrhythmia.
- The catecholamine surge is followed by loss of vasomotor tone and hypotension.
- Vasopressin is the preferred vasoconstrictor, as it does not deplete myocardial ATP supplies to the same extent as catecholamine-based vasopressors.
- Concurrent administration of hydrocortisone may reduce vasopressor requirements.
- Excess fluid resuscitation should be avoided in an attempt to avoid organ oedema—fluid resuscitation guided by cardiac output monitoring is included in the UK donor optimization bundle.

5.3.3 Respiratory

- Pulmonary oedema frequently occurs around the time of brain-stem death.
- Atelectasis and pneumonia may occur in the absence of coughing.
- Lung protective strategies should be employed; hyperoxia (which promotes free radical formation) should be avoided.
- Regular recruitment manoeuvres are recommended.

5.3.4 Endocrine

- Pituitary failure frequently accompanies brain-stem death.
- Consequences include:
  - Diabetes insipidus (with associated hypovolaemia and hypernatraemia):
    - Fluid replacement and administration of DDAVP
  - Hypothyroidism (which may impact upon cardiovascular function):
    - Liothyronine (T3) replacement
  - Depressed adrenal axis (with blunted stress response):
    - The routine administration of methylprednisolone is recommended in some national guidelines; it reduces vasopressor requirements and extravascular lung water, and may attenuate the inflammatory response.
  - Hyperglycaemia:
    - Target plasma glucose of 4–10 mmol.l^{-1} with insulin infusion
  - Deranged temperature control.

5.3.5 Renal

- Cardiovascular and endocrine changes may lead to profound fluid shifts.
- Care should be taken to optimize fluid status, avoiding, where possible, tissue oedema.

5.4 Donation after circulatory death (DCD)

- DCD was the original method of donation for transplantation.
- The practice of DCD has undertaken a recent resurgence as an alternative to the DBD donation pathway.

5.4.1 General

- DCD may occur in controlled or uncontrolled circumstances; these are outlined in the Maastricht Criteria (Table 11.1).
- The majority of DCD candidates have a severe neurological injury, are not expected to survive (or to make a recovery which they would accept), but have not met criteria for brain death.

Table 11.1 Maastricht classification of donation death after cardiac death

Category	Type	Circumstances	Typical location
1	Uncontrolled	Dead on arrival	Emergency Department
2	Uncontrolled	Unsuccessful resuscitation	Emergency Department
3	Controlled	Cardiac arrest follows planned withdrawal of life-sustaining treatments	Intensive Care Unit
4	Either	Cardiac arrest in a patient who is brain dead	Intensive Care Unit

5.4.2 Features of donation after circulatory death

- Consensus that:
    - Ongoing cardio-pulmonary support is not in the best interests of the patient
    - That cardio-pulmonary support should be withdrawn
    - That circulatory death will occur a short time after withdrawal of cardio-pulmonary support
- Support of potential donor physiology is continued whilst arrangements made:
    - Continuation of previous supports
    - Commencement of palliative care therapy
- Assessment for medical suitability
- Preparation for donation operation
    - Authorization by a designated officer
    - Mutually convenient time planned between ICU, theatre, and family
- Donation team pre-meeting prior to withdrawal of cardio-respiratory support
- Withdrawal of cardio-respiratory support
- Cessation of circulation (monitored)
- Period of observation (5 minutes)
- Diagnosis of circulatory death
- Transfer to operating room:
    - Conduct of donation operation
    - Re-intubation, if lung donation
- Aftercare of body and family

5.4.3 Family considerations

- The family should be aware that a DCD approach will allow them only limited time with their deceased relative; time will, however, be allowed post-retrieval.
- A prolonged death may preclude donation.

FURTHER READING

NHS Blood and Transplant. *Organ Donation: Resources for Professionals*. http://www.odt.nhs.uk/donation/deceased-donation/professional-resources/ (Accessed December 2015)

5.5 Tissue and eye donation

5.5.1 Potential tissues for donation

- Include:
    - Bone
    - Tendon
    - Meniscus
    - Skin
    - Heart valve
    - Pancreatic islets
    - Vascular tissue
    - Whole eye or cornea

5.5.2 Medical suitability

- Assessment of suitability for tissue donation occurs in a similar manner to organ donation.

- Donated tissue is different to organ donation in that it can be procured with, or separate to, organ procurement.
- A pre- or post-mortem medical suitability assessment can occur in patients not considered for organ donation.

5.5.3 Tissue procurement procedure

- Donated tissue can be procured up to 24 hours after cessation of circulation.
- Tissue donation may occur within the treating hospital or require transfer of the body to another specialized facility.
- Donated tissue often undergoes a period of further biomedical processing over weeks to months before being made available for human use, in some cases as medical products.
- This requires a higher level of process scrutiny and regulation.

6 Caring for organ donors and their family

6.1 Methods of managing the parallel processes of EOLC, and organ and tissue donation

6.1.1 Parallel care

- During donation processes, the principles of usual EOLC practice should be followed.
- If donation cannot occur, EOLC practice should continue unabated.
- In the setting of donation after circulatory death, the family may request activity that will accelerate death to enable donation within the appropriate warm ischaemic time; the family should be redirected to the treating intensive care team to discuss EOLC principles.

6.1.2 Division of care

- A method of managing the potential conflict of interest is to divide the care of a potential donor into the following roles:
  - End-of-life care:
    - Managed solely by treating intensive care team
    - Any issues raised about palliation are directed to this team
  - Organ and tissue donation:
    - Managed solely by the organ and tissue donation specialists—includes:
      - Consent for ante-/post-mortem assessment procedures
      - Delivery of pre-mortem interventions
      - Stewardship of donation process
      - Questions about donation process (ICU, operating theatre, after donation)
- This requires more communication and coordination, yet assists in clear clinical decision-making.
- In resource-limited circumstances where this role-separation is not possible, it may be of benefit to describe to the family the reasons around each decision and clinical process to minimize staff and family concern about the potential shared roles that may occur.

6.2 Separation of futility/EOLC discussions from donation discussions

- End-of-life conversations, and organ and tissue donation conversations need to be managed to prevent or minimize conflicts of interest.
- Ideally, the family, treating teams, and intensive care teams should reach consensus on the diagnosis of brain death or agreement to commence EOLC prior to discussion of organ and tissue donation.

- This also includes the rare circumstance of an ICU-based competent patient involved in their own decision-making (e.g. high cervical spinal injury without head injury).
- Once the consensus on withdrawal of cardio-respiratory support or brain death is achieved, it is appropriate to commence further discussion of EOLC, including organ and tissue donation.
- The donation conversation that follows may occur in the same conversation or in subsequent conversations around EOLC management.

6.3 Ideal donation conversations

An ideal organ and tissue donation conversations may the following features:

- Clear designation of the requestor's role in the donation process.
- Acknowledgement of the difficult circumstances.
- Provision of balanced information given about the risks and benefits for organ and tissue donation to enable an informed choice.
- Exploration of patient's previous discussions about organ and tissue donation.
- Review of the donor registry information with the next-of-kin.
- Information about the logistic processes and timelines during donation.
- A request for organ and tissue donation.
- Exploration of any concerns or misunderstandings.
- Permission to undertake testing or procedures that relate to donation that are normally in excess of EOLC practice.
- Acknowledgement that donation may not proceed, even if assented to, due to multiple medical, consent, and logistic reasons.
- Reassurance that standard EOLC practice continues in parallel.
- Expression of gratitude for consideration of this issue, regardless of donation consent outcome.

6.3.1 Modes of donation conversations

- Different approaches to the donation conversation exist and depend on clinician preference and local practice.
- It also depends on each party's concerns around minimizing conflicts of interest and emotional fatigue around ongoing EOLC and donation.
- Particularly, it may be useful to engage the organ and tissue donation services prior to this meeting for guidance and support in this potentially challenging conversation.
- It is preferable for the bedside intensive care nurse to be present as a patient advocate.
- Each conversational mode requires the consideration of the role of the treating intensivists and/or donation specialists in the conversation.
- In the UK, Specialist Nurses in Organ Donation (SN-OD) are frequently involved in, and may lead, the donation conversation.
- Options include:
  - Treating team request:
    - Treating team or intensive care representative makes the request for organ or tissue donation.
  - Designated request:
    - A clinician separate to the treating team/intensive care team (designated requestor) makes the request for organ or tissue donation at a family meeting without the treating or intensive care team.
    - This requestor may be a non-treating member of the hospital team or a local or external donation specialist.

- Meeting is commenced by the introduction of this independent practitioner by the treating team intensivist.
- Collaborative request
  - A clinician separate to the treating team/intensive care team (collaborative requestor) makes the request at a family meeting in continuing presence of the treating or intensive care team.
  - This requestor may be a non-treating member of the hospital team or a local or external donation specialist.
  - Meeting is commenced by the introduction of this independent practitioner by the treating team.
  - The requestor focuses solely on organ and tissue donation issues.
  - The treating team or intensivist focuses solely on the ongoing palliative care and EOLC issues.
- The utilization of the local organ donor registry information may be useful for inclusion in the donation request.
- Families are known to uphold their next-of-kin's wishes, if known.
- If a registration of donation intent has been made in the jurisdiction, this may facilitate improved discussion around donation.

6.3.2 Engagement of donation services

- Donation services vary in their capacity to be in attendance at the bedside.
- Awareness of local donation referral practice and availability of donation staff is helpful in planning donation conversations and processes.
- Donation services may be able to provide the following:
  - Information regarding current jurisdictional donation practice.
  - Comprehensive assessment for medical suitability of a potential donor.
  - Clinical management of a potential multiorgan and tissue donor:
    - Advice
    - Practical bedside assistance
  - Coordination of complex logistics of donation process.
  - Advocacy for potential donor during transition from intensive care to operating room and then to mortuary.
  - Support resource for grieving family of potential donor during and after donation process.

CHAPTER 12

Organizational issues

CONTENTS

1 Unit design, staffing, and levels of care

1.1 History of intensive care

1.1.1 Beginnings

- Intensive care medicine (ICM) is one of the newest medical specialties.
- The concept of a geographical and administrative separate area dedicated to the care of the sickest patients in the hospital has a number of historical precursors.
- During the Crimean War, Florence Nightingale is credited with reorganizing the sicker patients closest to the nursing station to facilitate more frequent observation and response to deterioration.
- In the poliomyelitis epidemic of the 1950s in Denmark, patients requiring ventilator support were placed in the same ward with dedicated staff (often medical students) used to supervise these patients, and to provide emergency assistance, and to raise the alarm for senior help, if required; this led to significant improvements in survival.

1.1.2 Evolution

- During the 1970s and 1980s, specialization became more formalized with separate medical and nursing training and professional development, as well as the dedicated units that are now ubiquitous in most hospitals in the developed world.

1.1.3 Present day

- ICM is now recognized as a specialty in its own right in Europe, North America, and Australasia; this has been reinforced by the creation of the College of Intensive Care Medicine of Australia and New Zealand, and the Faculty of Intensive Care Medicine in the UK.
- The organization of training and the physical space where patients are cared for has undergone a process of formalization designed to optimize training and care delivery.
- A number of 'minimum standards' relating to training, staffing, unit design, and service delivery are available—many of these are discussed throughout this chapter.

1.2 Levels of care

1.2.1 Intensive Care Society definition

- The UK Intensive Care Society's 'Levels of Critical Care for Adult Patients' (2002) (Table 12.1) provides a means of classifying critical care provision throughout the hospital.

Table 12.1 Levels of care for adult patients

Level 0	Patients whose needs can be met through normal ward care in an acute hospital.
Level 1	Patients at risk of their condition deteriorating, or those recently relocated from higher levels of care, whose needs can be met on an acute ward with additional advice and support from the critical care team.
Level 2	Patients requiring more detailed observation or intervention, including support for a single failing organ system or post-operative care, and those 'stepping down' from higher level of care.
Level 3	Patients requiring advanced respiratory support alone or support of at least two organ systems. This level includes all complex patients requiring support for multi-organ failure.

- Some larger units, when denoting the usage of critical care unit beds, will append letters depending on the subtype of area or patient, e.g. 'C' cardiac, 'N' neurological, 'T' trauma.
- Other, pre-designated areas of the hospital are sometimes used in times of high demand to deliver Level 3 surge capacity for a limited period of time (typically <24 hours in areas such as operating theatres or the emergency department resuscitation room).

1.2.2 Australian and New Zealand classification system

- The UK Intensive Care Society system should not be confused with the Level 1, 2, and 3 critical care unit descriptions used by the Australasian College of Intensive Care Medicine, which relate to the capabilities of intensive care units as a whole.
- The 'Minimum Standards for Intensive Care Units' (2011) describes these levels as:
  - A Level I ICU should be capable of providing immediate resuscitation and short-term cardio-respiratory support for critically ill patients.
  - A Level II ICU should be capable of providing a high standard of general intensive care, including complex multi-system life support, which supports the hospital's delineated responsibilities; where appropriate specialty support (e.g. neurosurgery and cardiothoracic surgery) is not available within the hospital, there should be an arrangement with a designated tertiary hospital so that patients referred can be accepted for specialty management (including ICU management).
  - A Level III ICU is a tertiary referral unit for intensive care patients and should be capable of providing comprehensive critical care, including complex multi-system life-support for an indefinite period.

1.3 Open and closed units

- ICUs can be described as 'open' or 'closed'.
- Open units:
  - Any doctor may admit to the ICU.
  - The 'home', 'admitting' team responsible for the patient, leads care with consultative input from the intensive care team for technical aspects.
  - This model is prevalent in North America.

- Closed units:
  - The intensive care specialist controls admission to the ICU.
  - Responsibility for the care of the patient transfers to the ICM consultant on entry to the unit.
  - Whilst consultation with admitting teams is ongoing, day-to-day decisions are made by the ICM team.
  - This is the most common model in Europe and Australasia.
- There is some evidence that the closed-unit model reduces mortality and length of ICU stay; this is difficult to interpret due to the many other confounding factors between the units compared in these studies.

1.4 Unit design

- New ICUs in the UK should be built in accordance with the Department of Health's 'Health Building Note 04–02' (2013); in Australasia, the standards are dictated by the College of Intensive Care Medicine's 'Minimum Standards for Intensive Care Units' (latest revision 2011).

1.4.1 Unit size

- Unit sizes vary but the number of beds usually lies between 5% and 10% of the total number of hospital beds, with a recommended minimum of six.
- Large units are often split into specialty-specific zones (e.g. medical/surgical).
- Large units benefit from being split into geographic cohorts or 'pods' of 8–15 patients.
- Capacity can be calculated using the Hill–Burton formula and allow planning for staffing and unit design:

$$\text{Calculated ICU capacity} = \frac{\text{number of admissions per year} * \text{average length of ICU stay (days)}}{365 * \text{ideal occupancy rate (expressed as fraction)}}$$

1.4.2 Bed space

- Each bed space should have a minimum area of 20 m^2 (25 m^2 for side rooms); this allows access to the bed from all sides and for multiple staff to attend at times of emergency.
- Adequate heating and ventilation.
- Compromise between staff visualization of the patient and privacy.
- At least one washbasin per two beds; one basin per bed is preferred.
- Bed:
  - Electric
  - Capable of Trendelenburg and chair positions
  - Equipped with a pressure-relieving mattress
- Chair:
  - Footrest and tilting facility
- Dual pendants for essential supply lines consisting of:
  - Electricity:
    - At least 28 single-socket outlets (unswitched)
    - At least some sockets must be uninterruptable power supply (UPS)
  - Gas supply:
    - Three to four oxygen outlets
    - Two 4-bar air outlets

- Consideration of 7-bar air outlet, if pneumatic surgical equipment is likely to be used
- Two to four medical vacuum outlets
- Anaesthetic gas scavenging, if use anticipated
  - Communication:
    - Up to four data outlets, networked to hospital record system
    - Patient and staff call system, including emergency call
    - Telephone outlet
    - TV outlet
- Equipment:
  - Computer
  - Patient monitoring equipment
  - Three to six infusion pumps
  - Four to ten syringe pumps
  - Blood warmer
  - Feeding pump
  - Ventilation and humidification equipment
- Storage space

1.4.3 Side rooms

- Side rooms increase patient privacy and reduce the risk of cross-infection; they also significantly increase the number of (nursing) staff required for safe and effective care.
- The precise number of side rooms required is dependent upon predicted case mix; units with high numbers of immunocompromised or infective patients will need a higher proportion.
- Minimum recommended for any unit is that 20% of beds should be side rooms.
- A lobby for gowning is desirable.
- Side rooms should be capable of simultaneous protective and source isolation.

1.4.4 Location within the hospital

- Priority areas that may impact on where an ICU is placed within a hospital include:
  - Operating theatres
  - Emergency department
  - Radiology
  - Other investigative or interventional areas (e.g. endoscopy and cardiac catheter laboratories)
  - Main clinical laboratory
  - Blood transfusion

1.5 Unit staffing

- Critical care staffing represents the bulk of costs attributable to ongoing ICU care.
- Approximately 60% of costs are related to staff, of which the nursing component is the largest component.
- Staffing levels will, to some extent, be dictated by the average severity of illness in the unit.

1.5.1 Nursing staff

- Levels of care are reflected in the nurse to patient (N:P) ratio.
  - In the UK, the N:P ratio at any given time is generally accepted as:
    - 1:4 for Level 1
    - 1:2.5 for Level 2

- 1:1 for Level 3 patients
- May be higher, for example, in patients undergoing extracorporeal membrane oxygenation (ECMO) where two nurses per patient may be needed.
- Extrapolating this from an individual shift, to round the clock nursing cover:
  - For a six-bed ICU with a 8-hour nursing shift pattern, then a total of 49 whole time equivalent nurses are required to staff the unit safely, accounting for leave/sickness and maintaining safe rest period during the shift.
- In addition to bedside nursing allocation:
  - A lead nurse not involved in patient care should act in a supernumerary capacity to assist and provide leadership.
  - Where more than ten beds are occupied, a second supernumerary nurse should be on shift to prevent loss of this role during breaks or times of surge (e.g. beginning and end of shift and new admissions).
  - In general, more than 50% of the nursing staff should have postgraduate qualifications in critical care nursing.
  - No more than 20% of the nursing staff should be from agency nurse banks.

1.5.2 Medical staff

- The ICM consultant body for a particular unit are expected to:
  - Lead the care of the patients in the intensive care unit.
  - Provide continuity through an appropriate rota system (5-day blocks of cover are recommended as a compromise between continuity of care and staff burnout).
  - Provide on-call cover 24 hours a day and be available to attend within 30 minutes; consultants should not have any other commitments whilst on call for ICU.
  - Lead two ward rounds per day (at least one of which should involve input from microbiology, nursing, physiotherapy, and pharmacy colleagues).
  - Organize units such that the consultant to patient cover is between 1:8 and 1:15.
  - Make sure a doctor with appropriate airway skills is available to attend at all times.
  - Work under the leadership of a clinical lead for ICU.
- Doctors in training within the ICU should work within an appropriate educational structure.
- Trainee doctor to patient ratio should not exceed 1:8.

1.5.3 Allied professionals

- Physiotherapists:
  - Role in respiratory therapy and rehabilitation
  - Recommended one whole time equivalent physiotherapist per four Level 3 ICU beds
  - Must be involved in at least one consultant-led ward round per day
  - An identifiable lead physiotherapist for critical care is desirable
- Pharmacist:
  - Role in optimizing pharmacotherapy and in medicine management
  - Each ICU must have at least one critical care pharmacist
  - Based upon availability Monday to Friday, 0.1 whole time equivalent pharmacist per Level 3 critical care bed (or per two Level 2 beds)
  - Must be involved on at least one consultant-led ward round per day
- Dietician:
  - Central to the management of complex nutritional needs on the ICU
  - A dietician should be part of the ICU multi-disciplinary team

- Occupational therapist:
  - A critical care lead for occupational therapy is desirable
  - Key role in the rehabilitation process
- Speech and language therapist:
  - Occupational therapist
  - Technician
  - Physician assistant (in some countries)

Allied medical professionals not related to the admitting teams who most interact with the intensive care team include microbiologists and radiologists. For both, regular meetings with senior physicians in these specialities are often organized within the weekly and even daily work of the ICM ward round.

FURTHER READING

College of Intensive Care Medicine. *Minimum Standards for Intensive Care Units*, 2011. http://www.cicm.org.au/Resources/Professional-Documents

Department of Health. *Critical Care Units: Planning and Design* (HBN 04–02), 2013. https://www.gov.uk/government/publications/guidance-for-the-planning-and-design-of-critical-care-units (Accessed December 2015)

Galley J and O'Riordan B. Guidance for nurse staffing in critical care. Royal College of Nursing. London. 2003. Available at: www.rcn.org.uk/__data/assets/pdf_file/0008/78560/001976.pdf (Accessed December 2015)

Intensive Care Society. *Guidelines for Provision of Intensive Care Services*, 2015. http://www.ics.ac.uk/ics-homepage/guidelines-and-standards/ (Accessed December 2015)

Valentin A, Ferdinande P. Improvement EWGoQ. Recommendations on basic requirements for intensive care units: structural and organizational aspects. *Intensive Care Medicine* 2011; 37(10): 1575–87.

---

2 Critical care outwith the ICU

2.1 Roles

2.1.1 Roles outwith the ICU

- Identification of deteriorating ward-based patients and early intervention.
- Identification of patients requiring formal admission to areas of high acuity.
- Follow-up of recently discharged patients to prevent early readmission.
- Support of ward staff where immediate care may be beyond their normal skill base.
- Rehabilitation of patients post-ICU.
- Institution of palliative care measures, where appropriate, on deteriorating patients.

2.1.2 Deteriorating patient systems

- This section will focus on deteriorating patient systems, which may be referred to by a number of terms including:
  - Critical care outreach team (CCOT)
  - Medical emergency team (MET)
  - Rapid response team (RRT)
  - Patient emergency response team (PERT)

2.2 Underlying principles

2.2.1 Principles

- Deteriorating patient systems have evolved out of the following principles:
  - Ward-based patients are at risk of physiological deterioration and preventable death.
  - Early identification of deterioration and early appropriate intervention to reverse that deterioration is likely to reduce the risk of unplanned ICU admission and death.
  - Certain groups of patients are at high risk of deterioration:
    - Recent step-down from critical care to wards
    - Recent major surgery
    - Certain diagnoses (e.g. severe sepsis)
  - Critical care staff are best placed to lead in the detection and management of deteriorating ward patients.
- As a consequence, the concept of 'ICU without walls' arose: the belief that critical care should not be delivered exclusively within the confines of the ICU.

2.2.2 Limbs of the deteriorating patient system

- A number of different outreach and deteriorating patient systems have evolved.
- These are often described in terms of limbs of a feedback system:
  - Afferent limb: the component of the system that identifies patient deterioration
  - Efferent limb: the component of the system that responds to patient deterioration
  - Administrative limb
  - Governance limb

2.3 Afferent limb

2.3.1 Track and trigger

- 'Tracks' patient physiology for evidence of deterioration and 'triggers' a response (track and trigger system, TTS).
- Based upon deviation of commonly recorded observations from a predetermined normal range.
- Broadly divided into single, multiple and aggregated systems.

2.3.2 Single parameter track and trigger systems:

- One severely aberrant variable triggers a response.
- Low sensitivity but reasonable specificity in identifying which patients will die during this admission.
- Commonly employed in Australia and New Zealand.

2.3.3 Multiple-parameter track-and-trigger systems:

- Lower 'abnormal' threshold but multiple abnormal parameters required to trigger.
- Lower thresholds should increase sensitivity, whilst need for multiple parameters maintains specificity.
- For example, the patient at risk team (PART) score.

2.3.4 Aggregated parameter track and trigger systems:

- Degree of physiological derangement is weighted and reflected in the score.
- For example, in the modified early warning score (MEWS) a heart rate of 40–49 beats per minute is awarded one point; a heart rate <29 beats per minute is awarded three points.
- Examples include the National Early Warning Score (NEWS); demonstrated to be good predictor of unexpected ICU admission.

2.3.5 Standardisation and non-physiological parameters

- There is a move in the UK to standardize the afferent limb to NEWS.
- In addition to objective, physiological parameters, many afferent limbs include the facility to activate on subjective, staff (or even family) concern; clinical intuition has been demonstrated to be an important contributor to patient assessment.

2.4 Efferent limb

- Efferent limbs vary; they may be broadly divided into:
  - Ramp-down systems
  - Ramp-up systems

2.4.1 Ramp-down systems

- Ramp-down systems deploy maximal response in the first instance.
- In the MET system, common in Australia and New Zealand, a critical care team typically consisting of a senior nurse and a doctor, capable of advanced intervention (e.g. rapid sequence induction), attend all calls; this is usually in addition to the patient's primary doctor and nurse.
- Following initial assessment, those staff not required for immediate patient care stand down.

2.4.2 Ramp-up systems

- Ramp-up systems typically deploy a sole member of medical or nursing staff; additional support is mobilized, as required.
- If a ramp-up system is utilized in combination with an aggregate track and trigger system, the magnitude of the initial response can be tailored to the score: patients activated with low scores are initially managed by sole, relatively junior staff; patients with high scores activate a full critical care team.
- This approach is common in the UK.

2.5 Underpinning evidence

- Uptake of deteriorating systems has been widespread; evidence demonstrating improved outcome is, however, lacking.

2.5.1 The MERIT study

- A multi-centre cluster randomized controlled trial conducted in Australia.
- Hospitals were randomized to implement a MET system or to continue with their current system.
- Findings:
  - Reduction in cardiac arrest and hospital mortality in both arms.
  - A difference in outcome emerged when 'as-treated' analysis rather than 'intention to treat' analysis was conducted.
  - These findings are believed to represent contamination of the control arm: widespread awareness of the MET concept during the trial caused those in control hospitals to utilize existing traditional systems (e.g. cardiac arrest teams) as MET.

2.5.2 The Priestly study

- A UK-based study, which randomized individual wards to critical care outreach or standard practice, demonstrated a significant reduction in hospital mortality within the intervention arm.

FURTHER READING

Hillman K, Chen J, Cretikos M, et al. Introduction of the medical emergency team (MET) system: a cluster-randomised controlled trial. *Lancet* 2005; 365(9477): 2091–7.

Jones DA, DeVita MA, Bellomo R. Rapid-response teams. *New England Journal of Medicine* 2011; 365(2): 139–46.

Kelly FE, Fong K, Hirsch N, Nolan JP. Intensive care medicine is 60 years old: the history and future of the intensive care unit. *Clinical Medicine* 2014; 14(4): 376–9.

National Early Warning Score (NEWS). Standardising the assessment of the acute illness severity in the NHS. Royal Colleague of Physicians, 2012.

National Institute for Clinical Excellence. Acutely ill patients in hospital: recognition of and response to acute illness in adults in hospital. *NICE, Guidance/Clinical Guidelines CG50* 2007.

Priestley G, Watson W, Rashidian A, et al. Introducing Critical Care Outreach: a ward-randomised trial of phased introduction in a general hospital. *Intensive Care Medicine* 2004; 30(7): 1398–404.

Vincent J-L. Critical care-where have we been and where are we going? *Critical Care* 2013; 17 (Suppl 1): S2–12.

3 Scoring systems and unit performance

3.1 Scoring systems

- Numerous scoring systems are employed in intensive care.

3.1.1 Basis of scoring systems

- Scoring systems are based upon:
  - Physiological variables
  - Therapeutic interventions being employed
  - Anatomical or radiological findings
  - Co-morbidities
- Most scoring systems have been developed from the logistic regression analysis of large population datasets; the predictive capacity is typically validated against a second dataset.

3.1.2 Types of scoring system

- Scoring systems may be subdivided (Fig. 12.1)

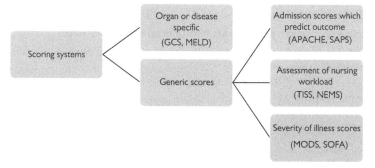

Fig. 12.1 Subdivision of scoring systems used on ICU.

3.1.3 Role of scoring systems

- Roles of scoring systems:
  - Common language for discussion
  - Comparator for clinical trials
  - Quantification of severity of illness:
    - Resource allocation
  - Estimators of prognosis:
    - Comparison of unit performance (actual versus predicted outcomes)
    - Rationing of care (controversial as no scoring system is a perfect predictor of outcome)

3.1.4 Assessment of scoring systems

- The performance of a scoring system can be assessed by means of:
- Discrimination:
  - Describes how effective a system is at predicting which patients will survive and which will die.
  - Commonly described in terms of area under the receiver operator curve (ROC):
    - A ROC is constructed by plotting the true-positive rate (sensitivity) of a system against the false-positive rate (1-specificity) for a range of score cut-offs.
    - Analysis of the area under the ROC provides an indication of the ability of a scoring system (or other predictive test) to discriminate between two outcomes (usually alive or dead in the context of ICU scores).
    - An area under the ROC of:
      - 1.0, represents perfect discrimination
      - 0.5, suggests the scoring system is no better than a coin toss in predicting the outcome
      - >0.7, is generally accepted as adequate discrimination for a clinical score or test
- Calibration:
  - Examines the correlation between the predicted outcome and actual outcome over a range of probabilities.
  - If a particular score predicts a mortality of 60%, then 60 out of 100 patients with that score would be expected to die; by comparing actual and predicted, the calibration is determined.
  - A scoring system can be calibrated to a given population; the Simplified Acute Physiology Score (SAPS) (section 3.2.2) is for example calibrated to different geographical regions.

3.2 Admission scores

3.2.1 Acute physiology and chronic health evaluation (APACHE)

- APACHE is an admission score and is based upon the most abnormal variables within the first 24 hours of ICU admission.
- Four versions of APACHE are currently in existence:
  - APACHE I
    - Developed in 1981.
    - Divided into acute physiology and chronic health status; 34 variables.
  - APACHE II
    - Developed in 1985.
    - Now most frequently used version of APACHE score.

- Reduced the number of physiological markers in comparison to original score.
- More specific definitions of chronic illness than the original score.
- Score integrated with diagnosis.
- The parameters that make up the APACHE II are outlined in Table 12.2; maximum score is 71.
- Area under the ROC for prediction of hospital mortality is 0.863.

- **APACHE III**
  - Developed in 1991.
  - More complex; increase in physiological parameters to 16 with more complicated weighting; maximum score 299; improvement in discrimination and calibration.
  - Also integrates the reason for ICU admission, treatment location prior to ICU, and differentiates surgical from non-surgical admissions.
  - Produces a daily updated score, which is a better predictor of outcome than the admission snapshot produced by earlier scores.
  - Length of stay predictor incorporated.
  - Less commonly used; predictive equations are commercially protected.

- **APACHE IV**
  - Developed in 1996.
  - Produced using different statistical modelling.
  - Infrequently used outwith North America.

Table 12.2 APACHE II score

Physiological variables (A)	Markers of 'severe organ system insufficiency' or 'immunocompromise' (C)
• Temperature • Mean arterial pressure • Respiratory rate • pH • P_aO_2 • Plasma Na$^+$ • Plasma K$^+$ • Plasma creatinine • White cell count • Haematocrit (Score between 0 and 4 for each variable depending upon degree of derangement)	• Liver: biopsy-proven cirrhosis with portal hypertension; episodes of past upper GI bleeding attributed to portal hypertension; or prior episodes of hepatic failure, encephalopathy, or coma. • Cardiovascular: New York Heart Association (NYHA) class IV heart failure. • Respiratory: chronic restrictive, obstructive, or vascular disease resulting in severe exercise restriction (i.e. unable to climb stairs or perform household duties); documented chronic hypoxia, hypercapnia, secondary polycythaemia, severe pulmonary hypertension (>40 mmHg); or respirator dependency. • Renal: receiving chronic dialysis. • Immunocompromised: the patient has received therapy that suppresses resistance to infection (e.g. immunosuppression, chemotherapy, radiation, long-term or high-dose steroids, or advanced leukaemia, lymphoma, or AIDS). (2 points for elective post-operative patient with immunocompromise or history of severe organ insufficiency; 5 points for non-operative patient or emergency postoperative patient with immunocompromise or severe organ insufficiency)
Age (B)	
Maximum of 6 points, proportional to age.	APACHE score = A+B+C Max score = 71

Adapted from *Critical Care Medicine*, 13, Knaus et al., 'APACHE II: a severity of disease classification system', pp. 818–829. Copyright (1985) with permission from Wolters Kluwer Health, Inc.

3.2.2 Simplified acute physiology score (SAPS)

- SAPS was developed in 1984 as a simplification of the APACHE system.
- SAPS II was produced in 1993.
- SAPS III arose in 1995 from a logistic regression analysis of a large international database (from 35 countries).
- SAPS III:
  - 20 variables:
    - Patient characteristics prior to admission
    - Circumstance of admission
    - Physiological derangement within *1 hour* of admission
  - Score customized to geographical region.
  - Area under the ROC for prediction of hospital mortality is 0.86.

3.2.3 Injury severity score (ISS)

- Illness severity scores, such as APACHE, have less predictive value in the context of major trauma, this may be because:
  - Traditional scores only reflect post-stabilization ICU physiology and not that immediately following injury.
  - The trauma population tends to be younger, with less co-morbidity and, therefore, differs from the 'typical' ICU population.
- The original trauma-specific score was the abbreviated injury scale, which developed into the ISS.
- The ISS is based upon the location and severity of injuries:
  - Six anatomical regions:
    - Head and neck (including cervical spine)
    - Face (including eyes, mouth, nose, and ears)
    - Thorax (including thoracic spine and diaphragm)
    - Abdomen and visceral pelvis (including lumbar spine)
    - Bony pelvis and extremities
    - External structures (including skin)
  - The most severe injury to each anatomical region is graded:
    - Minor: 1
    - Moderate: 2
    - Serious (non-life threatening): 3
    - Severe (life threatening—survival probable): 4
    - Critical (life threatening—survival uncertain): 5
    - Unsurvivable (despite treatment): 6
  - The ISS is calculated by adding the square of the score for the three most seriously injured regions:

$$ISS = A^2 + B^2 + C^2$$

  - The maximum score is 75
  - Any single region with a score of 6 (unsurvivable) automatically converts the ISS to 75

3.3 Severity of illness scores

3.3.1 Sequential organ failure assessment (SOFA) score

- Evolved as the consequence of a consensus conference in 1994.

- Six organ systems, score of 0–4 dependent upon degree of organ dysfunction or support required:
  - For each organ:
    - 0: no dysfunction
    - 1–2: organ dysfunction
    - 3–4: organ failure
- Organ systems are assessed on the following criteria:
  - Respiratory: $P_aO_2{:}F_iO_2$ ratio
  - Cardiovascular: a composite score that includes both the mean arterial blood pressure and the degree of pharmacological support (dobutamine, dopamine, adrenaline, or noradrenaline)
  - Neurological: the Glasgow coma scale
  - Renal: either plasma creatinine or daily urine output
  - Liver: plasma bilirubin
  - Coagulation: platelet count
- Allows for longitudinal evaluation of both individual organs and whole patient physiology.
- Worst value of the day recorded.
- Was not designed to predict mortality; however, increasing SOFA score over the first 48 hours of ICU admission is associated with a higher risk of death.
- A comprehensive description of the SOFA score, including the thresholds for each organ system, can be found in Ferreira et al. (2001).

3.3.2 Multiple organ dysfunction score

- Based on a literature review of 30 publications that characterized organ dysfunction.
- Seven systems identified, the variables selected based upon 'ideal descriptor'.
- Composite heart measure:

$$\text{Pressure adjusted heart rate} = \frac{\text{Heart Rate} \times \text{Central Venous Pressure}}{\text{Mean Arterial Pressure}}$$

- Scored 0–4 for each of the organ systems, based on first measurement of the day.
- Designed and validated on the population of one ICU.
- Not designed as a prediction score, there is however correlation with mortality.

3.4 Nursing workload scores

3.4.1 Therapeutic intervention scoring system (TISS)

- Developed in 1974.
- Assess severity of illness and compare patient care, based on nursing workload; based upon therapeutic interventions.
- Graded, based upon the complexity and time required.
- Initially 57 items, then increased to 76, most recently reduced to 28.
- Seven groups:
  - Basic activities, ventilatory support, cardiovascular support, renal support, neurological support, metabolic support, and specific interventions.
- Weighted to a total score of 78.
- One nurse can provide 46.35 TISS points worth of activity per shift.
- Each TISS point requires 10.6 minutes of the nurse's time.

3.5 Organ- or disease-specific scores

Organ- or disease-specific scoring systems include the following:

3.5.1 Respiratory

- Lung injury (Murray) score
- CURB -65score
- SMARTCOP score
- Pneumonia severity index

3.5.2 Liver and gastroenterology

- Model for end-stage liver disease (MELD) score
- Child–Pugh score
- Ranson score
- Glasgow–Imrie score
- West Haven score
- Blatchford score
- Rockall score

3.5.3 Neurological

- Glasgow coma score
- World Federation of Neurosurgeons' grading system
- Fischer scale
- Richmond agitation and sedation scale
- Full Outline of UnResponsiveness (FOUR) score

3.5.4 Renal

- RIFLE criteria
- AKIN system

3.6 Comparisons of unit performance

- Comparison of intensive care unit performance is an important aspect of quality control.
- Hospital mortality is the most commonly used comparator but other 'key quality indicators' include:
  - Early death (those occurring within 4 hours of ICU admission)
  - Late death (those occurring on the ICU after 7 days)
  - Out of hours discharge (patients discharged alive from ICU between 22.00 and 06.59 hours)
  - Delayed discharge (patients for whom time from being ready for discharge and departure is greater than 4 hours).
  - Unit-acquired infections (i.e. MRSA, *Clostridium difficile*, or bloodstream infection)
- When considering hospital mortality, the case mix and severity of illness of the ICU must be taken into account.
- Most commonly, the *standardized mortality ratio* is used to allow comparison.

3.6.1 Standardized mortality ratio

- Standardized mortality ratio (SMR) is the:
  - Ratio of the number of deaths in hospital, to the number that might be expected in a reference population.

$$SMR = \frac{Observed\ mortality\ rate}{Expected\ mortality\ rate\ \left(as\ predicted\ by\ a\ scoring\ system\right)}$$

- Expected deaths are typically predicted by applying a scoring system to the patient population; e.g. in ICU this might involve using the APACHE score to calculate the predicted mortality of the patients admitted during the observed period.
  - Score >1 worse than expected
  - Score <1 better than expected
- There are a number of limitations to SMR based on ICU scoring systems:
  - Does not account for pre- or post-ICU factors (poor performance in other areas of the hospital may impact upon the hospital mortality of ICU patients).
  - It Is not possible to control for all the factors that may contribute to the patient's risk of death.
  - Predicted mortality is only as accurate as the data collection.
  - Predicted mortality is only as accurate as the scoring model used (and no scoring model is perfect).
  - Small units are at greater risk of error and variation from the norm.
  - Death is not necessarily the most important factor.

3.6.2 Intensive Care National Audit and Research Centre (ICNARC)

- In the United Kingdom, large-scale data collection is coordinated by the Intensive Care National Audit and Research Centre (ICNARC).
- The Case Mix Programme (CMP) is the national clinical audit for adult critical care in England, Wales, and Northern Ireland.
- The Case Mix Programme Database (CMPD) contains pooled case mix, resource use, and outcome data on consecutive admissions to participating units (both intensive care and combined intensive/high-dependency units).
- Data are collected to precise rules and definitions, by trained data collectors, and undergo extensive local and central validation prior to pooling.
- The CMPD has been independently assessed to be of high quality and support for the collection, and use of patient-identifiable data without consent has been obtained under Section 251 of the NHS Act 2006.

3.6.3 Australia and New Zealand Intensive Care Society Centre for Outcome and Resource Evaluation (ANZICS-CORE)

- ANZICS-CORE has a similar role to ICNARC in Australia and New Zealand.
- It consists of four data registries:
  - Adult patient database
  - Paediatric intensive care registry
  - Critical care resources registry
  - Central line associated blood stream infection registry
- It provides peer-review and quality assurance across intensive care units and contributes to research and resource planning.

FURTHER READING

Bewick V, Cheek L, Ball J. Statistics review 13: receiver operating characteristic curves. *Critical Care* 2004; 8(6): 508.

Catalogue NI, Information Catalogue—Directory of Clinical Databases, 2007. http://www.icapp.nhs.uk/docdat/

Ferreira FL, Bota DP, Bross A, Melot C, Vincent JL. Serial evaluation of the SOFA score to predict outcome in critically ill patients. *JAMA: the Journal of the American Medical Association* 2001; 286(14): 1754–8.

Harrison DA, Brady AR, Rowan K. Case mix, outcome and length of stay for admissions to adult, general critical care units in England, Wales and Northern Ireland: the Intensive Care National Audit & Research Centre Case Mix Programme Database. *Critical Care* 2004; 8(2): R99–111.

Knaus WA, Zimmerman JE, Wagner DP, Draper EA, Lawrence DE. APACHE-acute physiology and chronic health evaluation: a physiologically based classification system. *Critical Care Medicine* 1981; 9(8): 591–7.

Knaus WA, Draper EA, Wagner DP, Zimmerman JE. APACHE II:a severity of disease classification system. *Critical Care Medicine* 1985; 13(10): 818–29.

Le Gall JR, Lemeshow S, Saulnier F. A new Simplified Acute Physiology Score (SAPS II) based on a European/North American multicenter study. *JAMA: the Journal of the American Medical Association* 1993; 270(24): 2957–63.

Vincent JL, Moreno R. Clinical review: scoring systems in the critically ill. *Critical Care* 2010; 14(2): 207.

4 Transfer

4.1 General

- Transfer of patients outside the ICU represents a significant risk to the patient; all efforts should be made to bring personnel and equipment to the patient.
- As a rule, the level and standard of care should be maintained at the same level throughout the transfer; this applies to:
  - Personnel
  - Monitoring
  - Therapy (where feasible)
- Whilst every transfer entails risk, the pre-hospital and inter-hospital environments typically present the greatest challenge; for this reason, this section focuses on transfer outwith the hospital; the principles are, however, applicable to transfers within the same facility.

4.1.1 Classification

- Transfers may be classified as:
  - Pre-hospital transfer: from scene of accident or illness to a healthcare facility.
  - Inter-hospital transfer:
    - Clinical: undertaken due to a lack of necessary resources or expertise at the referring hospital to safely and adequately managed patient condition
    - Non-clinical: undertaken due to lack of capacity at referring centre
  - Intra-hospital transfer:
    - Diagnostic: CT; MRI, nuclear medicine
    - Procedural: operating theatre; Interventional radiology
  - Intra-unit transfer:
    - Specialist bed-space: isolation room for infection control or protection of immunocompromised patient; bed-space with window for recovering patients; area with scavenging for those requiring anaesthetics gases.

4.1.2 Risks of transfer

- A recent study of 12 ICUs in France examined 3,006 intra-hospital transfers and found transfer to be associated with greater risk of:
  - Ventilator associated pneumonia
  - Pneumothorax
  - Atelectasis
  - Hypoglycaemia
  - Hyperglycaemia
  - Hypernatraemia
  - Increased length of stay
- Overall mortality was not, however, affected in this study.

4.1.3 Factors to consider

- When planning for any transfer, the following factors must be considered:
  - Perceived benefits of the transfer
    - Do the benefits exceed potential risk?
  - Urgency of transfer
    - Will delaying transfer impact negatively on patient outcomes (e.g. transfer to neurosurgical centre with extradural haematoma; cardiac centre for acute coronary reperfusion)?
  - Physiological stability of the patient
    - With the exception of time-critical transfers, the maximum degree of stability should be sought prior to transfer.
  - Expected trajectory of patient condition
    - If deterioration is anticipated, pre-emptive intervention prior to transfer is warranted (e.g. intubating a patient with fulminant hepatic failure expected to develop encephalopathy, prior to transfer to the liver centre).
  - Period of time out with a critical care environment
    - Important for calculation of consumables required (e.g. drugs, medical gases, and electricity).
  - Access to patient throughout transfer
    - If periods of relative inaccessibility are anticipated (e.g. helicopter transfer in which the airway may be relatively inaccessible; MRI where the patient will be isolated within the scanner), there is greater necessity to undertake procedures before departure.

4.2 Recommendations for transfer

- The College of Intensive Care Medicine (Australia and New Zealand) and the Intensive Care Society (United Kingdom) have both produced recommendations relating to the transfer of critically ill patients.

4.2.1 Organization

- A centralized regional co-ordination of inter-hospital transfer services is recommended.
  - Underpinned by agreed referral pathways, protocols, and governance processes.
- Regions may choose to create a dedicated transfer team.
- Staff involved in patient transfer should receive appropriate training; the extent and content of training will depend upon the patient group being transported and the vehicles being used.
- Equipment and vehicles should be standardized, where possible.

- A consensus decision regarding the suitability and timing of transfer should be reached between consultants in referring and receiving units; clinicians from other departments involved in the case should also be involved.
- A risk assessment should be undertaken prior to every transfer to identify potential problems and to determine the most appropriate mode of transport, accompanying personnel, and need for additional equipment.

4.2.2 Patient preparation

- With the exception of time-critical transfers (e.g. extradural haematoma for neurosurgical evacuation; acute myocardial infarction requiring emergency revascularisation), patients should be stabilized prior to transfer.
- Existing artificial airways should be secured; in the non-intubated patient at risk of airway compromise during transfer, endotracheal intubation should be undertaken prior to departure.
- Respiratory function should be optimized:
  - The patient may need to lie flat for prolonged periods of time
  - Transfer may be undertaken on a less sophisticated ventilator
  - Altitude will reduce the partial pressure of delivered oxygen
  - Altitude will cause expansion of non-drained pneumothoraces
  - Oxygen supply will be limited (and therefore devices with high oxygen consumption, such as high flow nasal prongs, may not be feasible)
- Haemodynamics should be optimized.
- A minimum of two points of venous access should be obtained and secured.
- Invasive arterial monitoring may be desirable to overcome the limitations of non-invasive blood pressure monitoring in high vibration vehicles.
- Appropriate level of sedation and analgesia.
- Nasogastric tube and urinary catheter placed if indicated and appropriately secured.
- Medical notes copied; transfer letter prepared.
- Patient and family informed of transfer.
- Stability should be reassessed once patient established on the transfer equipment.

4.2.3 Personnel

- The most appropriate personnel will be dependent upon:
  - The acuity and clinical needs of the patient at time of departure
  - The likelihood of deterioration and need for intervention *en route*
  - Duration of transfer
  - The mode of transport
- Normally at least two clinical staff.
- As a general rule:
  - Level 1 and some Level 2 patients—paramedic or ambulance technician and nurse
  - Some Level 2 patients will require a medical escort if deterioration or additional intervention anticipated
  - High acuity or complex Level 2 patients and all Level 3 patients will require nurse and medical escort; the doctor should be from an anaesthetic or critical care background and possess advanced airway skills

4.2.4 Equipment

- Basic and advanced airway equipment

- Means to ventilate:
    - Mechanical ventilator
    - Bag-valve-mask or other manual circuit
- Equipment for vascular access
- Selection of syringes and flushes
- Drugs, including:
    - All infusions and regular therapies (e.g. antibiotics) being received in the referring centre
    - Advanced life-support drugs
    - Anaesthetic agents
    - Cardiovascular agents (including intravenous fluids)

4.2.5 Consumables

- Care must be taken to ensure adequate supplies of consumables are taken on transfer:
    - Drug infusions
    - Oxygen
    - Electricity
- Calculating oxygen requirements
    - For the non-ventilated patient, hourly oxygen requirement may be calculated by:

$$\text{Oxygen flow per minute} \times 60$$

    - For the patient on mandatory ventilation, hourly oxygen requirement is calculated by:

$$(FiO_2 \times \text{minute volume} + \text{bias flow}) \times 60$$

    - Hourly oxygen requirement is then multiplied by the anticipated duration of the journey to calculate oxygen consumption.
- Anticipated journey time should take into account loading and unloading from vehicles and transfer within the hospital.
- It is advisable to take *double* the anticipated oxygen requirement to protect against unforeseen delays.
- The content of different sized oxygen cylinders are outlined in Table 12.3.

Table 12.3 Oxygen cylinder capacity

Cylinder	CD	D	E	F	G	H
Volume of oxygen	460 litres	340 litres	680 litre	1,360 litres	3,400 litres	6,800 litres
Duration at 15 litres per minute	30 minutes	23 minutes	45 minutes	91 minutes	227 minutes	453 minutes

4.2.6 Monitoring

- Full monitoring should be conducted throughout transfer.
- Observations should be documented.

4.3 Modes of transport

4.3.1 Road vs fixed wing vs helicopter

- Advantages and disadvantage of the different modes of transfers are discussed in Table 12.4.

Table 12.4 Comparison of modes of transport

	Advantages	Disadvantages
Road	Relatively cheap Widely available Less prone to weather disturbance	Length of time for longer distance Access to some areas (e.g. islands)
Fixed-wing aircraft	Speed (particularly over long distances)	Specific complications of reduced atmospheric pressure Relatively cramped and noisy environment Requires road transfer between airport and hospital Personnel require specific training Cost
Helicopter	Scene access for pre-hospital transfer Direct access to hospitals equipped with heli-pad Lower altitude than fixed-wing aircraft	Limited access to patient Very noisy environment Slower than fixed-wing aircraft. Personnel require specific training Cost

4.3.2 Impact of altitude

- Barometric pressure decreases with increasing altitude (Table 12.5).
- In a commercial fixed-wing aircraft, at standard cruising altitude of 36,000–40,000 feet, pressurization of the cabin will maintain pressure at 6,000–8,000 feet.
- A reduction in cruising altitude allows cabin altitude to be reduced to 'sea level'; lower cruising altitudes have however a detrimental impact upon speed and fuel efficiency.
- Falling barometric pressure has two major implications for aeromedical transfer:
- Decreased partial pressure of inspired oxygen (P_iO_2):

$$P_iO_2 = P_{ATM} \times F_iO_2$$

  - The effect of increasing altitude on inspired and arterial oxygen is demonstrated in Table 12.5

Table 12.5 Effect of altitude upon the partial pressure of inspired (P_iO_2) and arterial (P_aO_2) oxygen

Altitude	Sea level	12,000 feet	18,000 feet	24,000 feet	36,000 feet
Barometric pressure (kPa)	101.3	76	50.7	40	25.3
P_iO_2 (kPa)	18.7	10	8.3	6	2.8
P_aO_2 (kPa) (normal gas exchange)	13.3	7.3	6.1	4.4	2.1

- Expansion of gas filled cavities
  - Pneumothoraces may tension at altitude and must be drained.
  - Endotracheal cuffs will expand and should be filled with saline.
  - Gas within the gut lumen will expand and patients with gastrointestinal obstruction should avoid altitude, if possible (and have a nasogastric tube placed).
  - Pneumocephalus/pneumoperitoneum/pneumopericardium may also create pressure effects and should be drained, or altitude avoided, if possible.

FURTHER READING

Association of Anaesthetist of Great Britain and Northern Ireland. *Interhospital Transfer*, 2009. http://www.aagbi.org/publications/publications-guidelines

College of Intensive Care Medicine. *Guidelines for Transport of Critically Ill Patients*, 2013. http://www.cicm.org.au/Resources/Professional-Documents/

Intensive Care Society. *Guidelines for the Transport of the Critically Ill Adult* (3rd edn), 2011. http://www.ics.ac.uk/ics-homepage/guidelines-and-standards/

Schwebel C, Clec'h C, Magne S, et al. Safety of intrahospital transport in ventilated critically ill patients: a multicenter cohort study. *Critical Care Medicine* 2013; 41(8): 1919–28.

5 Extremes of age and weight

5.1 Paediatric anatomical and physiological differences
5.1.1 Airway

- Large head, short neck, prominent occiput, and relatively large tongue: head should be placed in the neutral position for airway management.
- Obligate nose breathers.
- High larynx with long stiff, U-shaped epiglottis; laryngoscopy typically undertaken with a straight-blade laryngoscope (e.g. Miller).
- The narrowest point of the upper airway is at the level of the cricoid cartilage (unlike adults, in whom the narrowest point is the glottis); uncuffed endotracheal tubes are used preferentially to avoid subglottic oedema.
- Endotracheal tube size may be estimated using the following standard formulae (guide only; clinical assessment should be undertaken and alternative tubes available):

$$\text{Internal diameter of endotracheal tube (mm)} = \frac{\text{age (years)}}{4} + 4$$

$$\text{Length of oral endotracheal tube (cm)} = \frac{\text{age (years)}}{2} + 12 \ (14 \text{ for nasal tube})$$

5.1.2 Breathing

- Children have limited respiratory reserve:
  - Lower functional residual capacity (FRC)
  - Closing volume exceeds FRC until age 8 years, therefore tendency to airway closure at end of expiration
  - Relatively high metabolic rate

- Ventilation is primarily diaphragmatic; gastric insufflation during mask ventilation may significantly impede ventilation and concurrent gastric decompression via a nasogastric tube is necessary.
- Tidal volume is relatively fixed; respiratory rate is the primary determinant of minute volume (and therefore CO_2 clearance).
- Anaesthetic equipment leads to a far larger relative increase in dead space in comparison to adults.

5.1.3 Circulation

- Infants have a fixed stroke volume and therefore cardiac output is rate-dependent.
- The normal range for systolic blood pressure changes over childhood:
  - Preterm 40–55 mmHg
  - Neonate 50–90 mmHg
  - Infant (1–11 months) 85–105 mmHg
  - >2 years 95–105 mmHg
  - >10 years 110–130 mmHg

5.1.4 Metabolism

- Infants adapt poorly to environmental extremes due to:
  - A large surface area to mass ratio, with increased heat gain or loss to the environment.
  - Poorly developed shivering, sweating, and vasoconstrictive mechanisms.
  - An inability to initiate behavioural changes (adding or removing clothing).
  - Brown fat provides a means of thermogenesis in infants.
- Liver enzymes are immature and metabolism of drugs is slower.
- Neonates are prone to hypoglycaemia.

5.1.5 Neurology

- Cerebral vasculature is immature and prone to rupture; shifts in P_aCO_2, P_aO_2, sodium, and blood pressure may result in spontaneous intracerebral haemorrhage.

5.2 Anatomical and physiological changes in old age

5.2.1 General

- Increased prevalence of co-morbidities.
- Increased likelihood of polypharmacy and therefore risk of side-effects and interactions.

5.2.2 Airway

- An edentulous state may make mask ventilation more difficult.
- Arthritic and osteoporotic changes may limit mobility of the cervical spine, with associated difficulty in laryngoscopy.
- Reduced soft tissue tone in the airway increases the likelihood of obstruction of the unsupported airway.

5.2.3 Breathing

- Loss of alveolar elastic recoil results in alterations in lung architecture sometimes described as 'senile emphysema'; gas exchange is impaired and progressive hyperinflation creates mechanical ventilatory disadvantage.
- The loss of elasticity results in increase in lung compliance, which coincides with a reduction in chest wall compliance; the consequence is reduction in FRC.

5.2.4 Circulation

- Decrease in the elasticity and compliance of the arterial system leads to systolic hypertension with associated increase in left ventricular afterload and resultant hypertrophy.
- Left ventricular hypertrophy is associated with sub-endocardial ischaemia and diastolic dysfunction; diastolic dysfunction increases the reliance on atrial contraction for ventricular filling.
- Age-related changes to the pacemaker and conduction system increases the propensity to arrhythmia.
- Baroreceptor response is impaired by aging: the response to vasodilation (with, for example, anaesthetic agents) may be delayed and less adequate than the younger population.

5.2.5 Neuromuscular

- Response to sedative agents is often more pronounced.
- There is an increased risk of delirium, particularly in the presence of long-term cognitive impairment.
- Loss of lean muscle mass reduces power.

5.2.6 Metabolism

- Reduced metabolism may prolong the actions of drugs.
- Temperature regulation may be less effective than in the younger population.

5.2.7 Renal

- Glomerular filtration rate declines with age.
- Changes in the renal–angiotensin–aldosterone system alters blood pressure control and response to vasoactive agents; it may also increase the risk of acute kidney injury.
- Loss of renal mass and reduced number of nephrons impairs the ability of the kidney to appropriately concentrate urine or manage sudden shifts in solute load.

5.2.8 Outcomes in the elderly on intensive care

- Older patients have a higher mortality than the young; however, this appears attributable to factors other than age alone (e.g. co-morbidities and severity of illness).
- Physical function is often significantly reduced in elderly survivors of intensive care.
- Predictive models and scoring systems have not usually been calibrated to the very elderly.

5.3 The obese patient on intensive care

5.3.1 General

- An increasing problem in intensive care; more than 30% of admissions to US intensive care beds are obese.
- On the intensive care unit, obesity is associated with an increased risk of morbidity and mortality, increased duration of mechanical ventilation, and increased duration of admission.
- Obesity is associated with a number of cardiovascular and metabolic co-morbidities.
- Risk to staff in terms of moving and handling.
- May require specialized equipment (beds, chairs, hoists, etc.).
- Consideration of maximum load on scanners, theatre tables, etc.
- Intra- and inter-hospital transfers are particularly problematic.

5.3.2 Airway

- Increased risk of difficult endotracheal intubation: the National Audit Project 4 identified obesity to be a common factor in serious adverse airway events.
- Percutaneous tracheostomy may be more challenging; standard length tracheostomy tubes may be too short if there is a thick layer of adipose tissue in the anterior neck.

5.3.3 Breathing

- Upwards displacement of the diaphragm leads to reduction in FRC and, therefore, decreased respiratory reserve; the time to desaturation during apnoea is shorter.
- Chest wall compliance is reduced by excess adipose tissue.
- A semi-recumbent position off loads the diaphragm and may improve respiratory mechanics.
- Care should be taken to calculate safe tidal volumes based upon *ideal* rather *actual* body weight.
- Consideration should be given to the impact of the chest wall and abdomen on airway pressures:
    - A significant proportion of airway pressure may be dissipated in the chest wall of obese patients.
    - It is the trans-pulmonary pressure (TPP) that is associated with ventilator-induced lung injury, rather than the airway pressure alone.
    - TPP = airway pressure – pleural pressure; obesity may lead to a high pleural pressure; failure to account for the positive pleural pressure common to obesity risks inadequate airway pressures and unnecessary under-ventilation.
    - Oesophageal pressure is an easily measurable surrogate for pleural pressure; measurement may allow safer and more effective titration of airway pressures.
    - It should be noted that in the spontaneously breathing patient, the physiological mechanics of spontaneous breathing generates a negative pressure (-2–3 cmH_2O); in the context of pulmonary pathology, the increased drive to breath may lead to the generation of excessively negative pleural pressures (pressures of less than -30 cmH_2O may be generated); on the basis that TPP dictates lung injury, very negative pleural pressures can create injurious TPP, even if airway pressures appear 'protective'.
- Increased incidence of obstructive sleep apnoea in the non-intubated patient; continuous positive airway pressure (CPAP) may be required during sleep, both in the hospital and in the community.

5.3.4 Circulation

- Increased risk of cardiovascular co-morbidities.
- Difficulty gaining vascular access.
- Non-invasive blood pressure monitoring is inaccurate if too small a cuff is used: the width of the cuff should be 40% of the circumference of the arm, and the bladder within the cuff should extend for 80% of the arm circumference.
- Increased risk of venous thrombosis; potential for under-dosing low molecular weight heparin, if standard regimens used.

5.3.5 Metabolism and nutrition

- A state of insulin-resistance typically exists with high circulating insulin levels.
- High insulin levels inhibit the mobilization of fat stores during times of stress, and therefore a tendency to metabolize protein stores; early nutrition is desirable and a higher protein intake is recommended.

5.3.6 Pharmacokinetics

- Increased volume of distribution, particularly for fat soluble drugs.
- Extrapolation of pharmacokinetic models (and dosing recommendations) developed from patients with normal body mass may not be accurate; the monitoring of plasma drug levels, where available, is recommended, particularly for anti-microbial agents.
- Care should be taken to differentiate between those drugs in which doses should be calculated on ideal (or lean) body weight (e.g. neuromuscular blocking agents) and those based on actual body weight (e.g. steroids).

FURTHER READING

de Rooij SE, Abu-Hanna A, Levi M, de Jonge E. Factors that predict outcome of intensive care treatment in very elderly patients: a review. *Critical Care* 2005; 9(4): R307.

Jamadarkhana S, Mallick A, Bodenham AR. Intensive care management of morbidly obese patients. *Continuing Education in Anaesthesia, Critical Care & Pain* 2013; 14(2): 73–78.

Macfarlane F. Paediatric anatomy and physiology and the basics of paediatric anaesthesia. 2006. www.frca.co.uk/documents/paedsphysiol.pdf

Murray D, Dodds C. Perioperative care of the elderly. *Continuing Education in Anaesthesia, Critical Care & Pain* 2004; 4(6): 193–6.

Roch A, Wiramus S, Pauly V, et al. Long-term outcome in medical patients aged 80 or over following admission to an intensive care unit. *Critical Care* 2011; 15(1): R36.

Saber A. Perioperative care of elderly surgical patients. *American Medical Journal* 2013; 4(1): 63–77.

---

6 Discharge from the intensive care

6.1 Surviving ICU

6.1.1 Survival

- Mortality from ICU has now fallen to such an extent that for all comers to ICU, approximately 80% are expected to survive to hospital discharge.

6.1.2 The post-intensive care syndrome

- It is now well recognized that survival from a stay in ICU is not without price: patients may be left with cognitive, cardiorespiratory, musculoskeletal, and/or functional impairment in later life.
- A proportion (up to one-half) of ICU survivors will experience cognitive, psychological, and physical changes in the months and years following discharge.
- This collection of symptoms is frequently described as the 'post-intensive care syndrome'.

6.2 Post-intensive care syndrome: cognitive

6.2.1 Features

- Memory difficulties
- Reduced attention span
- Impaired executive function

6.2.2 Risk factors

- Previous cognitive defect
- Acute respiratory distress syndrome (ARDS)
- Sepsis
- Delirium

6.2.3 Outcome

- Improvement variable
- Many do not recover to baseline

6.3 Post-intensive care syndrome: psychological

6.3.1 Risk factors

- As for cognitive sequelae
- Previous psychiatric illness
- Female
- Under 50 years
- Low educational level
- Prolonged duration of sedation and benzodiazepine administration in ICU

6.3.2 Features

- Post-traumatic stress disorder (PTSD):
  - Behavioural disturbance; avoidance behaviour
  - Nightmares and hallucinations
- Anxiety and depression
  - Irritability, fatigue, restlessness, anorexia
- Sexual dysfunction

6.3.3 Outcomes

- Improvement in symptoms in most patients
- May persist for months to years

6.4 Post-intensive care syndrome: physical

6.4.1 Risk factors

- Prolonged mechanical ventilation
- Multiple organ failure
- Sepsis
- Hyperglycaemia
- Prolonged bed rest

6.4.2 Features: respiratory

- Patients recovering from severe respiratory failure often suffer respiratory symptoms post-ICU; investigation demonstrates:
  - Restrictive lung function
  - Reduced carbon monoxide diffusion capacity
  - Reduced 6-minute walk test

- In addition to lung parenchymal changes, other contributing factors include:
    - Tracheomalacia
    - Neuromuscular dysfunction
    - Malnutrition
- The long-term respiratory consequences of ICU admission are illustrated in a series of follow-up studies of the 'ARDSnet' population.

6.4.3 Features: musculoskeletal

- Numerous factors contribute to weakness post ICU (for discussion see: chapter 5, section 8)
- May be exacerbated by contractures
- Reduced physical QOL scores

6.4.4 Outcomes

- Respiratory function test typically return to ≥85% of baseline
- Exercise tolerance does not return to baseline at 12 months, in a significant minority of patients; this is the consequence of:
    - Neuromuscular weakness
    - Large joint immobility
    - Dyspnoea

6.5 Post-intensive care syndrome: family

6.5.1 Risk factors

- Poor relationship with healthcare staff during relatives admission
- Perceived lack of control or involvement in decision making

6.5.2 Features

- Family members may report:
    - Anxiety
    - Depression
    - PTSD
    - Complex grief

6.6 Interventions on ICU

6.6.1 Facilitate early rehabilitation

- Minimization of sedation.
- Early mobilization.
- Avoidance of known risk factors.
- Early assessment of rehabilitation needs by therapists; frequent reassessment throughout the ICU stay and beyond.
- Rehabilitation plan with short- and medium-term goals from the outset of ICU stay.
- Where feasible, family should be involved in rehabilitation.
- Information regarding the patient's condition and support required should be provided to patient and family.

6.6.2 Patient diary

- Patient diaries have been demonstrated to reduce the incidence of PTSD, possibly by replacing the factual memories lost by patients during their ICU stay.

6.7 Interventions post-ICU

6.7.1 Follow-up clinics

- The follow-up of survivors of critical illness after discharge from hospital is recommended by NICE (UK).
- NICE recommend that follow-up clinics be arranged 2, 6, and 12 months following hospital discharge, depending on the severity of illness, length of stay, and need for follow-up.
- Furthermore active assessment for common problems during rehabilitation (e.g. weakness, post-traumatic stress disorder, or sexual dysfunction) with an appropriate planned response is required.

FURTHER READING

Herridge MS, Cheung AM, Tansey CM, et al. One-year outcomes in survivors of the acute respiratory distress syndrome. *The New England Journal of Medicine* 2003; 348(8): 683–93.

Herridge MS, Tansey CM, Matte A, et al. Functional disability 5 years after acute respiratory distress syndrome. *The New England Journal of Medicine* 2011; 364(14): 1293–304.

Needham DM, Davidson J, Cohen H, et al. Improving long-term outcomes after discharge from intensive care unit: report from a stakeholders' conference. *Critical Care Medicine* 2012; 40(2): 502–9.

National Institute for Clinical Excellence. Rehabilitation after critical illness, 2009. Available at https://www.nice.org.uk/guidance/cg83. (Accessed December 2015).

Wilcox ME, Herridge MS. Lung function and quality of life in survivors of the acute respiratory distress syndrome (ARDS). *Presse Medicale* 2011; 40(12 Pt 2): e595–603.

Wade DM, Howell DC, Weinman JA, et al. Investigating risk factors for psychological morbidity three months after intensive care: a prospective cohort study. *Critical Care* 2012; 16: R192.

CHAPTER 13

Ethics, law, and communication

CONTENTS

1 Ethical and legal principles

1.1 Ethical principles

1.1.1 Biomedical ethics

- The intensive care community has increasingly become the steward of ethical and legal decision-making around futility and end-of-life care based on the tenets of biomedical ethics:
    - Respect for autonomy
    - Beneficence
    - Non-maleficence
    - Justice

1.1.2 Disproportionate care

- Limiting the under-provision or over-provision of medical care (disproportionate care) is an increasing challenge.
- Disproportionate care has effects at the bedside on patient, family, and healthcare staff, along with systematic effects at hospital, healthcare system, and societal levels.

1.2 Legal principles

1.2.1 Legal frameworks

- The legal context of the interaction of the patient and healthcare system is important in providing care.
- The application of legal frameworks at a local hospital level need to be understood in relation to:
    - Human rights' charters
    - Coronial or forensic medicine matters
    - Competency
    - Refusal of therapy
    - Surrogate decision-making

- Withdrawal of cardiorespiratory support
- 'Do not attempt' resuscitation decisions
- Palliative care and euthanasia

FURTHER READING

Beauchamp T, Childress J. *Principles of Biomedical Ethics*, 7th edn. Oxford University Press, USA, 2013.

Kompanje EJ, Piers RD, Benoit DD. Causes and consequences of disproportionate care in intensive care medicine. *Current Opinion in Critical Care* 2013; 19(6): 630–5.

2 Capacity, competence, and consent

2.1 General

2.1.1 Legal and medical interaction

- Patients must have mental *capacity* (a medical assessment) to be deemed to have the *competence* (a legal term) to provide *consent* for any intervention.
- Competence and capacity are relative terms and relate to specific decisions; in general, the greater the magnitude of a decision (and associated implications), the greater the level of capacity required to provide consent.

2.1.2 Statute

- In the UK, the key statutes relating to competence, capacity, and consent are the Mental Capacity Act 2005 (England and Wales) and the Adults with Incapacity Act 2000 (Scotland).
- The legislation sets out the criteria and procedures to be followed in making decisions when patients lack capacity to make these decisions for themselves.
- It also grants legal authority to certain people to make decisions on behalf of patients who lack capacity.

2.2 Capacity

- Patients are assumed to have capacity unless proven otherwise.
- All efforts must be taken to help patients participate in decisions.
- Bizarre or risky decisions don't mean patients lack capacity.
- Assumptions regarding lack of capacity due to age, disability, appearance, behaviour, medical condition, beliefs, or apparent inability to communicate are dangerous and actively prohibited.

2.2.1 Assessment of capacity

- In order to have mental capacity a patient must be able to:
    - Understand the information provided
    - Retain the information for long enough to make a decision
    - Use or weigh the information
    - Communicate that decision
- Capacity is decision-specific: a patient may have capacity to make a decision for a simple decision (e.g. consent for intravenous access) but not for a complex decision with significant implications (e.g. consent for colectomy for cancer).
- If there is doubt or dispute regarding capacity:
    - Delay procedure (if possible)

- Discuss with:
  - Friends and family
  - Nursing staff
  - Psychiatrists
  - Neurologists
  - Speech and language therapists
- Seek an external second opinion
- Involve an independent advocate
- Formal case conference
- Go to mediation

2.2.2 Acting in best interests

- If a patient lacks capacity, medical staff should act in their best interests.
- In order to do so, the clinician should, if time allows, consult:
  - Close relatives
  - Anyone the patient has named as an advocate
  - Anyone caring for the patient
  - Anyone with an interest in the patient's welfare
  - If none of the above are available, then an Independent Mental Capacity Advocate (IMCA) (in England and Wales) should be consulted.
- This applies to unconscious patients in whom urgent life-saving procedures may be performed without consent.

2.3 Consent

2.3.1 General

- Consent may be:
  - Implied
  - Verbal
  - Written

2.3.2 Written consent

- Written consent is necessary for interventions associated with significant risk; when there may be repercussions for employment, social or personal life; or if treatment is innovative, or part of a research activity.
- If the patient cannot give written consent but the procedure is required, the agreement of the patient should be written in the notes.

2.3.3 Validity

- In order for consent to be valid it must be:
  - Voluntary (free from coercion by family, friends, or healthcare staff)
  - Informed
  - Provided by a patient with capacity

2.3.4 Provision of information

- The consent procedure should provide information regarding:
  - The nature of the procedure
  - The benefits
  - Potential complications
  - Alternative options

2.3.5 The 'reasonable patient' test

- The particular risks discussed will depend to some degree on the situation; legally, doctors are obliged to discuss potential adverse events with a degree of risk to which a 'reasonable patient' would attach relevance; this is likely to include:
  - Common minor risks (e.g. minor insertion site bleeding post-tracheostomy)
  - Uncommon major risks (e.g. loss of airway and death during tracheostomy)

FURTHER READING

Appelbaum PS. Assessment of patients' competence to consent to treatment. *New England Journal of Medicine* 2007; 357(18): 1834–40.

Buchanan A. Mental capacity, legal competence and consent to treatment. *Journal of the Royal Society of Medicine* 2004; 97(9): 415–20.

White S, Baldwin T. The Mental Capacity Act 2005—implications for anaesthesia and critical care. *Anaesthesia* 2006; 61(4): 381–9.

---

3 Specific circumstances

3.1 Advanced directives

- The premise of advanced care planning is for a person to ensure autonomy over their future medical care by providing a written statement (advanced care directive) regarding acceptable and unacceptable treatment options, whilst in a competent state.

3.1.1 Contents of advanced directive

- This document may include:
  - 'Do not resuscitate' orders
  - Maximal intensity of care requested
  - Treatments that are deemed unacceptable
  - A statement on the acceptable quality of life after therapy
- The burden of decision-making in next-of-kin has been shown to be reduced in advanced care directives or prior discussions about these issues.

3.1.2 Legality of advanced directives

- Different jurisdictions have varying levels of legality or enforcement of advanced care directives.
- An intensivist is required to elicit the formality of these discussions and incorporate these appropriately into the future care plan of a patient.
- In the UK, an advanced directive must be evaluated to determine whether it is:
  - Valid, that is:
    - When the decision was made:
      - The patient was an adult
      - The patient had capacity
      - The patient was not subject to undue influence
      - The decision was made on the basis of adequate information

- If the decision relates to refusal of potentially life-prolonging treatment, it must be in writing, signed, and witnessed, and include a statement that it is to apply 'even if life is at risk'.
- It has not subsequently been withdrawn, or that more recent action and decisions of the patient suggest that they have changed their mind.
  - Applicable to the current situation, that is:
    - The directive is clearly applicable to the patient's current situation.
    - The directive specifies no circumstances in which decisions would be invalid that are relevant to the current situation.
    - There are no reasonable grounds to believe that circumstances exist that the patient did not anticipate and would have changed their decision if anticipated (e.g. relevant clinical developments, changes to patient circumstances).
- If any doubt regarding the validity or applicability of an advanced directive exists, clarity should be sought and, if necessary, the courts involved.
- In an emergency, the presumption should be to prolong life and provide treatment.

3.2 Lasting power of attorney

- A lasting power of attorney (LPA) is a legal document that allows an individual (donor) to grant decision-making powers to one or more nominated 'attorney'.

3.2.1 Scope

- LPAs may relate to:
  - Health and welfare
  - Property and financial affairs
- In general, LPAs are created by competent adults who expect to lose capacity in the future; patients lacking capacity cannot appoint an LPA; however, the courts may designate a Court Appointed Deputy with similar powers.
- The LPA document may specify limitations to the attorney's decision-making powers; the power to refuse life-sustaining treatment must be explicitly stated.

3.2.2 Role of the attorney

- The attorney must themselves fulfil criteria for capacity.
- The attorney only has decision-making power if the donor lacks capacity at the time of a decision; if lack of capacity is transient, the decision-making power of the attorney is withdrawn on return of capacity.

3.3 Independent mental capacity advocates (IMCA)

3.3.1 Role of the IMCA

- For patients who lack capacity and have no representative, an IMCA may be appointed.
- An IMCA is an individual, distinct from health and social care staff, who provides advocacy for those individuals lacking capacity.
- An IMCA will provide a patient perspective during best-interest decisions.
- The IMCA has no decision-making powers but may challenge healthcare staff regarding the appropriateness of decisions.

3.4 Deprivation of liberty

3.4.1 Background

- The Deprivation of Liberty Safeguards (DoLS) were added to the Mental Capacity Act in 2009; this introduction was to create a safeguard for adults lacking capacity, who may be unjustly deprived of liberty to enact medical treatment.

3.4.2 The 'acid test'

- The 'acid test' relating to deprivation of liberty is:
  - If a person is under continuous supervision and is not free to leave, this a deprivation of liberty. If the person is unable to consent to the deprivation of liberty, an authorization is required under the DoLS regime or from the Court of Protection, if the deprivation of liberty is to be lawful.

3.4.3 Appropriateness of deprivation of liberty

- Deprivation of liberty may be considered appropriate:
  - If it is in their best interests to protect them from harm
  - If it is a proportional response when compared with the potential harm faced by the person
  - If there is no less-restrictive alternative
- Deprivation of liberty is unlikely to be a concern if the patient:
  - Has the capacity to decide to be admitted to intensive care
  - Has consented to the restrictions applied to them
  - Has given consent for intensive care admission prior to losing capacity—for instance, prior to surgery
  - Is expected to be deprived of liberty for a short period of time (although the specific time period is unclear)

3.4.4 Practical undertakings

- For the patient lacking capacity in whom deprivation of liberty is being undertaken:
  - An application for a Deprivation of Liberty Authorization should be made.
  - An assessment of the appropriateness of deprivation of liberty will be conducted.
  - If granted, a representative will be nominated to oversee and review the deprivation of liberty.

3.5 Decisions surrounding resuscitation

3.5.1 Background

- Recent court cases in the UK have highlighted the importance of advance decision-making around cardiopulmonary resuscitation and the communication of these decisions to patient and family.

3.5.2 Guidance

- Subsequent guidance issued by the British Medical Association, the Royal College of Nursing, and the UK Resuscitation Council recommend:
  - Anticipatory decisions regarding the appropriateness of CPR in the event of cardiac arrest should be made for every patient being admitted to hospital.
  - Decisions should be based upon a patient's individual circumstances.
  - Changes in the patient's condition, or a request from the patient or family, should prompt a review of resuscitation decisions.
  - Every effort should be made to discuss decisions with the patient and/or their family.
  - If it is the belief of the healthcare team that the patient is dying from an irreversible underlying disease and that resuscitation will not be effective, then CPR should not be undertaken; this does not require patient consent but should be communicated.

- A decision not to attempt resuscitation does not override clinical judgement at the time of a cardiac arrest if (a) a clearly reversible cause is underlying the deterioration and (b) the circumstances do not match those anticipated at the time of the original decision.
- All discussions and decisions should be clearly documented.

3.5.3 *Tracey versus Cambridge University Hospital NHS Trust*

- The importance of discussing decisions surrounding resuscitation with patients and their relatives was highlighted by the case of Tracey versus Cambridge University Hospital NHS trust (2014):
  - Mrs Tracey—a lady with lung cancer who sustained serious injuries in a motor vehicle accident—was admitted to intensive care.
  - Staff judged that an attempt at resuscitation in the event of cardiac arrest would not be in her best interests and instituted a 'Do not attempt' resuscitation order.
  - The family contested the right of the hospital to undertake such a decision without consultation with patient or family.
  - The courts, whilst not disputing the underlying decision, ruled that the failure of the hospital to undertake this consultation was a breach of her human rights.
  - The implications are:
    - It is the duty of the doctor to consult with the patient when making decisions relating to CPR.
    - There is, however, no legal right to resuscitation (if medical staff believe it to be futile).
    - Nor is there a legal right to a second opinion (although this may clearly be desirable).

FURTHER READING

Crews M, Garry D, Phillips C, et al. Deprivation of liberty in intensive care. *Journal of the Intensive Care Society* 2014; 15(4): 320–4.

Etheridge Z, Gatland E. When and how to discuss "do not resuscitate" decisions with patients. *British Medical Journal* 2015; 350: h2640.

Joint statement by the British Medical Association, Royal College of Nursing and the Resuscitation Council (UK). *Decisions Relating to Cardiopulmonary Resuscitation* (3rd edn), October 2013. https://www.resus.org.uk/dnacpr/decisions-relating-to-cpr/

---

4 Decision-making

4.1 Key principles

In the UK, guidance is available in the General Medical Council publication *Treatment and Care Towards the End of Life: Good Practice in Decision Making*. There are five principles that underpin decision-making:

- *Equalities and human rights*—all patients are entitled to be treated with dignity, respect, and compassion.
- *Presumption in favour of preserving human life*—initial presumption should be that all reasonable steps will be taken to prolong life.
- *Presumption of capacity*—initial presumption is that all adult patients have the capacity to make decisions regarding care.

- *Maximizing capacity to make decisions*—all reasonable efforts must be taken to maximize the patient's ability to participate in decision-making.
- *Overall benefit*—if capacity is absent, medical decision-makers should choose the option likely to provide the greatest benefit to the patient and least likely to restrict future choices.

4.1.1 Patient-centred decision-making

- Decision-making in intensive care medicine requires ongoing conversation and discussion between:
  - Patient
  - Next-of-kin
  - Family, friends, and support persons
  - Treating or 'bedcard' units
  - Intensive care team
- Patient-centred decision-making is best facilitated through the formation of patient-centred treatment goals of care from the time of admission to intensive care unit.

4.1.2 Considerations in intensive care decision-making

- Patient:
  - Competency in decision-making (see Section 1.2 for further information regarding competence and capacity)
  - Previously expressed wishes for acceptable level of intervention or subsequent function after recovery:
    - Verbal statements
    - Written statements
    - Advanced care orders
    - Previous resuscitation orders
- Previous history of illness:
  - Current and previous level of co-morbidity
  - Trajectory of impairment in preceding 3–12 months:
    - Cognitive
    - Functional:
      - Personal activities of daily living (PADLs)
      - Domestic activities of daily living (DADLs)
      - Community activities of daily living (CADLs)
  - Previous engagement in self-care
  - Previous engagement in healthcare
- Current acute illness:
  - Level of reversibility of acute medical problems which could be supported by intensive care therapy
  - Element of chronicity to any acute illness
  - Likelihood of survival with intensive care support
  - Likelihood of long-term rehabilitation or dependent care
- Intensive care support:
  - Resuscitation status:
    - For CPR
    - Not for CPR

- Level of intensive care support deemed suitable:
  - Mechanical ventilation
  - Non-invasive ventilation
  - Inotropic or vasopressor support
  - Extracorporeal support:
    - ECMO
    - RRT
    - Other
- Intent of intensive care support:
  - Restorative to previous level of previous function
  - Restorative to a lower level of function
  - Palliative
- Surrogate decision-makers:
  - Hierarchy of decision-makers
  - Powers of attorney
  - Guardianship orders
- Family and support persons:
  - Level of involvement or engagement with patient
  - Disputes or disagreements which may change decision-making
- Spiritual or religious beliefs about acceptable interventions.

4.1.3 Getting help with difficult decisions

- Treatment limitations and end-of-life care issues can be complex.
- When making treatment withdrawal or end-of-life decisions, it is recommended that, in addition to the patient or their surrogate, the treating/referring team are involved, as are intensive care colleagues.
- Disagreement may be become evident and a clinician must be able to draw on assistance from the following:
  - Treating team colleagues
  - Intensive care colleagues
  - Internal or external second opinions from:
    - Treating team disciplines
    - Intensivists
  - Clinical ethicist
  - Patient advocate (either a relative, friend, or IMCA (UK))
  - Medicolegal team
  - Designated officer
  - Administrative support
  - Religious or spiritual leaders
- Understanding barriers to effective decision-making by involving appropriate support persons for clinicians and patients early, improves dispute resolution and provision of patient-centred care.

4.1.4 Documentation of decision-making

- All appropriate intensive care therapy relies on effective, high-fidelity transmission of important information to all staff across the 24-hour cycle.

- Ideally, documentation of all decision-making, both simple and complex, should be contemporaneously documented in the medical record and include:
  - Clinical scenario
  - Details of involved parties concerning decision
  - Reasons for clinical decision
  - Resuscitation status
  - Maximum level of offered intensive care support
  - Intensive care supports deemed not appropriate
  - Changes in any reportable observations
  - Ongoing plans for further planned therapy
  - Ongoing plans for comfort care
- These decisions should be documented in appropriate existing health service documents, such as:
  - Resuscitation status form
  - Advanced care directive forms
  - Medical record

FURTHER READING

Donaldson J, Tapley M, Jolley D. *Treatment and Care Towards the End of Life: Good Practice in Decision Making*. BMJ Publishing Group, London, 2012.

5 Communicating with families

- The care of the family as the patient's advocate and likely surrogate decision-maker is arguably as important as the care of the patient.
- Family dynamics are frequently complex; meetings often relate to complicated situations.
- The communication skills-set can be learned and honed, based on principles outlined.

5.1 Family meeting planning

- Discussion of family meetings for families of critically ill patients require detailed understanding of the patient's circumstances in a 'biopsychosocial model'.
- Preparation for a family meeting with all stakeholders in the family meeting is mandatory to ensure patient- and family-centric communication.
- A '*pre-meeting meeting*' with all healthcare staff prior to the family meeting is advisable to ensure an agreed consistency of message and to enable anticipation of any patient or family concerns.

5.1.1 Preparation

- Considerations in preparation for a family meeting include:
  - Time-frame available for discussion and information exchange
  - Objectives of the family meeting:
    - Update of patient condition and further history-taking
    - Exploring complex decision-making and choices
    - Open disclosure
    - Conflict resolution
    - Second opinions
    - Change in therapeutic goals and expectations

- ▣ Discussion of palliation
- ▣ Discussion of organ and tissue donation
- ■ Plan for further family meetings
- ■ Environment:
  - ▣ Rooms available for privacy and quiet
  - ▣ Family comfort:
    - – Sufficient seating
    - – Drinks, snacks
    - – Box of facial tissues
- ■ Patient:
  - ▣ Possible engagement of patient (if bedside meeting appropriate)
  - ▣ Knowledge:
    - – Previous history
    - – Previous statements of choices around medical care
    - – Current ICU treatment course
    - – Treating unit therapeutic plans
    - – Likelihood of recovery
- ■ Family
  - ▣ Presence of legal surrogate decision-makers and important people
  - ▣ Spiritual or religious support
  - ▣ Interpreters of appropriate language
  - ▣ Awareness of family disputes
  - ▣ Risk of violence or abuse
  - ▣ Members affected by acute mental illness or intoxication
- ■ Intensive care team:
  - ▣ Ensure safe care of intensive care department during family meeting
  - ▣ Bedside nurse availability as family advocate
  - ▣ Social worker
  - ▣ Pastoral care
- ■ Treating team:
  - ▣ Representative to present therapeutic options, recommendations or opinion
- ■ Family dynamics
- ■ Specific communication issues:
  - ▣ Teleconference or videoconference
  - ▣ Language or communication needs of patient or family:
    - – Availability of interpreters (local or telephony)
    - – Avoidance of family as interpreters

5.1.2 Family meeting delivery

A family meeting requires consideration of the following:
- ● Punctual attendance of healthcare staff to planned meetings
- ● Communication in a respectful and private space
- ● Pre-meeting of healthcare staff for understanding the purpose and outcomes of the meeting:
  - ■ Also roles of intensive care and treating staff:
    - ▣ 'Giver' of bad news
    - ▣ Advocates
    - ▣ Support

- Provision of appropriate supports for family:
  - Personal comfort
  - Appropriate support persons
- Introduction of all members in the family meeting at each family meeting, if appropriate
- Discussion of the purpose of the family meeting
- Request for family to recap their understanding of current progress
- Clarification of any misunderstandings
- Provision of overview of intensive care stay
- Current description of current supports
- Delivery of new information
- Discussion of parallel care goals and processes:
  - Care aimed at recovery
  - Care aimed at comfort
- Request for any further questions or clarification from family
- Offer of any further practical, financial, or spiritual supports
- Summary of meeting and plan for care
- Close of family meeting:
  - Provision of expectations:
    - Bedside visitation rules
    - Description of usual local ICU communication patterns between family meetings
    - Request for a family spokesperson to coordinate and streamline family communication to and from the healthcare staff
    - Processes in the event of patient deterioration
  - Timing of next planned family meeting

5.1.3 Family meeting follow-up

- Family meetings can triggers significant distress and acute grief within a patient and family.
- Enabling open and transparent communication through agreed departmental practice and communication rules is important.
- Provision of support in between formal family meetings can be achieved by:
  - High quality of documentation and handover of family meeting outcomes
  - Proactive provision of social work and pastoral care
  - Empowerment of junior staff and bedside staff to address family issues
  - Escalation of difficult communication or conflict early to senior staff for management
  - Further attendance of family meetings in a similar punctual, respectful, and structured manner

CHAPTER 14

Perioperative care

CONTENTS

1 Perioperative intensive care

1.1 General

1.1.1 Background

- The past decade has seen growing interest in the care of surgical patients and the development of perioperative medicine.
- This interest has been driven by the following findings:
  - Static mortality rates for non-cardiac surgery.
  - The identification of a high-risk surgical group, which accounts for 80% of surgical mortality but only 12.5% of surgical procedures—patients in this group are older, have more co-morbidities, and undergo emergency and GI surgery.
  - Under-utilization of critical care beds in the high-risk surgical group: <15% of such patients admitted to ICU.
  - High complication rates—up to 50% for common procedures.
  - Significant costs associated with high-risk surgery and its complications.
  - Marked variation in both local, regional, national, and international surgical outcomes.
  - Marked variation in surgical outcomes according to time of presentation, e.g. weekend vs weekdays.
  - Survivors of surgery affected by complications have worse adverse long-term outcomes.
- This has led to a coordinated and collaborative approach between clinicians and researchers in surgery, anaesthesia, and critical care.

1.1.2 The high-risk surgical patient

- The Royal College of Surgeons (RCS) (England): *Higher Risk General Surgical Patient Report 2011* recommended:
  - Clear pathway for emergency general surgical patients, including appropriately skilled clinicians and prompt access to investigations and interventions.
  - Clear escalation strategy following identification of emergencies and complications.

- A mortality risk assessment (e.g. P-POSSUM score) should be undertaken for every patient prior to procedure:
    - Those with predicted mortality ≥5% should have consultant involvement at every step of the care pathway.
    - Those with predicted mortality ≥10% should have their case performed under direct supervision of both consultant surgeon and consultant anaesthetist.
- Use of 'end of surgery bundle' to reassess risk of death and determine optimal location for ongoing patient care:
    - All high-risk patients should be considered for admission to critical care.
    - Patients with a predicted risk of death ≥10% should be admitted to critical care as a matter of routine practice.
- National audit of surgical outcomes
- The UK multi-centre cluster randomized EPOCH study is ongoing and aims to assess the utility of a modified version of the RCS pathway applied to patients requiring emergency laparotomy using quality improvement methodology.

1.2 Risk prediction for general surgery

- Risk may be estimated by a number of means.
- Online calculators can be found at: www.riskprediction.org.uk

1.2.1 American Society of Anesthesiologists Physical Status Classification System (ASA)

- A simple, five-point system in widespread use amongst anaesthetists (Table 14.1).
- A sixth category (ASA VI) is used to identify brainstem-dead patients in theatre for organ retrieval.
- The suffix 'E' is used to identify emergency cases in which delay to surgery would increase risk of loss of life or limb.
- ASA score correlates with post-operative hospital mortality with one historical British series of 6,300 patients finding rates of 0.1% for ASA I, 0.7% for ASA II, 3.5% for ASA III, 18.3% for ASA IV, and 93.3% for ASA V.

1.2.2 Portsmouth physiological and operative severity score for the enumeration of morbidity and morbidity (P-POSSUM)

- Uses information on patient demographic, co-morbidities, functional status, acute physiology, and biochemistry, and intra-operative factors to calculate risk of morbidity and mortality.
- Easy to use and validated; can be calculated on an online portal.
- Generates a prediction of mortality.

1.2.3 Royal College of Surgeons' clinical criteria for major gastrointestinal and vascular surgery

- Patients with any of the following features are estimated to have a predicted mortality of ≥5%:
    - Age >50 years and:
        - Emergency, urgent, or re-do surgery
        - Or have acute kidney injury or chronic kidney disease with serum creatinine >130 µmol.l^{-1}
        - Or have diabetes
        - Or strong suspicion of or risk factors for cardiorespiratory disease
    - Age >65 years
    - Shock of any cause in all age groups

1.2.4 Hospital episode statistics procedure groups

- The following *emergency* procedures have a mortality of ≥10% (this doesn't take into account co-morbidities or acute organ dysfunction):
  - Laparotomy for peritonitis
  - Bowel or rectal resection
  - Therapeutic upper gastrointestinal endoscopy
  - Peptic ulcer surgery
  - Gastrectomy
  - Splenectomy
- Other high-risk groups include those with the following features:
  - Dialysis-dependent
  - Immunosuppressed
  - Long-term steroid use
  - Long-term beta blocker use
  - High ASA score
  - Massive transfusion
  - High lactate (>4 mmol.l^{-1}) or significant organ dysfunction (e.g. P_aO_2/F_iO_2 ratio <40 kPa) post-operatively

1.2.5 Cardiopulmonary exercise testing (CPET/CPEX)

- CPET offers a means of quantifying cardio-respiratory reserve by determining the anaerobic threshold; this correlates with perioperative risk.
- Patients are exercised on a fixed cycle; inspired and expired gases, SpO_2, blood pressure, and ECG are continuously monitored.
- Numerous variables are measured or derived, including oxygen consumption (VO_2), CO_2 production (VCO_2), anaerobic threshold (AT), and respiratory exchange ratio (RER).
- AT does not vary with patient effort and is a reliable measure of baseline cardio-respiratory function.
- An AT of <11 ml.kg^{-1}.min^{-1} is associated with increased risk of adverse outcomes and such patients should be admitted to critical care following major surgery.
- Given the need to be able to use a fixed cycle, CPET is only utilized in the elective population; patients with limitation of musculoskeletal mobility may not be able to perform CPET.

Table 14.1 American Society of Anesthesiologists' physical status classification system

ASA score	Description
ASA I	A normal, healthy patient.
ASA II	A patient with mild systemic disease without substantial functional limitations (e.g. current smoker, mild obesity, well-controlled hypertension).
ASA III	A patient with severe systemic disease with substantial functional limitations (e.g. poorly controlled COPD, morbid obesity, history of myocardial infarction or stroke (>3 months previously).
ASA IV	A patient with severe systemic disease, which is a constant threat to life (e.g. recent myocardial infarction (<3 months previously), severe valve disease, severe sepsis, ARDS).
ASA V	A moribund patient who is not expected to survive without the operation (e.g. ruptured abdominal aortic aneurysm, ischaemic bowel, multiple-organ dysfunction syndrome).

Adapted from *ASA Physical Classification System* with permission from the American Society of Anaesthesiologists, 2014. http://www.asahq.org/resources/clinical-information/asa-physical-status-classification-system

FURTHER READING

Agnew N. Preoperative cardiopulmonary excercise testing. *Continuing Education in Critical Care, Anaesthesia, and Pain* 2010; 10(2): 33–7.

American Society of Anaesthesiologists House of Delegates. *ASA Physical Classification System.* Last approved October 2014. http://www.asahq.org/resources/clinical-information/asa-physical-status-classification-system

Pearse RM, Harrison DA, James P, et al. Identification and characterisation of the high-risk surgical population in the United Kingdom. *Critical Care* 2006; 10: R81.

The Royal College of Surgeons of England and Department of Health. *The Higher Risk General Surgical Patient: Towards Improved Care for a Forgotten Group*, The Royal College of Surgeons of England 2011.

Smith JJ and Tekkis PP. *Risk Prediction in Surgery: P-POSSUM Scoring.* http://www.riskprediction.org.uk/pp-index.php. Accessed January 2016.

Wolters U, Wolf T, Stützer H, Schröder T. ASA classification and perioperative variables as predictors of post-operative outcome. *British Journal of Anaesthesia* 1996; 77(2): 217–22.

Pearse RM, Moreno RP, Bauer P, et al. Mortality after surgery in Europe: a 7 day cohort study. *Lancet* 2012; 380 (9847): 1059–65.

1.3 Perioperative haemodynamic optimization

1.3.1 Haemodynamic optimization

- Perioperative optimization of haemodynamics, in particular fluid status, has been demonstrated to improve outcomes.

1.3.2 The National Institute for Clinical Excellence (NICE) guidelines

- NICE in the UK make the following recommendations:
  - Intra-operative use of the Deltex Medical® Oesophageal Doppler Cardiac Output monitor to guide fluid therapy during major and high risk surgery.
  - This recommendation is based on evidence from clinical trials that use of this tool reduces the amount of invasive monitoring used, reduces length of stay and complications, and therefore also reduces cost.

1.3.3 OPTIMISE study

- OPTIMISE was a UK multi-centre randomized control trial comparing protocolized cardiac output guided fluid and inotropic therapy both intra-operatively and for 6 hours post-operatively versus usual care in patients undergoing major abdominal surgery.
- It showed no reduction in complications or 30-day mortality; however when combined in a meta-analysis with historical data rate of perioperative complications was reduced.

1.3.4 The post-anaesthetic care unit (PACU)

- The identification of the high-risk surgical patient and the recent focus on surgical outcomes has led the RCS to recommend an expansion in critical care facilities to facilitate management of these patients; this has driven the development of the PACU.
- The PACU is designed to provide dedicated Level 2 and Level 3 care for post-operative patients for the first 24 hours following surgery.

- This focus on post-operative patients allows high-quality protocolized care to be delivered, including haemodynamic optimization, respiratory support, analgesia, and advanced monitoring.
- The aim is to prevent complications and enhance outcomes—with associated socio-economic benefits.

1.4 Enhanced recovery after surgery (ERAS) programmes

1.4.1 The ERAS approach

- The ERAS approach was first adopted by Professor Henrik Kehlet in Denmark in the early 1990s.
- There has recently been an expansion in the utilization of ERAS in major elective surgery in the UK following a Department of Health initiative driven by large local and regional variation in both practice and outcomes—the enhanced recovery partnership (ERP).
- ERAS has been shown consistently to safely reduce length of stay for surgical patients; this has obvious advantages for both the patient, in terms of speed and extent of recovery, and for society, in terms of cost.
- The UK ERP scheme has been rolled out in elective major surgery in colorectal, urological, orthopaedic, and gynaecological surgery.
- The basic principles of the UK ERP follow:

1.4.2 Pre-operatively

- Work up:
  - Ensure general condition and co-morbidities optimized, including investigation and correction of anaemia
  - Plan estimated date of discharge and set discharge criteria
  - Carbohydrate loading
  - Avoid bowel preparation
- Admission:
  - Admit on day of surgery
  - Maintain hydration and intake of carbohydrate drinks

1.4.3 Intra-operatively

- Fluid and haemodynamic therapy guided by minimally invasive methods, e.g. oesophageal Doppler
- Use of balanced crystalloid solutions, e.g. Hartmann's, Ringers lactate
- Use minimally invasive surgical techniques, if possible
- Avoid hypothermia
- Use regional anaesthesia techniques, if possible, and epidural analgesia

1.4.4 Post-operatively

- Avoid iv fluids, if possible
- Push both oral fluid and nutritional intake early
- Avoid NG tubes and drains
- Avoid systemic opiate analgesia in favour of simple oral analgesia
- Early mobilization
- Remove catheters, etc., early
- Robust rehabilitation plan

1.4.5 Discharge/follow-up

- Discharge on planned date or when discharge criteria met
- Ensure robust multi-disciplinary team (MDT) follow-up
- Ensure patient has access to methods of accessing members of MDT, e.g. phone numbers, etc.

FURTHER READING

Kehlet H. Multimodal approach to control post-operative pathophysiology and rehabilitation. *British Journal of Anaesthesia* 1997; 78: 606–17.

Mythen MG, Swart M, Acheson N, et al. Perioperative fluid management: consensus statement from the enhanced recovery partnership. *Perioperative Medicine* 2012; 1: 2.

NHS Enhanced recovery partnership programme. *Delivering Enhanced Recovery, Helping Patients to Get Better Sooner After Surgery.* Department of Health, 2010. http://webarchive.nationalarchives.gov.uk/20130107105354/http://www.dh.gov.uk/prod_consum_dh/groups/dh_digitalassets/documents/digitalasset/dh_119382.pdf.

NICE Medical Technology Guidance 3: CardioQ-ODM Oesophageal Doppler Monitor. National Institute for Health and Clinical Excellence. March 2011. Available at https://www.nice.org.uk/guidance/mtg3 (Accessed December 2015).

Paton F, Chambers D, Wilson P, et al. Effectiveness and implementation of enhanced recovery after surgery programmes: a rapid evidence synthesis. *British Medical Journal Open* 2014; 4: e0050515.

Pearse RM, Harrison DA, MacDonald N, et al. (for the OPTIMISE group) Effect of a perioperative, cardiac output guided hemodynamic therapy algorithm on outcomes following major gastrointestinal surgery. *Journal of the American Medical Association* 2014; 311(21): 2181–90.

Pearse R. *Enhanced Peri-Operative Care for High Risk Patients (EPOCH) Trial: Trial Protocol Version 1*, September 2013. http://www.epochtrial.org/docs/EPOCH%20Protocol%20v1%20Ofinal.pdf

Simpson JC and Moonesinghe SR. Introduction to the postanaesthetic care unit. *Perioperative Medicine* 2013; 2: 5.

2 Major cardiac surgery

2.1 General

2.1.1 Procedures

- For the purposes of this chapter, 'major cardiac surgery' refers to coronary artery bypass grafting (CABG) and valve replacement.
- Most major cardiac surgical procedures require cardiopulmonary bypass (CPB) intra-operatively; this is not however universal and increasingly, 'off-pump' techniques are being utilized.
- The most frequently used surgical approach is via sternotomy but a less invasive thoracotomy approach is possible for some procedures.

2.1.2 Perioperative cardiac care

- Post-operative care of the cardiac surgery patient usually occurs in a specialist cardiac post-operative care unit or the cardiac ICU.

- Cardiac surgical units have pioneered healthcare improvement strategies such as open access publication of unit outcomes as a way of benchmarking practice and identifying units that require targeted improvement.
- Outcomes for major cardiac surgery continue to improve and mortality at present is approximately 2%.

2.1.3 Cardiopulmonary bypass (CPB)

- CPB is an extracorporeal circuit which draws blood from the great veins and right atria, oxygenated the blood and returns it to the aorta; the heart and lungs are thereby 'bypassed', and the heart can be arrested to provide a still and bloodless surgical field.
- Exposure of blood to this extracorporeal circuit has a number of consequences including activation of the clotting system, precipitation of an inflammatory response, significant perioperative fluid shifts, and the risk of embolic events. In addition it requires administration of high doses of anticoagulation, usually in the form of heparin.
- Many of the complications described later are directly related to CPB.

2.2 Significant complications of major cardiac surgery

2.2.1 Bleeding

- Some pleural and mediastinal drain output is normal during the first few hours post-cardiac surgery; as a general rule, acceptable limits are:
    - 400 ml in the first hour or
    - 200 ml.h^{-1} for the first 2 hours or
    - 100 ml.h^{-1} for the first 4 hours
- 'Medical' (i.e. relating to impaired coagulation):
    - Residual heparinization following CPB; reflected in prolonged ACT, APTT, or R-time on TEG; reversed with protamine (protamine promotes histamine release and may precipitate systemic hypotension, pulmonary hypertension, and bronchospasm).
    - Absolute thrombocytopaenia and impaired platelet function:
        - CPB consumes platelets and a drop in absolute count is expected.
        - Patients undergoing emergent coronary surgery may be recently exposed to anti-platelet agent and have platelet dysfunction not reflected in the absolute count.
        - Functional platelet mapping may be of use.
        - Clotting factors, including fibrinogen, may be consumed by CPB-related activation of the coagulation system; fluid shifts on CPB may result in dilution of clotting.
- 'Surgical' (i.e. failure of haemostasis).

2.2.2 Myocardial dysfunction (post-CPB 'stunning')

- CPB deprives the coronary arteries of blood flow from the aorta (as the aorta is typically clamped distal to their origin); this results in an ischaemia-reperfusion injury.
- Ischaemia-reperfusion injury manifests as systolic and diastolic dysfunction, arrhythmias, and endothelial dysfunction.
- Interventions designed to minimize the impact of ischaemia-reperfusion injury include:
    - *Cardioplegia*: a blood-based solution with high potassium content, which renders the heart asystolic, conserving ADP, and improving the surgical field
    - *Hypothermia* (reducing metabolic demand)
    - *Use of hyperosmotic buffer cardioplegic solutions*: to minimize myocardial oedema and acidosis
- Duration of CPB is an important determinant of the impact of ischaemia-reperfusion injury.

- In addition, patients undergoing coronary artery bypass graft will, by definition, have ischaemic heart disease with associated systolic and diastolic dysfunction; this may be exacerbated by time on CPB.
- Deteriorating cardiac function should not be attributed to ischaemia-reperfusion injury without consideration of other possible aetiology; coronary ischaemia may occur in the post-cardiac surgical patient due to:
  - Kinking or compression of coronary grafts
  - Spasm of native coronary arteries or grafts
  - Air embolus into the coronary arteries

2.2.3 Systemic inflammatory response syndrome

- Occurs post-CPB as a consequence of ischaemia-reperfusion injury and exposure to an extra-corporeal circuit

2.2.4 Arrhythmia

- Very common in the post-cardiac surgical period.
- Distension of the chambers, inflammation, and enhanced sympathetic activity are all contributing factors.
- Atrial fibrillation is most frequently encountered, affecting around 35% of patients and typically occurring on the second or third post-operative day.
- Amiodarone and beta blockers are the mainstay of management for tachyarrhythmias.
- Bradyarrhythmias are also common, particular in surgery to the aortic or mitral valves (which are located in close proximity to the atrioventricular node; many patients will have temporary epicardial pacing wires sited intra-operatively (pacing is discussed in chapter 2, section 4.5).

2.2.5 Cardiac tamponade

- Localized pericardial collections may have a significant haemodynamic impact.
- Transthoracic echocardiography is of limited value in detecting tamponade as drains, dressings and air in the mediastinum allow for poor windows.
- Transoesophageal echocardiography is likely to provide better image quality; however, a 'negative' echo does not exclude tamponade and there should be a low threshold for surgical exploration, if there is suspicion.

2.2.6 Hypothermia

- Patients are rewarmed as they are liberated from CPB; post-operative hypothermia is, however, common due to the open chest cavity, relatively cold operating theatres, and anaesthetic inhibition of warming reflexes.
- Hypothermia leads to:
  - Peripheral vasoconstriction with subsequent increase in afterload
  - Shivering and increased oxygen demand
  - Impaired coagulation
- Hypothermia should, therefore, be avoided with the use of warmed fluids, heater humidifiers in the ventilator circuit, and forced air warming blankets.

2.2.7 Pericarditis

- Post-cardiotomy pericarditis is common; this manifests as global concave ST segment elevation on the ECG.

2.2.8 Other potential complications
- Atelectasis
- ARDS
- Acute kidney injury
- Delirium
- Stroke

2.3 Routine post-operative management following major cardiac surgery

2.3.1 General
- Most patients will only require a brief stay in intensive care following elective major cardiac surgery; in uncomplicated cases, patients can be extubated within 6 hours of the end of the procedure.
- Patients requiring ongoing mechanical ventilation should have a lung protective strategy employed.
- Normothermia and the avoidance of shivering should be ensured.
- The causes of, and approach to, hypotension following cardiac surgery are outlined in Table 14.2.

2.3.2 Fluid management
- Fluid therapy should be optimized:
  - Fluid therapy and haemodynamics should be optimized using cardiac output monitoring, e.g. pulmonary artery catheter, pulse contour analysis, and echocardiography.
  - After initial stabilization, a conservative approach to fluid management is recommended and diuretics may be indicated.

2.3.3 Bleeding
- Vigilance for **bleeding** is essential:
  - Try to ascertain if bleeding is medical or surgical: significant blood loss (i.e. >400 ml in first post-op hour in chest drain) in the presence of normal clotting (i.e. normal TEG/ROTEM trace and normal platelet count) is suggestive of surgical cause.
  - Patients with suspected surgical bleeding should be taken back to theatre for definitive therapy.
  - Treatment of medical bleeding should be guided by TEG/ROTEM results.

2.3.4 Vigilance for tamponade
- Vigilance for pericardial tamponade is essential:
  - Requires high index of suspicion.
  - Low blood pressure, low cardiac output, and rising filling pressures (central venous pressure (CVP), pulmonary artery occlusion pressure (PAOP)) is suggestive of tamponade but the diagnosis should be considered in any unstable patient following cardiac surgery.
  - Transoesophageal echocardiography is the most sensitive means of detecting tamponade in cardiac ICU patients; sensitivity is not, however, perfect and haemodynamically significant localized pericardial collections can be missed.
  - There should be a low threshold for emergency re-sternotomy.

2.3.5 Blood products

- Haemoglobin should be maintained >90 g.l^{-1}: a recent randomized control trial demonstrated an increase in post-operative mortality with more restrictive haemoglobin targets (although this was not the primary outcome of the study).

2.3.6 Rhythm management

- Maintenance of heart rate according to targets should be achieved and heart rhythm maintained:
    - Epicardial atrial and ventricular pacing leads, if present, can be used to titrate heart rate to a haemodynamically optimal setting.
    - Chronotropic agents (both positive and negative) may be used to achieve target heart rate.
    - Potassium and magnesium levels should be kept within the upper limits of the normal range.
    - Beta blockade should be considered in cases where tachyarrhythmia is anticipated.

2.3.7 Cardiac function

- Maintenance and optimization of cardiac function:
    - Fluid volume state should be optimized.
    - Inotropes and vasopressors should be considered, depending on the clinical picture.
    - Echocardiography is a valuable tool.
    - Pulmonary artery catheter should be considered, particularly in cases where right ventricular (RV) dysfunction is thought to play a major role.
    - Mechanical assistance, such as intra-aortic balloon pump, ECMO, and ventricular assist devices, can be considered in cases where conventional measures have failed.

2.3.8 Post-operative medications

- Anti-platelet therapy (e.g. post-CABG) and anticoagulation (e.g. post-valve replacement) may be required—this should be agreed with the surgical team.
- Beta blocker and ACE inhibitors should be commenced, or reintroduced as appropriate.

FURTHER READING

Aranki S, Cutlip D, Aroesty JM. *Early Cardiac Complications of Coronary Artery Bypass Graft Surgery*, August, 2014. www.uptodate.com.

Hett DA. Anaesthesia for off pump coronary artery surgery. *Continuing Education in Anaesthesia, Critical Care, and Pain* 2006; 6(2): 60–62.

Melanson P. *Management of Post-Operative Cardiac Surgery Patients*. McGill University Ontario ICU protocols, 2001. https://www.mcgill.ca/criticalcare/teaching/protocols/cardiac (Accessed December 2015)

Murphy GJ, Pike K, Rogers CA, et al. Liberal or restrictive transfusion after cardiac surgery. *New England Journal of Medicine* 2015; 372(11): 997–1008.

Roekaerts, PMHJ and Heijmans, JH. Early Post-operative Care After Cardiac Surgery, Perioperative Considerations in Cardiac Surgery. In: Cuneyt Narin (Ed.) InTech, 2012. Available from: http://www.intechopen.com/books/perioperative-considerations-in-cardiac-surgery/-earlypost-operative-care-after-cardiac-surgery

Rosser JH, Parnell AD, Massey NJ. Post-operative care of the adult cardiac surgical patients. *Anaesthesia and Intensive Care Medicine* 2012; 13(10): 503–9.

Table 14.2 Hypotension post cardiac surgery

Aetiology	Features	Investigation	Management
Bleeding (medical) Incomplete reversal of intra-operative heparin Thrombocytopaenia Perioperative antiplatelet agents Coagulopathy of other causes (e.g. liver dysfunction)	HR↑ CVP/PAOP↓ CI↓ Blood in drains (usually, can be occult, e.g. in pleural space)	Activated clotting time (ACT) TEG produces faster results than formal coagulation studies; provides additional functional information Full blood count Coagulation screen	Correction of hypovolaemia and anaemia with fluids and packed red cells Protamine to reverse residual heparinization Blood products to correct coagulopathy and thrombocytopaenia
Bleeding (surgical) Bleeding from coronary anastomosis Bleeding from CPB cannulation sites Injury to mediastinal vessels	HR↑ CVP/PAOP↓ CI ↓ Blood in drains (tends to be brisker than medical bleeding)	As for bleeding (medical) to exclude a medical component to the haemorrhage Surgical exploration	Correction of hypovolaemia and anaemia with fluids and packed red cells; correction of clotting abnormalities Surgical exploration and repair
Post-operative vasodilation Post-CPB systemic inflammatory response Anaesthesia related	HR↑ CVP/PAOP↓ CI ↑ Minimal blood in drains	Exclusion of other causes Cardiac output monitoring	Vasoconstrictor agents (e.g. noradrenaline); care not to generate excessive afterload or coronary vasoconstriction
Myocardial dysfunction Post-cardiotomy 'stunning' Coronary graft failure Acute valve dysfunction May be a pre-existing element of dysfunction	HR↑ CVP/PAOP↑ CI → Minimal blood in drains	ECG to look for regional ischaemia Echo to look for regional ischaemia and assess valve function Calcium levels	Optimize electrolytes Commence inotropes (e.g. milrinone) Consideration of mechanical support (e.g. IABP) Surgical correction of graft or valvular problems

continued

Table 14.2 *continued*

Aetiology		Features	Investigation	Management
Pericardial tamponade	Undrained bleeding into the pericardium; may be very localized and still cause haemodynamic compromise	HR↑ CVP/PAOP↑↑ CI↓ Minimal blood in drains	Echo (transoesophageal echo often required); a negative echo does not however exclude a localized tamponade in the post-cardiac surgical patient.	Surgical re-exploration.
Arrhythmia	Bradyarrhythmia are common post-aortic and mitral valve surgery (but can occur in any) Tachyarrhythmias also occur	HR↑↑or ↓↓ CVP/PAOP↑ CI↓ Minimal blood in drains	Check electrolytes Check temporary pacing system (if present)	As outlined in chapter2, section 4.
Other	Sepsis Anaphylaxis Tension pneumothorax Failure of monitoring (e.g. malposition of transducer) Failure of drug delivery (e.g. kinked central line; pump failure)			

CI, cardiac index; CVP, central venous pressure; PAOP, pulmonary artery occlusion pressure; HR, heart rate; CPB, cardiopulmonary bypass; ECG, electrocardiogram; TEG, thromboelastogram; IABP, intraaortic balloon pump.

3 Aortic surgery

3.1 Procedures

3.1.1 Open thoracic aneurysm repair

- Complex procedure associated with significant morbidity and mortality.
- Depending on location of aneurysm, may have following surgical approach:
  - Median sternotomy
  - Left thoracotomy
  - Left thoracotomy extended across costal margin for retroperitoneal access
- May require cardiopulmonary bypass.
- May require interruption of cerebral circulation and use of intra-operative cerebral protection techniques, e.g.:
  - Selective cerebral perfusion
  - Retrograde cerebral perfusion
  - Hypothermic circulatory arrest with cardiopulmonary bypass
- Significant complications of open thoracic aneurysm repair:
  - Acute kidney injury (AKI)
  - Spinal cord ischaemia and resultant neurological deficit
  - Bleeding and coagulopathy
  - Cardiovascular complications, e.g. stroke or myocardial infarction

3.1.2 Open abdominal aneurysm repair

- Associated with significant mortality:
  - 36% if emergency repair of ruptured aneurysm
  - 6% mortality of elective aneurysm repair
- Accessed via laparotomy.
- Intra-operative cross-clamping of the aorta is associated with increased afterload during cross-clamping, and ischaemia-reperfusion injury +/− cardiovascular collapse after restoration of circulation at the cross clamp site.
- Significant complications of open aortic aneurysm repair:
  - AKI—cross-clamping/ischaemia
  - Ischaemia-reperfusion injury and multiple-organ failure
  - Ischaemia distal to cross-clamp site in absence of collateral circulation
  - Myocardial infarction
  - Cholesterol emboli to extremities
  - Bleeding and coagulopathy
  - Abdominal compartment syndrome

3.1.3 Endovascular aneurysm repair (EVAR)

- EVAR is a minimally invasive method of aneurysm repair—it can be used in both the elective and emergency setting.
- Requires collaborative working between vascular surgeons and interventional radiology.
- Involves image-guided insertion of a graft via an access vessel. Once *in situ*, the folded graft is deployed from its delivery sheath and allowed to expand—the aim is that the graft enables blood flow to be maintained though the aorta while excluding the aneurysm sac.

- Advantages of endovascular approach are as follows:
  - Minimally invasive
  - Avoids cross clamping of aorta
  - Reduction in perioperative mortality
  - Reduction in perioperative complications
  - Can be done using regional/local anaesthesia with conscious sedation
  - Can facilitate aneurysm repair in patients in whom open repair would have been contra-indicated due to co-morbidities
- Disadvantages of EVAR:
  - Technically challenging
  - Anatomical considerations mean many aortic aneurysms are not amenable to endovascular repair
  - Some EVAR cases will require conversion to open techniques
- Significant complications of EVAR:
  - Endoleak—persistent flow within aneurysm sac
  - Requirement for conversion to open procedure
  - Bleeding and coagulopathy
  - Embolic and ischaemic complications:
    - Stroke
    - Limb ischaemia
    - Spinal cord ischaemia (particularly with thoracic EVAR)
  - Aneurysm rupture or dissection
  - AKI:
    - Flow related (e.g. embolization, related to guidewire)
    - Contrast induced
  - Post-implantation syndrome—SIRS type response in absence of infection, treated with NSAIDs

3.2 Routine post-operative management following aortic surgery

3.2.1 General

- Management in the critical care unit or post-anaesthetic care unit (PACU) is appropriate.
- Standard perioperative critical care measures including:
  - Analgesia
  - Routine bundles of care, including DVT prophylaxis
  - Maintenance of normothermia
  - Ventilatory support, if required
  - Critical care monitoring, including invasive arterial blood pressure monitoring

3.2.2 Blood pressure management:

- Blood pressure management in the aortic surgical patient can be complex; see Chapter 2, Section 6.3.1 for a discussion on preoperative blood pressure management for aortic dissection.
- An appropriate post-operative blood pressure target should be agreed between the surgical, anaesthetic, and intensive care teams.
- Blood pressure must be sufficient to achieve adequate organ perfusion (accepting that intra-abdominal pressure may be elevated).
- Excessive blood pressure may place strain on new grafts and should be avoided; the use of beta blockers reduces the force of cardiac ejection and reduces shear force on the aorta.

3.2.3 Coagulation management:

- Monitor for signs of haemorrhage and maintain target haemoglobin.
- Monitor and correct coagulopathy.

3.2.4 Spinal protection

- Thorough and frequent neurological assessment (especially when thoracic aortic surgery).
- Maintain spinal perfusion pressure (i.e. MAP-spinal pressure >80 mmHg).
- In some cases a spinal drain will be inserted intra-operatively to drain CSF in order to decrease pressure around the cord and maintain blood flow—any issues such as blood tinged CSF within the drain or new neurological findings should be brought to the attention of the responsible surgeon immediately.

3.2.5 Abdominal and urinary care

- Monitor urine output and renal function; renal replacement therapy may be required.
- Be vigilant for abdominal compartment syndrome (particularly post-emergency AAA repair); this may require laparostomy.

3.2.6 Rehabilitation

- Physiotherapy and rehabilitation—including early mobilization in appropriate cases (this is often possible on Day 1 post op in EVAR cases).

FURTHER READING

Al-Hashimi M, Thompson J. Anaesthesia for elective open abdominal aortic aneurysm repair. *Continuing Education in Anaesthesia, Critical Care, and Pain* 2013; 13(6): 208–12.

Chaer RA. *Endovascular Repair of Abdominal Aortic Aneurysm*. UpToDate. http://www.uptodate.com/contents/endovascular-devices-for-abdominal-aortic-repair uptodate.com. February 2015

Kasipandian V, Pichel AC. Complex endovascular aortic aneurysm repair. *Continuing Education in Anaesthesia, Critical Care, and Pain* 2012; 12(6): 312–6.

Katzen BT, Dake MD, MacLean AA, et al. Endovascular repair of abdominal and thoracic aortic aneurysms. *Circulation* 2005; 112: 1663–75.

Leonard A and Thompson J. Anaesthesia for ruptured abdominal aortic aneurysm. *Continuing Education in Anaesthesia, Critical Care, and Pain* 2008; 8(1): 11–15.

Nataraj V and Mortimer AJ. Endovascular abdominal aortic aneurysm repair. *Continuing Education in Anaesthesia, Critical Care, and Pain* 2004; 4(3): 91–94.

Wang GJ and Fairman RM. *Endovascular Repair of the Thoracic Aorta*. In: UpToDate, Waltham, MA. Accessed June 2015.

Woo YJ and Mohler ER. *Management and Outcome of Thoracic Aortic Aneurysm*. In: UpToDate, Waltham, MA. Accessed June 2015.

4 Intracranial surgery

4.1 Procedures

4.1.1 Common procedures

- *Craniotomy* refers to a neurosurgical intervention where a skull bone flap is temporarily removed to facilitate access to the brain.

- *Craniectomy* refers to cases where the skull bone flap is not replaced at the end of the procedure—this is to allow swelling of the brain and hence avoid raised ICP; the skull flap can be replaced at a later date when swelling resides.
- The *trans-sphenoidal* route may be used for pituitary surgery.
- The majority of elective neurosurgery is performed for intracranial mass lesions.
- Emergency neurosurgery is frequently performed in cases of intracranial haemorrhage/haematoma—both spontaneous and as result of trauma.
- Patients require care in critical care or a post-anaesthetic care unit—in many elective cases this will be a short stay.

4.1.2 Significant complications of intracranial surgery

- Bleeding and haematoma
- Cerebral ischaemia
- Raised intracranial pressure (ICP)
- Seizures
- Cerebral oedema
- Pneumocephalus (with potential for tension and pressure effect)
- CSF leak (with potential for infection)
- Neurogenic pulmonary oedema
- Diabetes insipidus and endocrine disturbance—commonly after pituitary surgery

4.2 Routine post-operative management following intracranial surgery

4.2.1 Ventilation

- In stable patients, rapid extubation and recovery from anaesthesia is desirable: assessment of conscious level and neurological status in the awake patient is much more accurate and straightforward; sedation/anaesthesia can mask new neurological deficits.
- Extubation can lead to increased cerebral blood flow, increased ICP, and hyperaemia—these issues can in turn lead to haemorrhage and cerebral oedema; as such, the following measures are required to minimize the physiological stress of extubation and emergence from anaesthesia:
  - Analgesia and anti-emetics are essential as pain and nausea are common.
  - Shivering should be avoided by use of perioperative warming measures.
  - Patient should be stable from the cardio-respiratory perspective.
- In more complex patients (e.g. those with more significant disease/injury, prolonged procedure, significant bleeding, oedema, or low pre-procedure GCS), deep sedation and delayed extubation may be required to facilitate neuroprotective measures: sedation should be targeted to a standardized sedation score.
- Ongoing mechanical ventilation may be required:
  - If conscious level is reduced to the extent where the airway is compromised.
  - If there are concerns around the potential for raised ICP.
  - P_aO_2 and P_aCO_2 should be maintained within normal ranges and lung protective strategies followed.

4.2.2 Cardiovascular

- Haemodynamic stability is essential—instability is associated with excess morbidity and mortality in the post-neurosurgical patient:
  - Both hypotension and hypertension have significant deleterious effects post-neurosurgery.

- The multi-disciplinary team should set an acceptable target range specific to the patient's circumstances.
- Beta blockers are first agents in hypertension as they do not directly affect ICP; cerebral vasodilators, such as glyceryl trinitrate (GTN), should be avoided as they may increase cerebral blood flow.
- Vasopressors, such as noradrenaline, should be considered in the fluid-replete hypotensive patient.

4.2.3 Fluid and electrolytes

- Maintenance of intravascular volume and serum electrolytes is desirable:
  - Adequate intravascular volume is required to maintain CPP.
  - Negative fluid balance is associated with adverse outcomes in traumatic brain injury and should be avoided where possible in this patient group.
  - The ideal fluid in neurosurgical patients is not known; however, it is widely believed that isotonic fluids, such as 0.9% saline, are preferable.
  - Sodium and serum osmolality should be maintained within the normal range where possible as low osmolality and significant sodium shifts can lead to cerebral oedema.
  - Some metabolic consequences of neurosurgery may manifest in changes in sodium concentration, e.g. diabetes insipidus, syndrome of inappropriate ADH secretion, or cerebral salt wasting.

4.2.4 Neurological monitoring

- In the conscious patient regular neurological and systemic examination is essential to detect complications and deterioration.
- In the sedated and ventilated patient, the following is required in addition to routine care and examination:
  - Standard ICU monitoring, including invasive arterial blood pressure monitoring and end tidal CO_2 monitoring.
  - ICP monitoring may be required—neuroprotective measures can be targeted to a set ICP target.
  - Some institutions use regular (e.g. daily) CT imaging instead of ICP monitoring; there is no outcome difference in traumatic brain injury TBI) when intracranial pressure (ICP) targeted therapy is compared to regular imaging directed therapy.
  - Other monitoring, such as transcranial Doppler, CSF microdialysis, jugular bulb venous saturation monitoring, continuous or compressed EEG monitoring, may be used (neurological monitoring on the intensive care unit is further discussed in Chapter 5, Section 3).

FURTHER READING

Chestnut RM, Tempkin N, Carney N, et al. A trial of intracranial-pressure monitoring in traumatic brain injury. New England Journal of Medicine 2012; 367: 2471–81.

Zacko C, LeRoux P, et al. Perioperative Neurosurgical Critical Care. Neurocritical Care Society practice update, 2013. www.neurocriticalcare.org (Accessed December 2015)

5 Free flap surgery

5.1 Procedure

5.1.1 Common procedures

- Refers to the surgical method where a vascularized area of tissue and its neurovascular bundle are removed from a donor site and transferred to a new region with microvascular reanastomosis.
- Generally used in reconstructive surgery, e.g. following removal of tumour (e.g. breast, head/neck, melanoma), trauma, and burns.
- Hypoperfusion and subsequent flap failure is the primary specific concern.

5.1.2 Flap failure

- The free flap may fail due to:
  - Thrombosis (which in turn may be related to low flow)
  - Ischaemia/hypoperfusion:
    - Hypotension, e.g. post-operative SIRS, hypovolaemia, sedation/analgesia, epidural
    - Vasoconstriction, e.g. hypothermia, pain, hypovolaemia, inappropriate use of vasopressors
  - Flap oedema:
    - Excess administration of crystalloid
    - Marked haemodilution
    - Ischaemia

5.2 Routine post-operative management following free flap surgery

5.2.1 Flap monitoring

- Monitor flap closely:
  - Clinically—colour, temperature, capillary refill, texture (clinical assessment requires significant clinical experience and training).
  - Ultrasound Doppler techniques may also be used, particularly in the context of buried flaps.
  - Observations should be charted regularly, e.g. hourly for the first 48 post-operative hours; every 4 hours for the next 5 days; once daily until discharge.
  - Any changes in the condition of the flap should be brought to the attention of the relevant surgical team urgently.

5.2.2 Optimization of oxygen delivery to the flap

- Ensure adequate oxygenation.
- Maintain normothermia and maintain difference between peripheral and core temperature at < 1°C—hypothermia leads to vasoconstriction.
- Optimize haemodynamics and maintain blood pressure, avoiding hypotension and hypertension (targets specific to the patient should be agreed with the multidisciplinary team).
- Vasoconstrictors must be used with extreme caution; whilst pharmacological vasoconstriction may be required to offset the effects of sedation and a SIRS response, and to maintain adequate systemic perfusion pressure, care must be taken to impede microcirculation to the flap.
- Maintain haematocrit at approximately 30%, i.e. avoid excessive haemodilution.
- Smooth emergence from anaesthesia and extubation:
  - Excessive coughing and surges in blood pressure may have deleterious effects on the flap.
  - Optimize analgesia and maintain comfort.

FURTHER READING

Adams et al. Anaesthesia for microvascular free tissue transfer. *Continuing Education in Anaesthesia, Critical Care, and Pain* 2003; 3(2): 33–37.

Banks et al. Aintree University Hospitals NHS Foundation Trust. *Guidelines on Microvascular Free Flap Monitoring*, 1st edn, 2010. http://www.headandneckcancer.co.uk/File.ashx?id=9026

6 Pneumonectomy

6.1 Procedure

6.1.1 Pneumonectomy

- Pneumonectomy is the surgical resection of an entire lung.
- The most frequent indication is bronchial carcinoma; other indications include trauma and massive haemoptysis.

6.1.2 Risks

- Mortality is high:
  - Recent 30-day mortality has been quoted to be as high as 11%.
  - Right-sided pneumonectomy is associated with a higher mortality than the left—the reasons underlying this are unclear.
  - Emergency surgery (e.g. trauma and massive haemoptysis) carries a significantly higher mortality than elective.

6.2 Anatomical and physiological changes post pneumonectomy

- A number of anatomical and physiological changes occur post pneumonectomy.

6.2.1 Immediate anatomical changes

- The post-pneumonectomy space (PPS) fills with air (routine intercostal drain insertion is not indicated in pneumonectomy; if a drain is inserted it should not be placed on suction as this may precipitate mediastinal shift towards the PPS with associated haemodynamic compromise).

6.2.2 Late anatomical changes

- Raised hemidiaphragm.
- Mediastinum shifts towards PPS.
- Remaining lung hyper-inflates.
- CXR reveals complete opacification of affected hemithorax at around 4 months post resection.

6.2.3 Changes in lung function

- Lung volumes, forced vital capacity, and carbon monoxide transfer all reduce typically by <50%.

6.3 Significant complications of pneumonectomy

6.3.1 Pulmonary oedema of the remaining lung

- The entire cardiac output passes through one lung; an increase in hydrostatic pressure may precipitate pulmonary oedema, with a very high mortality.

6.3.2 Haemothorax

- Suspect if there is radiological evidence of a large volume of fluid within the PPS within 24 hours of surgery.
- Requires surgical exploration.

6.3.3 Chylothorax

- Usually develops within the first three post-operative weeks.

6.3.4 Bronchopleural fistula

- Discussed in Chapter 1, Section 12.3.

6.3.5 Post-pneumonectomy syndrome

- Manifests as breathlessness, recurrent infection, and stridor.
- Caused by compression of trachea and main stem bronchus of remaining lung by post-resection mediastinal shift.
- Requires operative intervention to alleviate.

6.3.6 Other

- Empyema in PPS
- Contralateral pneumothorax
- Arrhythmia
- Myocardial infarction
- Cardiac herniation:
  - Movement of heart into PPS through pericardial defect
  - Can lead to twisting of great vessels and subsequent cardiovascular collapse
- Scoliosis
- AKI
- Paralysis—secondary to disruption of spinal blood supply
- Patients with advanced age, BMI>30, COPD, co-morbidities, and current smoker status are at increased risk of pulmonary complications

6.4 Post-operative management following pneumonectomy

6.4.1 Respiratory

- Many patients are extubated shortly after the procedure.
- Lung protective measures should be used in those requiring ongoing mechanical ventilation.
- Adequate analgesia is required to facilitate deep breathing and coughing to protect the remaining lung—epidural is an effective method in this setting.
- Physiotherapy should be used to help maintain function in the remaining lung.
- Vigilance and prompt treatment required for complications such as haemothorax, contralateral pneumothorax, chylothorax, and empyema.

6.4.2 Cardiovascular and fluid balance

- Fluid therapy and cardiovascular optimization guided by cardiac output monitoring; excessive fluid may precipitate potentially disastrous pulmonary oedema of the remaining lung.

FURTHER READING

Agostinin et al. Post-operative pulmonary complications following thoracic surgery: are there any modifiable risk factors? *Thorax* 2010; 65: 815–18.

Kopec SE and Irwin RS. *Sequelae and Complications of Pneumonectomy*, UpToDate. In: UpToDate, Waltham, MA. Accessed June 2015.

Pedoto A and Heerdt PM. Post-operative care after pulmonary resection: postanesthesia care unit versus intensive care unit. *Current Opinion in Anaesthesiology* 2009; 22: 50–55.

Key papers

3CPO

Gray A, Goodacre S, Newby D.E, et al. Noninvasive ventilation in acute cardiogenic pulmonary edema. *New England Journal of Medicine* 2008; 359(2): 142–51.

6S

Perner A, Haase N, Guttormsen AB, et al. Hydroxyethyl starch 130/0.42 versus Ringer's acetate in severe sepsis. *New England Journal of Medicine* 2012; 367(2): 124–34.

ABC

Girard TD, Kress JP, Fuchs BD, et al. Efficacy and safety of a paired sedation and ventilator weaning protocol for mechanically ventilated patients in intensive care (Awakening and Breathing Controlled trial): a randomised controlled trial. *Lancet* 2008; 371(9607): 126–34.

ABLE

Lacroix J, Hebert P, Fergusson D, et al. Age of transfused blood in critically ill adults. *New England Journal of Medicine* 2015; 372, 1410–8.

ACURASYS

Papazian L, Forel J-M, Gacouin A, et al. Neuromuscular blockers in early acute respiratory distress syndrome. *New England Journal of Medicine* 2010; 363(12): 1107–16.

ALBIOS

Caironi P, Tognoni G, Masson S, et al. Albumin replacement in patients with severe sepsis or septic shock. *New England Journal of Medicine* 2014; 370(15): 1412–21.

Annane study

Annane D, Sebille V, Charpentier C, et al. Effect of treatment with low doses of hydrocortisone and fludrocortisone on mortality in patients with septic shock. *JAMA: the Journal of the American Medical Association* 2002, 288(7), 862–71.

ARDSnet study

The Acute Respiratory Distress Syndrome Network. Ventilation with lower tidal volumes as compared with traditional tidal volumes for acute lung injury and the acute respiratory distress syndrome. The Acute Respiratory Distress Syndrome Network. *New England Journal of Medicine* 2000; 342(18): 1302–130g.

ARISE

Peake SL, Delaney A, Bailey M, et al. Goal-directed resuscitation for patients with early septic shock. *New England Journal of Medicine* 2014; 371(16): 1496.

BALTI 2

Smith FG, Perkins GD, Gates S, et al. Effect of intravenous β-2 agonist treatment on clinical outcomes in acute respiratory distress syndrome (BALTI-2): a multicentre, randomised controlled trial. *Lancet*; 379(9812): 229–35.

Berlin definition

The ARDS Definition Task Force. Acute respiratory distress syndrome: the Berlin definition. *JAMA: the Journal of the American Medical Association* 2012; 307(23): 2526–33.

CALORIES

Harvey SE, Parrott F, Harrison DA, et al. Trial of the route of early nutritional support in critically ill adults. *New England Journal of Medicine* 2014; 371: 1673–84.

CESAR

Peek GJ, Mugford M, Tiruvoipati R, et al. Efficacy and economic assessment of conventional ventilatory support versus extracorporeal membrane oxygenation for severe adult respiratory failure (CESAR): a multicentre randomised controlled trial. *Lancet* 2009; 374(9698): 1351–63.

CHEST

Myburgh JA, Finfer S, Bellomo R, et al. Hydroxyethyl starch or saline for fluid resuscitation in intensive care. *New England Journal of Medicine* 2012; 367(20): 1901–11.

CORTICUS

Sprung CL, Annane D, Keh D, et al. Hydrocortisone Therapy for Patients with Septic Shock, *New England Journal of Medicine* 2008; 358: 111–24.

CRASH I

CRASH I Investigators. Effect of intravenous corticosteroids on death within 14 days in 10 008 adults with clinically significant head injury (MRC CRASH trial): randomised placebo-controlled trial. *Lancet*; 364(9442): 1321–8.

CRASH II

Shakur H, Roberts I, Bautista R, Caballero J, Coats T. Effects of tranexamic acid on death, vascular occlusive events, and blood transfusion in trauma patients with significant haemorrhage (CRASH-2): a randomised, placebo-controlled trial. *Lancet* 2010; 376(9734): 23–32.

CRISTAL

Annane D, Siami S, Jaber S, et al. Effects of fluid resuscitation with colloids vs crystalloids on mortality in critically ill patients presenting with hypovolemic shock: The cristal randomized trial. *JAMA: the Journal of the American Medical Association* 2013; 310(17): 1809–17.

CRYSTMAS

Guidet B, Martinet O, Boulain T, et al. Assessment of hemodynamic efficacy and safety of 6% hydroxyethylstarch 130/0.4 vs. 0.9% NaCl fluid replacement in patients with severe sepsis: the CRYSTMAS study. *Critical Care* 2012; 16(3): R94.

DECRA

Cooper DJ, Rosenfeld JV, Murray L, et al. Decompressive craniectomy in diffuse traumatic brain injury. *New England Journal of Medicine* 2011; 364(16): 1493–502.

Dopamine trial

Bellomo R, Chapman M, Finfer S, Hickling K, Myburgh J. Low-dose dopamine in patients with early renal dysfunction: a placebo-controlled randomised trial. Australian and New Zealand Intensive Care Society (ANZICS) Clinical Trials Group. *Lancet* 2000; 356(9248): 2139–43.

EDEN

Rice TW, Wheeler AP, Thompson BT, et al. Initial trophic vs full enteral feeding in patients with acute lung injury: the EDEN randomized trial. *JAMA: the Journal of the American Medical Association* 2012; 307: 795–803.

FACCT

ARDSnet group. Pulmonary-Artery versus Central Venous Catheter to Guide Treatment of Acute Lung Injury. *New England Journal of Medicine* 2006; 354(21): 2213–24.

FEAST

Maitland K, Kiguli S, Opoka RO, et al. Mortality after fluid bolus in African children with severe infection. *New England Journal of Medicine* 2011; 364(26): 2483–95.

HARP

Craig TR, Duffy MJ, Shyamsundar M, et al. A randomized clinical trial of hydroxymethylglutaryl-coenzyme a reductase inhibition for acute lung injury (The HARP Study). *American Journal of Respiratory and Critical Care Medicine* 2011; 183(5): 620–6.

IABP-SHOCK

Thiele H, Zeymer U, Neumann F-J, et al. *Intraaortic Balloon Support for Myocardial Infarction with Cardiogenic Shock. New England Journal of Medicine* 2012; 367(14): 1287–96.

ISAT

Molyneux A, Group ISATC. International Subarachnoid Aneurysm Trial (ISAT) of neurosurgical clipping versus endovascular coiling in 2143 patients with ruptured intracranial aneurysms: a randomised trial. *Lancet* 2002; 360(9342): 1267–74.

IVOIRE

Joannes-Boyau O, Honoré PM, Perez P, et al. High-volume versus standard-volume haemofiltration for septic shock patients with acute kidney injury (IVOIRE study): a multicentre randomized controlled trial. *Intensive Care Medicine* 2013; 39(9): 1535–46.

Kumar study

Kumar A, Roberts D, Wood KE, et al. Duration of hypotension before initiation of effective antimicrobial therapy is the critical determinant of survival in human septic shock. *Critical Care Medicine* 2006; 34(6): 1589–96.

LIDO

Follath F, Cleland J.G, Just H, et al. *Efficacy and safety of intravenous levosimendan compared with dobutamine in severe low-output heart failure* (the LIDO study): *a randomised double-blind trial. Lancet* 2002; 360(9328): 196–202.

Meduri paper

Meduri GU, Headley AS, Golden E, et al. Effect of prolonged methylprednisolone therapy in unresolving acute respiratory distress syndrome: a randomized controlled trial. *JAMA: the Journal of the American Medical Association*1998; 280(2): 159–65.

MERIT

Hillman K, Chen J, Cretikos M, et al. Introduction of the medical emergency team (MET) system: a cluster-randomised controlled trial. *Lancet* 2005; 365(9477): 2091–7.

NICE-SUGAR

The NICE-SUGAR Study Investigators. Intensive versus conventional glucose control in critically ill patients. *New England Journal of Medicine* 2009; 36013: 1283–97.

OSCAR

Young D, Lamb SE, Shah S, et al. High-Frequency Oscillation for Acute Respiratory Distress Syndrome. *New England Journal of Medicine* 2013; 368(9): 806–13.

OSCILLATE

Ferguson ND, Cook DJ, Guyatt GH, et al. High-frequency oscillation in early acute respiratory distress syndrome. *New England Journal of Medicine* 2013; 368(9): 795–805.

OPTIMISE

Pearse RM, Harrison DA, MacDonald N, et al. Effect of a perioperative, cardiac output-guided hemodynamic therapy algorithm on outcomes following major gastrointestinal surgery: a randomized clinical trial and systematic review. *JAMA: the Journal of the American Medical Association* 2014; 311(21): 2181–90.

PAC-Man

Harvey S, Harrison D.A, Singer M, et al. *Assessment of the clinical effectiveness of pulmonary artery catheters in management of patients in intensive care* (PAC-Man): *a randomised controlled trial*. *Lancet* 2005; 366(9484): 472–7.

PEITHO

Meyer G, Vicaut E, Danays T, et al. Fibrinolysis for patients with intermediate-risk pulmonary embolism. *New England Journal of Medicine* 2014; 370(15): 1402–11.

PRODEX/MIDEX

Jakob S, Ruokonen E, Grounds R, et al. Dexmedetomidine for Long-Term Sedation Investigators: Dexmedetomidine vs midazolam or propofol for sedation during prolonged mechanical ventilation: two randomized controlled trials. *JAMA: the Journal of the American Medical Association* 2012; 307(11): 1151–60.

ProCESS

Yealy DM, Kellum JA, Huang DT, et al. A randomized trial of protocol-based care for early septic shock. *New England Journal of Medicine* 2014; 370(18): 1683–93.

ProMISe

Mouncey PR, Osborn TM, Power GS, et al. Trial of early, goal-directed resuscitation for septic shock. *New England Journal of Medicine* 2015; 372(14): 1301–11.

PROSEVA

Guérin C, Reignier J, Richard J-C, et al. Prone Positioning in Severe Acute Respiratory Distress Syndrome. *New England Journal of Medicine* 2013; 368(23): 2159–68.

PROWESS

Bernard GR, Vincent J-L, Laterre P-F, et al. Efficacy and safety of recombinant human activated protein C for severe sepsis. *New England Journal of Medicine* 2001; 344(10): 699–709.

PROWESS-SHOCK

Ranieri VM, Thompson BT, Barie PS, et al. Drotrecogin alfa (activated) in adults with septic shock. *New England Journal of Medicine* 2012; 366(22): 2055–64.

RENAL

The RENAL Replacement Therapy Study Investigators. Intensity of continuous renal replacement therapy in critically ill patients. *New England Journal of Medicine* 2009; 361: 1627–18.

Rivers' study

Rivers E, Nguyen B, Havstad S, et al. Early goal-directed therapy in the treatment of severe sepsis and septic shock. *New England Journal of Medicine* 2001; 345(19): 1368–77.

SAFE

Finfer S, Bellomo R, Boyce N, French J, Myburgh J, Norton R. A comparison of albumin and saline for fluid resuscitation in the intensive care unit. *New England Journal of Medicine* 2004; 350(22): 2247–56.

SEPSISPAM

Asfar P, Meziani F, Hamel J-F, et al. High versus low blood-pressure target in patients with septic shock. *New England Journal of Medicine* 2014; 370(17): 1583–93.

SLEAP

Mehta S, Burry L, Cook D, et al. Daily sedation interruption in mechanically ventilated critically ill patients cared for with a sedation protocol: a randomized controlled trial. *JAMA: the Journal of the American Medical Association*2012; 308(19): 1985–92.

SOAP II

De Backer D, Biston P, Devriendt J, et al. *Comparison of dopamine and norepinephrine in the treatment of shock. New England Journal of Medicine* 2010; 362(9): 779–89.

STICH

Mendelow AD, Gregson BA, Fernandes HM, et al. Early surgery versus initial conservative treatment in patients with spontaneous supratentorial intracerebral haematomas in the International Surgical Trial in Intracerebral Haemorrhage (STICH): a randomised trial. *Lancet* 2005; 365(9457): 387–97.

SURVIVE

Mebazaa A, Nieminen M.S, Packer M, et al. Levosimendan vs dobutamine for patients with acute decompensated heart failure: the SURVIVE randomized trial. *JAMA: the Journal of the American Medical Association* 2007; 297(17): 1883–91.

TracMan

Young D, Harrison DA, Cuthbertson BH, Rowan K. Effect of early vs late tracheostomy placement on survival in patients receiving mechanical ventilation: the TracMan randomized trial. *JAMA: the Journal of the American Medical Association* 2013; 309(20): 2121–9.

TRICC

Hebert PC, Wells G, Blajchman MA, et al. A multicenter, randomized, controlled clinical trial of transfusion requirements in critical care. *New England Journal of Medicine* 1999; 240: 409–17.

TRISS

Holst LB, Haase N, Wetterslev J, et al. Lower versus higher hemoglobin threshold for transfusion in septic shock. *New England Journal of Medicine* 2014; 371: 1381–91.

TTM

Nielsen N, Wetterslev J, Cronberg T, et al. Targeted temperature management at 33°C versus 36°C after cardiac arrest. *New England Journal of Medicine* 2013; 369(23): 2197–206.

Van den Berghe study

Van den Berghe G, Woulters P, Weekers F, et al. Intensive insulin therapy in the critically ill patients. *New England Journal of Medicine* 2001; 34519: 1359–67.

VASST

Russell JA, Walley K.R, Singer J, et al. *Vasopressin versus norepinephrine infusion in patients with septic shock. New England Journal of Medicine* 2008; 358(9): 877–87.

VISEP

Brunkhorst FM, Engel C, Bloos F, et al. Intensive Insulin Therapy and Pentastarch Resuscitation in Severe Sepsis. *New England Journal of Medicine* 2008; 358(2): 125–39.

Index

Tables, figures and boxes are indicated by an italic, *t*, *f* and *b* following the page number.